Heart Transplantation - New Insights in Therapeutic Strategies

Edited by Norihide Fukushima

Published in London, United Kingdom

Heart Transplantation - New Insights in Therapeutic Strategies
http://dx.doi.org/10.5772/intechopen.98028
Edited by Norihide Fukushima

Contributors
Payam Akhyari, Yukiharu Sugimura, Sebastian Bauer, Moritz Immohr, Arash Mehdiani, Hug Aubin, Ralf Westenfeld, Udo Boeken, Artur Lichtenberg, Estela Azeka, Minoru Ono, Soo Yong Lee, Samuel Jacob, Si M. Pham, Anthony N. Pham, Yasumasa Tsukamoto, Takuya Watanabe, Hiroki Mochizuki, Masaya Shimojima, Tasuku Hada, Satsuki Fukushima, Tomoyuki Fujita, Osamu Seguchi, Megumi Ikura, Kazuki Nakagita, Takaya Uno, Hiromi Takenaka, Sachi Matsuda, Miho Yoshii, Rikako Nagata, Ichiro Nakakura, Naoki Hayakawa, Tsutomu Nakamura, Kyoichi Wada, Andrea Székely, Andras Szabó, Balazs Szécsi, Massimo Baraldo, Francesco Lo Re, Ugolino Livi, Sandro Sponga, Chiara Nalli, Antonella Zucchetto, Jacopo Angelini, Dawn E. Bowles, Michelle Mendiola Pla, Yuting Chiang, Jun-Neng Roan, Elena Sandoval, Daniel Pereda, Norihide Fukushima

First published in London, United Kingdom, 2022 by IntechOpen
IntechOpen is the global imprint of INTECHOPEN LIMITED, registered in England and Wales, registration number: 11086078, 5 Princes Gate Court, London, SW7 2QJ, United Kingdom

British Library Cataloguing-in-Publication Data
A catalogue record for this book is available from the British Library

Additional hard and PDF copies can be obtained from orders@intechopen.com

Heart Transplantation - New Insights in Therapeutic Strategies
Edited by Norihide Fukushima
p. cm.
Print ISBN 978-1-80355-432-7
Online ISBN 978-1-80355-433-4
eBook (PDF) ISBN 978-1-80355-434-1

For EU product safety concerns:
IN TECH d.o.o., Prolaz Marije Krucifikse Kozulić 3, 51000 Rijeka, Croatia,
info@intechopen.com or visit our website at intechopen.com.

Meet the editor

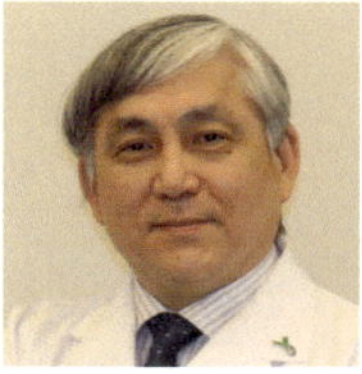

Dr. Norihide Fukushima is a professor at Graduate School of Nursing, Senri Kinran University, Japan, a visiting director at the National Cerebral and Cardiovascular Center, Japan, and a recruit professor in the Department of Surgery, Graduate School of Medicine, Osaka University, Japan. After graduating from the Graduate School of Medicine, Osaka University, he finished clinical training in the 1st Department of Surgery, Osaka University Hospital, and obtained his Ph.D. in Prolonged Cardiac Immersion storage in 1992. Dr. Fukushima worked at Loma Linda University, California, USA as a research and clinical fellow from 1991 to 1994. His team underwent the first heart transplantation in Japan in 1999. He and his colleagues made a revision to the Transplant Act in 2010 to increase deceased organ donation and heart transplantation in Japan.

Contents

Preface

Since the first heart transplantation was performed by Dr. Christiaan Barnard in South Africa in 1967 [1], there has been steady progress in terms of recipient selection, donor selection and management, surgical technique, preoperative management, immunosuppression regimens, and mechanical circulatory support during waiting for heart transplantation. The rapid progress in all these areas has been associated with steady improvement in outcomes before and after heart transplantation.

Until the early 1980s, even before cyclosporine became available, progress in the endomyocardial biopsy method and histological definition of acute cellular rejection as well as the addition of rabbit anti-thymocyte globulin to steroids and azathioprine as a method of immunosuppression increased post-heart transplant patient survival at one year to 65% [2].

Between 1981 and 1985, the use of cyclosporine reduced acute cellular rejection as well as lethal infection early after heart transplantation and patient survival rate at one year increased to more than 80%. This resulted in the widespread acceptance of heart transplantation in adults. However, acceptance of infantile heart transplantation was relatively slow in coming because there was no definition of brain death in children younger than 5 years of age until 1987 in the United States. After xenogeneic heart transplantation using a baboon heart was performed by Dr. Leonard L. Bailey in 1984 [3], the number of pediatric heart transplants slowly but steadily increased. In pediatric heart transplantation, we need to consider growth and development, the influence of steroids, non-compliance in adolescents, and the abilities of a transplanted heart to grow.

Medical therapy has improved the lives of most end-stage heart failure patients who will not receive heart transplants. The development of mechanical circulatory support also changed therapeutic strategies for Stage D heart failure patients. After the first total artificial heart as a bridge to transplant (BTT) was performed at the Texas Heart Institute in 1972 [4], the extracorporeal left ventricular assist device (LVAD) was introduced to BTT in 1978 and the Novacor LVAD (Baxter Health Corp., Oakland, CA) was first implanted at Stanford for BTT [5]. The Randomized Evaluation of Mechanical Assistance for the Treatment of Congestive Heart Failure (REMATCH) Study [6] revealed that implantable pulsatile LVAD had clinically meaningful survival benefits as well as improved the quality of life in Stage D heart failure patients in 1999, and thus destination therapy began worldwide. The development of continuous-flow LVAD further changed the feature of therapeutic strategies for Stage D heart failure patients. These LVADs had less morbidity such as pump thrombus and infection than pulsatile implantable LVAD. The CE Mark trial follow-up results of HeartMate 3 (Abbott, North Chicago, IL) implantation showed high patient survival rates of 98%, 92%, 81%, and 74% at 1 month, 6 months, 1 year, and 2 years post-implantation, respectively [7]. Temporary support with the Impella 5.0 (Abiomed, Danvers, MA) may allow for an effective bridge to decision strategy for hemodynamic stabilization and multidisciplinary heart team assessment of critically ill patients with heart failure [8].

This book presents recent information in the field of heart transplantation. It includes thirteen chapters that address such topics as novel immunosuppression therapy and the role of transplant pharmacists, donor management and intervention for primary graft failure, mechanical circulatory, diagnostic modalities for cardiac allograft vasculopathy, surgical techniques, pediatric heart transplantation, and gene therapy. We hope that readers will find this book a useful resource because of its summarization of relevant details and issues that will facilitate the acquisition of emerging new information in each area of heart transplantation.

I would like to thank the contributors for their help in making this useful and interesting book.

Norihide Fukushima
Professor,
Visiting Director at National Cerebral and Cardiovascular Center,
Senri Kinran University Graduate School of Nursing
Suita, Japan

References

[1] Cooper DK. Christiaan Barnard and his contributions to heart transplantation. Journal of Heart and Lung Transplantation. 2001;**20**(6):599-610

[2] Zhu Y, Lingala B, Baiocchi M, et al. The Stanford experience of heart transplantation over five decades. European Heart Journal. 2021;**42**(48):4934-4943

[3] Chinnock RE, Bailey LL. Heart transplantation for congenital heart disease in the first year of life. Current Cardiology Reviews. 2011;**7**(2):72-84

[4] Cooley DA. Heart substitution: transplantation and total artificial heart. The Texas Heart Institute experience. Artificial Organs. 1985;**9**(1):12-16

[5] Starnes VA, Oyer PE, Portner PM, et al. Isolated left ventricular assist as bridge to cardiac transplantation. Journal of Thoracic and Cardiovascular Surgery. 1988;**96**(1):62-71

[6] Rose EA, Moskowitz AJ, Packer M, et al. The REMATCH trial: rationale, design, and end points. Randomized Evaluation of Mechanical Assistance for the Treatment of Congestive Heart Failure. Annals of Thoracic Surgery. 1999;**67**(3):723-30

[7] Mehra MR, Naka Y, Uriel N, et al. A Fully Magnetically Levitated Circulatory Pump for Advanced Heart Failure. New England Journal of Medicine. 2017;**376**:440-50

[8] Lima B, Kale P, Gonzalez-Stawinski GV, et al. Effectiveness and Safety of the Impella 5.0 as a Bridge to Cardiac Transplantation or Durable Left Ventricular Assist Device. American Journal of Cardiology. 2016 May 15;**117**(10):1622-1628

Section 1

Donor Selection

Chapter 1

Donor Assessment and Management for Heart Transplantation

Norihide Fukushima

Abstract

For many years, heart transplantation has been an established procedure for patients with end-stage heart failure using the so-called "Standard Criteria" for an optimal heart donor. However, annually listed patients for heart transplantation greatly increased worldwide, and the use of extended criteria donor hearts has been utilized as many as possible in many countries. In this chapter, firstly, pathophysiology of brain death is explained. Secondly, donor assessment and issues of extended criteria donors are introduced. Then, donor management to maximize the heart graft availability, and the Japanese donor assessment and evaluation system and its outcome are reviewed.

Keywords: heart transplantation, donor assessment, donor management, anti-diuretic hormone (ADH), denervation, brain death

1. Introduction

Heart transplantation (HTx) has been established as the definitive therapeutic strategy in end-stage organ failure patients and results in satisfying long-term results. However, this surgical therapy is extremely limited by severe donor organ shortages worldwide, especially in Japan [1]. Therefore, adequate, and optimal assessment and management for deceased organ donors are mandatory to increase heart graft availability [2].

As the revised Japanese Transplant Act was issued on 17th July 2010 and organs can be donated after brain death (BD) with their family's consent if he or she does not deny organ donation since this revision [1], BD organ donation increased from 13 cases in 2009 to 97 cases in 2019. However, the number of HTx was still extremely smaller than in other developed countries. The extraordinarily severe organ shortage and long waiting time for HTx had made Japanese transplant programs consider using extended criteria donor (ECD) hearts.

The most troublesome issue facing HTx is primary allograft dysfunction (PGD) [3, 4]. This complication is the leading cause of early post-HTx death in the world. The use of ECD hearts may increase the PGF rate. Therefore, it is essential to establish a special donor evaluation and management system to maximize donor heart utilization. Maximizing donor heart availability is also the last wish of donors and donor families. However, if a transplant recipient dies soon after HTx due to PGD, the donor family feels the loss of their lover again. Therefore, donor management strategies to improve heart graft function and reduce early post-HTx mortality are very important for the donor family as well as for recipients [2–4].

Disease-transmitted disease (DTD) is also an inherent risk of heart transplantation as well as other solid organ transplantation [5]. The Ad Hoc Disease Transmission Advisory Committee (DTAC) reported that unanticipated DTD occurred only in 0.18% of recipients, with 0.23% of proven or probable DTD to at least one recipient. DTD was related to significant morbidity and mortality with about 33% of graft loss or recipient death. The recipient death in malignancy occurred significantly higher than that in infection. Therefore, the procurement transplant coordinator (PTC) should carefully listen to the clinical course, data, and history of medical staff and family to rule out these absolute contraindications prior to obtaining informed consent for organ donation from the relatives.

Full-scale donor management begins after the potential donor is sentenced brain dead and his or her family's consent to organ donation is obtained [2–4]. Basic therapeutic strategies for donor management consist of interventions for impaired heart and lung function to optimize the patient's hemodynamics, increase oxygen delivery to peripheral tissue, and finally improve the function of other organs, such as the liver and kidney. The hemodynamic targets are arterial blood pressure greater than 90 mmHg, central venous pressure (CVP) between 6 and 10 mmHg, urine output around 100 ml/h (0.3 to 3 ml/kg/h), and heart rate between 80 and 120/minutes. As there are only about 15 to 20 hours between the start of full-scale interventions for donor assessment and management and the start of organ retrieval surgery in Japan, we need to establish specific therapeutic strategies to optimize patient's hemodynamics and restore the function of damaged organs as many as possible in such short period [2], which are extremely different from those in standard intensive that usually take several days to accomplish. Moreover, the donor management physicians need to understand the pathological and physiological mechanisms and characteristics of brain death from the initiation to the completion period.

2. Pathological and physiological mechanism and characteristics of brain death

2.1 Pathological and physiological changes from the initiation to completion of brain death

Many investigators [3, 4] have reported that a short-lived catecholamine (CA) storm derived from acute intracranial hypertension caused systemic hypertension, acute left ventricular (LV) failure, and acute transient mitral valve regurgitation, leading to a rise in left atrial pressure in animal experiments. These events led to ischemic myocardial damage of LV associated with pulmonary edema. Histological examination of myocardial tissue exposed to CA storm shows widespread ischemic damage and necrosis in animal experiments. However, in the human clinical situation, a broad spectrum of adverse hemodynamic instability is observed and may depend on the speed of development of BD.

Soon after the initial surge of the CA storm, CA levels decreased to levels below the baseline and pituitary failure developed [6, 7]. In addition, the lung is also impaired by an acute systemic inflammatory response, neurogenic pulmonary edema, aspiration, hemopneumothorax, atelectasis, and later pneumonia.

2.2 Absent or decreased secretion of anti-diuretic hormone (ADH) after brain death

The anti-diuretic hormone (ADH) is principally produced by neurosecretory cells that have their cell bodies in the supra-optic and paraventricular nuclei of the hypothalamus, and the ADH storage vesicles are transported down the axon via the hypothalamic-hypophysial tract, released into a portal system in the posterior pituitary and finally enter the body's systemic circulation (**Figure 1**).

ADH is the primary hormone to maintain tonicity homeostasis by promoting water reabsorption in the kidneys and causing vasoconstriction. Briefly, ADH binds to the V receptor on the renal principal cells within the late distal tubule and collecting ducts and promotes reabsorption of water guided by the osmotic gradient established by sodium chloride and urea in the kidney. This action makes concentrated, or hyperosmotic, urine, and keeps our body to conserve water in times of dehydration or blood volume loss [8]. ADH also binds to V receptors on vascular smooth muscle and activates the G protein signaling cascade, which leads to a contraction of vascular smooth muscle leading to increases in total peripheral resistance and thus maintaining sufficient arterial blood pressure and tissue perfusion [8].

BD causes profound supraventricular and paraventricular hypothalamic nuclei ischemia and secondary loss of ADH secretion into the posterior lobe of the pituitary gland, which results in diabetes insipidus. As ADH is also secreted from peripheral tissues, undetectable levels of ADH have been noted in 75% of BD. As water reabsorption action of ADH is decreased, the kidneys cannot concentrate urine and make large amounts of dilute urine, which leads to hyponatremia associated with high serum osmolality and hypovolemia. As the vasoconstrictive effect of ADH is decreased, the vascular tone of systemic arteries is decreased and leads to hypovolemia. Therefore, the absence or decreased secretion of ADH after BD causes hemodynamic instability and compromised transplanted organ function.

Administration of ADH [9–11], in addition to treating diabetes insipidus by volume supply, reduces inotropic requirements and has been associated with improved heart graft function. Pure vasopressors, such ADH, are less likely to cause reduced tissue perfusion, metabolic acidosis, or pulmonary hypertension and may be more appropriate medicine than noradrenaline for vasoplegic shock syndrome, especially after BD

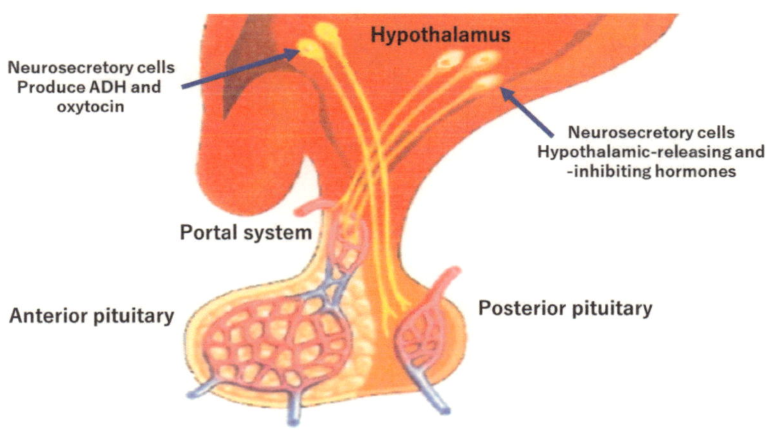

Figure 1.
Hypothalamo-hypophyseal portal system.

2.3 Cessation of autonomic nerve regulations on circulation

After BD, the brain-heart connections are definitively interrupted and autonomic cardiovascular regulation mainly thorough baroreflex is gone. Therefore, the hemodynamics of BD persons become unstable [4]. For example, a decrease in the blood return to the heart due to blood loss, hypovolemia, and putting pressure on the upper abdomen or postural change may rapidly cause low blood pressure in BD persons. After 20 to 30 seconds of the hypotension phase, the somatically induced adrenal sympathetic reflex responses result in an increase in adrenaline secretions from the adrenal medulla, which induces subsequent high blood pressure usually higher than 150 mmHg and tachycardia. In BD patients who are poorly controlled, arterial blood pressure and heart rate may go up and down. This phenomenon is often observed in hypovolemic patients derived from reduced ADH secretion due to BD. The subsequent increase in serum adrenaline decreases the myocardial density of beta-adrenergic receptors (BAR), which leads to PDG early post-HTx.

Disrupted brain-heart connections, so-called denervation, are also observed in HTx recipients. The authors [12] previously described that the heart graft could not augment cardiac performance rapidly in response to an acute decrease in the preload due to the cessation of autonomic nerve regulation on the graft. In normal individuals, if a preload of the heart rapidly decreases, autonomic sympathetic nerves are activated through vagal reflexes increasing heart rate and left ventricular contractility. Therefore, LV Emax after releasing occlusion of vena cava inferior (VCIO) is significantly higher than LV Emax during VCIO (**Figure 2A**). However, as the heart graft cannot autonomically increase heart rate or LV contractility soon after a rapid decrease in LV preload, LV Emax after releasing VCIO is not different from LV Emax during VCIO (**Figure 2B**). The heart graft performance may be augmented only after elevated serum adrenaline levels by secretion of adrenaline from the adrenal gland. Thus, the denervated heart, such as the heart graft as well as the heart of a BD person, cannot rapidly enhance its performance in response to a rapid decrease in the LV

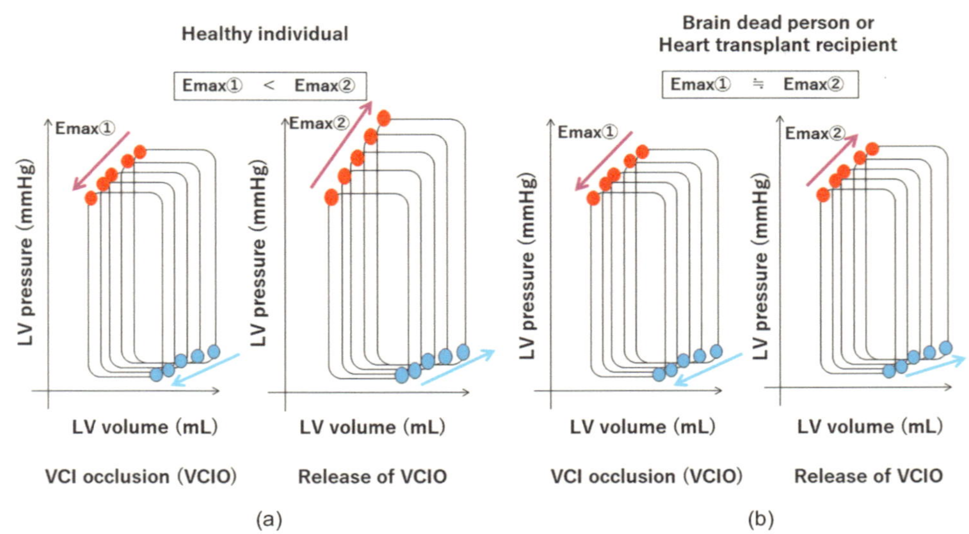

Figure 2.
Changes in left ventricular Emax during and after releasing vena cava inferior (VCI): A. Healthy individuals, B. Brain dead persons or heart transplant recipients.

preload, such as sudden blood loss or a sudden decrease in cardiac return. Therefore, denervation also causes hemodynamic instability in a BD person.

3. Donor assessment

3.1 Rule out of absolute contraindications for deceased donor eligibility

Although absolute contraindications for deceased donor eligibility depend on the organ procurement organization (OPO), most OPO provided a list of absolute contraindications for donor eligibility (**Table 1**).

As mentioned above, DTD is an inherent risk of heart transplantation [5]. Although DTAC reported that unanticipated DTD occurred only in 0.23% of proven or probable DTD to at least one recipient, DTD was related to significant graft loss or recipient death. It is important for PTC to carefully get information associated with DTD to rule out these absolute contraindications for heart transplantation.

3.1.1 Infection

3.1.1.1 Viral infection

Almost all OPOs determine that a positive test for human immunodeficiency virus infection and acquired immunodeficiency syndrome is an absolute contraindication, and most OPOs determined that hepatitis B virus (HBV) surface antigen (HBsAg), human T cell lymphotropic virus types I and II and determined or suspected prion-related disease are absolute contraindication.

Infection
Positive tests for
Anti-HIV-1 or anti-HIV-2
Hepatitis B or C* virus
Human T cell lymphotropic virus types I and II
History or evidence of HIV high-risk behaviors, even if HIV antibody negative
Prion-related disease
Creutzfeldt-Jakob disease (CJD)
family history of CJD
recipient of human-derived pituitary hormone or dura mater
Active systemic bacterial, viral, or fungal infections
Malignancies
Leukemias, lymphomas, and active malignancies

**Most organs from donors with a positive test for hepatitis C virus (HCV) can be transplanted to a recipient with a positive test for HCV.*
HIV: human immunodeficiency virus.

Table 1.
Absolute contraindications for donor heart eligibility.

Transplantation of donor hearts with anti-HBV core antibody (HBcAb) is associated with a small risk of virus transmission. In fact, Huprikar et al [13] reported that the risk of HBV transmission from HBcAb + HBsAg− donors are observed mainly in liver transplant recipients and that transmission is significantly lower in kidney transplant recipients and essentially negligible in thoracic transplant recipients. Even in liver transplantation, many investigators have reported that anti-hepatitis-B immunoglobulin (HBIg) or lamivudine can prevent HBV transmission by HBcAb + HBsAg− donors. In our institute, HBIg is routinely used in heart transplantation from anti-HBc + HBsAg− donors.

Most organs from donors with positive tests for hepatitis C virus (HCV) can be transplanted to a recipient with a positive test for HCV [5]. In the field of thoracic transplantation, transplantation of HCV + donor grafts to HCV + recipients is unacceptable, mainly because there are multiple strains of hepatitis C virus, and the presence of antiviral antibody in the recipient does not guarantee immediate immunity to HCV after heart transplantation.

3.1.1.2 Other pathogen infection

Regards bacterial or yeast infection, sepsis or infectious vegetation in the heart are contraindications for heart transplantation. Although the donor organ contamination (DOC) rate is high, infections due to DOC are rare after heart transplantation if adequate perioperative antibiotic prophylaxis and aseptic organ procurement are strictly performed [14]. The heart from a donor with positive blood culture without any signs of systemic infection can be transplanted if the proven bacteria are Gram-positive cocci and sensitive to common antibiotics.

3.1.2 Malignancies

Of the 335 donors who transmitted proven or probable disease to at least one recipient being reported to UNOS from 2008 to 2017, 70 transmitted malignancies and kidney, lung, and liver cancers were the most common malignancies, with 18, 10, and 10 donors, respectively, transmitting to at least one recipient. Fifteen donors with potential donor disease transmission events involving breast cancer and 28 involving thyroid cancer were reported by either transplant centers or OPOs with no proven/probable transmissions.

Regards to central nervous system (CNS) tumors, Hynes et al. [15] analyzed a cohort of 58,314 adult thoracic organ recipients from the UNOS database and reported none of 337 recipients who received organs from the donor documented CNS tumor, developed CNS tumors at a median follow-up of 72 months and that Kaplan-Meier curves indicate no significant difference in the time to death between patients with and without receiving from the donor with CNS tumor.

Donors with past histories of certain types of cancers may be considered as donors, including certain types of primary CNS tumors. Desai et al. [16] reported that the use of organs from selected donors with a history of cancer had a potential overall benefit in survival. But a small, yet real, risk of cancer transmission is present, of which the recipient should be informed. Although the transmitted risk can be reduced by sophisticated evaluation, it cannot be no risk.

3.2 Viability assessment of donor heart

The real goal of donor heart assessment is not to evaluate the donor heart function just prior to the heart procurement but rather to predict the transplanted heart graft performance after weaning from the cardiopulmonary bypass in the operating room and through the postoperative period. One also should consider the preexisting myocardial damage as well as myocardial damage due to BD-related stress.

3.2.1 Assessment of Hemodynamics and Heart Function

To accomplish optimal donor management, we need to obtain clinical information, such as the cause of BD, pathophysiological mechanism and findings of BD, past and family history, underlying disease, therapeutic interventions, especially inotrope dosage, ADH, thyroid hormone, and antibiotics, water and blood valance, and parameters of preload and afterload on the heart, such as systemic and pulmonary arterial pressure, CVP and pulmonary capillary wedge pressure, cardiac output, and/or mixed-venous oxygen saturation [2, 4].

Multicenter analysis (1719 consecutive primary HTx) reported that donor hearts requiring inotropic support of up to 6 mcg/kg/min of dopamine or dobutamine had satisfactory results [17]. Even if the donor experiences cardiopulmonary resuscitation (CPR) > 5 minutes, the donor heart might be acceptable to transplant, if optimal donor management stabilizes the donor's hemodynamics, improve left ventricular wall motion, and restore ischemic myocardial changes in ECG [2].

3.2.2 Evaluation tools for donor heart viability

3.2.2.1 Chest X-ray

As in usual clinical settings. cardiomegaly, chest trauma, or pleural effusions are checked by chest X-ray.

3.2.2.2 Electrocardiogram (ECG)

As most BD donors have some degree of myocardial damage caused by combined pre-underlying heart disease and BD events, ECG usually shows some degree of abnormality in ST segments and QRS waves. Sustained abnormalities in ST segments and QRS and multifocal ventricular ectopic beats under optimal donor management are considered high risks.

Even in an elderly donor with a history of cardiac arrest, the heart was acceptable for transplantation if hemodynamics becomes stable with a minimum dosage of inotrope administration and ischemic ECG changes disappear after optimal donor treatment.

3.2.2.3 Echocardiography

Echocardiography is the most reliable assessment tool to determine donor heart suitability. Echocardiography can evaluate cardiac valve function and myocardial hypertrophy as well as the existence of congenital malformations. Even if global and even regional ventricular dysfunction may be induced by the BD event, these wall motion abnormalities can be reversible within hours. Therefore, serial echocardiography should be done before a heart graft is abandoned to use due to myocardial dysfunction

In the presence of LV underfilling, LV seems to be hypertrophic or to have suitable LV systolic function. Therefore, circulatory blood volume should be estimated by central venous pressure (CVP), pulmonary capillary wedge pressure (PCWP), or the size and respiratory movement of inferior vena cava (IVC), as well as the required dosage of inotropes prior to undergoing echocardiography to assess heart function.

3.2.2.4 Coronary angiography

As asymptomatic coronary atherosclerosis is found even in children and young people, coronary angiography, at least in donors >45 years or according to the donor risk factors, is routinely performed in western countries. However, it has not been elucidated which type or level of donor coronary atherosclerosis really impairs the post-transplant outcome, which suggested that angiography in donors <60 years might not be necessary. Of course, recent myocardial infarction especially during the completion of BD and diffuse coronary sclerosis are absolute contraindications for heart transplantation, but single stenosis with good myocardial performance in the responsible region is acceptable, especially if it can be treated by percutaneous cardiac intervention or concomitant bypass surgery during transplantation [18, 19].

3.2.2.5 Chest computed tomography (CT)

For several social reasons in Japan, we do not routinely perform coronary angiogram before procurement. Therefore, we often check for coronary artery calcification (CAC) on conventional chest computed tomography (CT) to estimate the risk of pre-existing coronary artery disease in the donor heart. But we previously reported that the pre-existing CAC in a donor heart is significantly associated with the maximum intimal thickness of the coronary artery greater than 0.5 mm after transplantation, but that it was not a significant predictor for cardiac events in the future, probably due to the higher use of everolimus in the CAC group post-transplant [20].

In the future, contrast CT scan, especially cardiac CT scan, might be useful to rule out coronary arterial disease in the donor heart.

4. Extended donor criteria and how to decide the suitability of ECD hearts

To expand the cardiac donor pool, ECD hearts should be used. In this section, extended donor criteria are shown and how to select and deal with ECD hearts are discussed (**Table 2**).

4.1 Myocardial damage

The donor myocardium is damaged to a greater or less extent, for many reasons, such as massive CA secretion at the BD completion, heart arrest, chest trauma, and the CPR maneuver.

As the brain-damaged patients are often maintained on the dry side to reduce brain edema, the heart appears to move with vigor due to reduced preload on the heart. To evaluate the precise cardiac systolic function, central venous pressure at the time of evaluation should be 8–10 mmHg. It is also important to adjust hemoglobin concentration, electrolyte balance, and acid-base equilibrium at that time. As Swan-Gatz catheterization or coronary angiography are not routinely able to perform in the procurement hospital in Japan for several social reasons, myocardial damage and underlying heart diseases are determined by hemodynamics, requirement doses of

1. Myocardial damage
   - Injury of the heart (history of chest trauma, maneuver of cardiopulmonary resuscitation, and open cardiac massage)
   - Cardiac arrest with cardiopulmonary resuscitation (> 5 minutes)
2. High-dose requirement of inotrope administration (dopamine >15 mcg/kg/min)
3. Underlying heart disease defined by echocardiography (without a history of open-heart surgery)
   - Correctable valvular dysfunction
   - Correctable congenital heart anomaly
4. Left ventricular hypertrophy (wall thickness > 15 mm)
5. Prolonged total ischemic time(> 4 hours)
6. Elderly age
   - 55 years (especially without coronary angiography)
   - Bypassable one- or two-vessel coronary arterial disease
7. Body size and gender mismatch
   - Undersizing or oversizing by more than 20% body weight
   - Female to male (especially undersized donor by more than 20% body weight)

Table 2.
Extended criteria donor (ECD) for heart transplantation.

inotropes and ADH administration, the LV wall motion and morphology by echocardiogram, and electrocardiogram (ECG) findings.

It is very important to evaluate donor cardiac function after treating diabetes insipidus, adjusting the tone of peripheral vessels, and recovering the affinity of the β-adrenergic receptor for adrenaline in the myocardium by administrating ADH via the central venous line and optimizing circulating blood volume [2].

The heart with a history of cardiac arrest with cardiopulmonary resuscitation can be transplanted if the cardiac function is recovered and the heart has no significant underlying disease or ischemic ECG changes [2, 21]. Recently, the ISHLT registry report 2020 also reported that recipients of donors who died from anoxia or head trauma had the highest 1-year survival (89.9%), whereas the lowest 1-year survival (84.1%) was seen in recipients of donors who died from cerebrovascular accident/stroke [22].

4.2 High-dose requirement of inotrope administration

Even hemodynamics or cardiac systolic function are well maintained, the myocardium is considered damaged if a high dose of inotrope administration is required to stabilize hemodynamics. Therefore, an assessment of LV function should be done after reducing dosages of inotropes as less as possible.

As high serum adrenaline concentration, as well as a high dose of intravenous adrenaline administration, has a significant relationship with a decrease in the myocardial density of β-adrenergic receptors [23, 24], the use of adrenaline should be used as less as possible. Less than 0.05 mcg/kg/min of adrenaline is acceptable. Regards to the dose of dopamine and others, the donor heart requiring greater than 15 mcg/kg/min of dopamine is considered ECD heart, especially with abnormal ECG and echocardiographic findings. Mostly, less than 15 mcg/kg/min of dopamine is acceptable.

4.3 Underlying heart disease

The hearts with the most valvular and congenital cardiac abnormalities are not eligible for transplantation. Therefore, pre-existing heart diseases should be carefully assessed by the echocardiogram and the chest CT scan before procurement surgery.

In donors with acceptable heart function, however, a simultaneous repair can be done on a donor heart with simple congenital heart disease (e.g., atrial septal defect, ventricular septal defect, or patent ductus arteriosus), mild or moderate valvular regurgitation in the mitral and/or tricuspid valve or normally functioning bicuspid aortic valve.

4.4 LV hypertrophy

As the hypertrophic myocardium is susceptible to ischemia-reperfusion injury, the hypertrophic heart with left ventricular wall thickness greater than 13 mm should be decided carefully to use. The hypertrophic heart with ECG criteria for LVH and total ischemic time (TIT) longer than 4 hours is inadvisable to transplant.

4.5 Prolonged total ischemic time (TIT)

It has been reported that prolonged total ischemic time (TIT) was a significant correlation with the early post-transplant death after HTx. The acceptable safe preservation time limit for HTx might be less than 4 hours. In fact, the report of the International Society for Heart and Lung Transplantation (ISHLT) showed that the relative risk of 1-year mortality was affected by TIT for longer than 6 hours [23]. However, pediatric hearts with TIT longer than 8 hours were reported to be safely transplanted [21].

To prolong the safe limit of preservation period in immerse heart preservation method, many studies were carried out. The author of the chapter reported that the modification of preservation solution and the application of terminal leukocyte-depleted blood cardioplegia preserved good function of orthotopically transplanted cardiac grafts after 24-hour immersed preservation in the canines and goats [25].

4.6 Elderly age

As aging increases the risk to have the myocardial damage due to coronary arterial disease, left ventricular hypertrophy, and valvular disease, donors older than 50 years of age were generally considered to be ECD. In fact, older donor age is associated with decreased survival after heart transplantation, especially within the first month after transplantation [23]. Moreover, the relative risk of developing cardiac allograft vasculopathy within 8 years is also affected by donor age. Therefore, meticulous evaluation of coronary arteries with coronary angiography as well as left ventricular wall motion with echocardiography are essential to assess the heart of elderly persons.

Although coronary arterial interventions are applicable in the recipient after heart transplantation, several cases of simultaneous coronary arterial grafting have been reported to use the donor hearts with significant coronary artery disease [18, 19]. Overall graft patency at 2 years was reported to be 82%.

One may consider completion of BD as a certain kind of stress test on the myocardium such that if subsequent ECG or echocardiography is favorable, the chance of an elderly donor having significant CAD is probably low. This screening strategy without the use of coronary angiography is thought to make an efficient selection of elderly donor hearts for transplantation with a good outcome. But if the donor has left ventricular hypertrophy and/or significant ECG changes, the heart is not eligible for transplantation [2].

4.7 Body size and gender

Although a small donor size relative to the recipient may increase a survival risk post-transplantation, a normal-sized adult male is suitable for most recipients. Russo et al. [26] demonstrated that transplanting a female donor heart into a male recipient is associated with a significantly higher risk of PGD. On the other hand, the risk of CAV universally increased with increasing donor age [22]. However, recipients of male allografts had an increased risk of CAV development, regardless of the recipient's gender [22].

5. Donor management

To manage a donor optimally, hemodynamics, cardiac and respiratory function, infection, and other organ functions of the donor should be assessed precisely. As there are no specialized therapeutic strategies for liver or renal dysfunction during a short period of donor management usually less than 20 hours, cardiopulmonary management to improve organ perfusion and blood gas supply, and metabolic management are the main therapeutic strategies for ECD management.

5.1 Circulatory management

The repeated assessment and optimal management of donor left ventricular (LV) dysfunction offer a tremendous potential to increase cardiac donor utilization as a significant proportion of hearts are declined for reasons of "poor ventricular function." However, it has been reported that in younger donors, left ventricular dysfunction can completely recover to normal overtime prior to procurement in a donor and after transplantation in a recipient. Although echocardiography is a very effective tool to assess heart anatomy, especially valvular anomalies, the use of a single echo assessment of ventricular function is not recommended to decide the functional suitability of a donor heart graft.

The goals of hemodynamic management are to achieve normovolemia, minimize vasoconstrictors and vasodilators to keep a normal cardiac afterload and optimize cardiac output with minimal doses of inotropes, which increase myocardial oxygen demands, deplete high-energy phosphates and the density of BAR in the myocardium. The targets of hemodynamic parameters are systemic blood pressure > 90 mmHg, central venous pressure (CVP) 6 to 10 mmHg, urine output 100 ml/h (0.5 to 3 ml/kg/h), and heart rate 80 to 120/minutes with a minimum dosage of inotrope administration.

5.2 Respiratory management

The use of low-tidal-volume ventilation is recommended because a mechanical ventilator with high tidal volumes is potentially harmful and may exacerbate donor lung injury already damaged during the completion of BD. Recruitment maneuvers are an important component of donor optimization, especially when the oxygenation is subnormal and pulmonary abnormalities are visible on the chest x-ray. Repeated bronchoscopy (6 to 8 hours interval) is also important to improve donor lungs.

5.3 Administration of ADH

Administration of low-dose arginine vasopressin in conjunction with correction of hypovolemia due to diabetes insipidus reduces inotropic requirements and improves kidney, liver, and heart graft function, as shown previously [2]. As ADH increases both vascular tone and the affinity of BAR, ADH is effective even in patients with reduced urine output. ADH may stabilize hemodynamics, increase renal blood flow, and finally increase urine output.

Although desmopressin is mostly beneficial for the primary treatment of diabetes insipidus, it does not usually reduce inotrope requirements in organ donors [2]. Furthermore, desmopressin is reported to increase the incidence of thrombotic events.

ADH should be continuously given through a central venous line with a dose of 10–2o microU/Kg/h or 0.5–1 U/h. In case of hypotension, a loading bolus dose of ADH 0.5 to 1U is effective. If hemodynamics is stabilized by ADH administration, noradrenaline, and then adrenaline can be discontinued. If serum adrenaline level comes within a normal range, the heart rate is converged to an intrinsic heart rate between individuals of the same age, usually into a range of 90 to 120/minutes which is higher than the resting heart rate, because the autonomic regulation on the heart is gone in a BD patient. To optimize hemodynamics throughout procurement surgery, ADH should be continuously infused until the insertion of perfusion cannulas for all procured organs become ready and heparin is given [2].

Reduced ADH secretion due to BD may increase urine output, serum sodium, and osmolality, as well as reduce serum potassium, which decreases circulatory blood volume and intracellular fluid and cause hepatic or renal dysfunction and arrhythmia. Therefore, ADH administration can restore these consequences and is considered a key medication for donor management. Adjusting serum sodium and potassium with 135–150 and 3.8–4.5 mEq/l, respectively, hematocrit greater than 30%, blood sugar with 120–180 mg/dl, and body temperature with 35.5–36.5°C, are also important for optimal donor management.

6. Japanese strategies for donor evaluation and management

6.1 Medical consultant system in Japan

Since BD organ transplantation was started on 28th February 1999 in Japan, every organ procurement team has taken its own staff physicians to the procurement hospital. They evaluated the donor heart function by performing echocardiography by themselves in ICU prior to procurement operation.

Since November 2002, special transplant management doctors (a medical consultant; MC), who used to be cardiac transplant surgeons and are currently cardiac transplant cardiologists, have been sent to the procurement hospital. They estimate donor heart function and determine whether the heart is useful for transplantation. They also intensively manage the donor by giving ADH as shown above, minimizing the dose of intravenous inotropes, and improving the donor organ function until the procurement heart team arrives at the procurement hospital.

Management strategy of lungs has been modified after the 50th organ procurement from a BD donor in December 2006. After then, in addition to routine bronchial toileting and posture change, repeated broncho fiberscope and frequent bronchial toileting were performed, if there were symptoms and/or signs of atelectasis or pneumonia in the chest x-ray and CT chest scan, After changing the lung management strategy, not only lung availability but also patient survival rate after lung transplantation significantly increased [27]. Then, since 2011, lung transplant surgeons played a role in evaluating and managing lungs as lung MC [28].

6.2 1st step donor evaluation

PTC of Japan Organ Tx Network (JOT) is sent to a hospital if there is a potential BD organ donor. They evaluate the patient clinical course and check clinical records to rule out the absolute contraindications, shown above. They obtain informed consent for BD organ donation from his or her relatives. After then, two times of legal examination for BD is carried out.

6.3 2nd step donor evaluation

After completion of 1st legal examination for BD determination, MCs come to the hospital. They and JOT PTC obtain the donor's clinical data such as past history, family history, clinical course during the completion of BD and after BD, such as the history of cardiopulmonary resuscitation and pulmonary aspiration, medication given, such as inotropes, ADH and antibiotics, transfusion, blood examination, blood gas examination, hemodynamic parameters, ECG findings, and data of image examination such as the chest x-ray and the abdominal and chest CT scan. MCs also perform ultrasound examinations for heart and abdominal organs and broncho fiberscope. Rule out malignancies by findings of the CT scan and ultrasound examination and support of making donor evaluation sheets by JOT PTCs are is also an important job of MC.

After 2nd legal examination for BD determination, the patient has declared dead and donor evaluation sheets and images of sequential ECGs, chest x-rays, echocardiography, and chest CT scans are sent to the heart transplant centers of potential recipients using a mobile system, called a donor data delivery system (DDDS) established by JOT. Then transplant center decides whether the recipient undergo heart transplantation from this BD donor and the procurement team is sent to the hospital

According to their assessment of donor hemodynamics and respiration, MCs proposed individualized donor management strategies to physicians taking care of the donor in the procurement hospital.

6.4 3rd step donor evaluation

After arriving at the donor hospital, the procurement team also evaluates the donor heart function with echocardiography by themselves in ICU and determines whether the heart can be transplanted to their recipient. They send this information to their transplant team.

6.5 Pre-procurement meeting and management of the procurement operation

Before starting the procurement operation, all procurement surgeons, anesthesiologists, and operating room nurses gathered in the meeting room. They negotiated on the types of organs procured, the organ transportation method, the method of each organ procurement (e.g., organ dissection/perfusion technique, incision lines, blood drainage technique, etc), what kinds of samples (e.g., blood, lymph nodes, and spleen) were needed, and how to manage the donor during operation. A heart procurement surgeon also supports anesthesiologists to stabilize the patient's hemodynamics throughout the procurement operation.

Skillful staff surgeons, not resident surgeons, harvests the donor heart. As it was reported that increased intraoperative colloid infusion was significantly associated with poor allograft function post-lung transplantation, maintenance of circulating blood volume and blood osmolality by infusing packed red blood cells and albumin during procurement operation are very important to improve lung graft function posttransplant. To achieve good organ perfusion with preservation solution, the dosage of inotropes should be kept to the minimum to dilate the procured organ vessels and ADH is continuously given until heparin sulfate (400 U/Kg) is given.

6.6 Final donor evaluation

After opening the chest, the procurement team will evaluate the heart by inspection and palpation to decide to use the heart. They also look out for unexpected malignancies in the pleural and abdominal cavities.

7. Discussion

For many years, heart transplantation has been an established treatment strategy for end-stage heart failure patients using the so-called "Standard Criteria" donor heart. However, over the past three decades, the number of annually listed patients for heart transplantation greatly increased worldwide, and the strict use of the "Standard Criteria" hearts has enhanced severe donor heart shortage, significantly prolonged waiting times and increased the death rate of listed patients prior to heart transplantation. Therefore, the use of ECD hearts has increased worldwide. However, even in 2020, only 3,658 hearts of 9,364 BD donors (39.1%) were transplanted in the USA. As only 760 BD donors have been available in Japan for more than 20 years until the end of 2020 because of the very strict Japanese Organ Transplant Act, only 297 donor hearts would have been transplanted if the rate of heart utilization from the BD donors in Japan is same as in the USA. These extraordinary pressures of donor heart shortage had made Japanese heart transplant programs use a much greater number of ECD donor hearts than in developed countries. Therefore, an original and sophisticated donor evaluation and management system have been established in Japan, such as MC and pre-procurement meetings and so on.

To elucidate the role of this Japanese donor evaluation and management system, consecutive 775 BD donors since the Act was issued until the end of August 2021 in Japan, were reviewed. A total of 611 hearts (78.8%) were transplanted, and organ transplanted per donor was 5.1 (3,985 organs from 775 donors). The number of heart donor $\geq$ 60 years of age was 63 (10.3%). In the heart donors who had information about the cause of death, the cause of BD was subarachnoid hemorrhage in 160, hypoxic brain damage in 126, other cerebrovascular disorders in 120, head trauma in 100, post-cardiopulmonary resuscitation in 29, and asphyxias in 23. Overall survival rates of cardiac recipients at 1 year, 5, 10, and 20 years were 93.3, 88.3, 79.1, and 75.3%, respectively. Patient survival at 10 years with donor aged 10–19 years, 20–29 years, 30–39 years, 40–49 years, 50–59 years, and 60–69 years were 100, 61.6, 95.5,

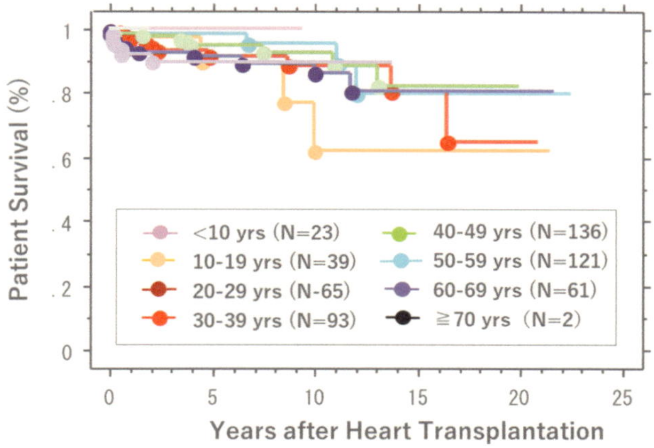

Figure 3.
Cumulative patient survival rate of heart transplant recipients by donor age group (up to August 31, 2021). yrs: years.

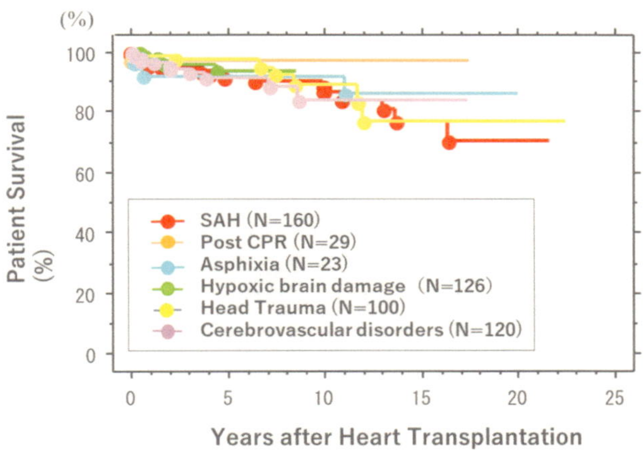

Figure 4.
Cumulative patient survival rate of heart transplant recipients by donor cause of death group (up to August 31, 2021). SAH: subarachnoid hemorrhage, Post-CPR: post-cardiopulmonary resuscitation.

88.4, 92.7, 85.9, and 89.3%, respectively (**Figure 3**). Patient survival at 10 years from a donor with subarachnoid hemorrhage, hypoxic brain damage, other cerebrovascular disorders, head trauma, post-cardiopulmonary resuscitation, and asphyxias were 87.7, 93,2 (at 8.6 years), 82.9, 88.3, 96.6, and 85.2%, respectively (**Figure 4**). These values were not significantly different.

8. Conclusion

As deceased organ donation has not increased compared to an increase in listed candidates for heart transplantation worldwide, extended criteria donor hearts have been used in many countries. However, in most countries, only 20–30% of donor hearts from BD donors have been used. Therefore, in Japan where donor shortage has been extremely sever than in other developed countries, special strategies for maximizing heart availability should be established. By establishing the MC system in Japan, the availability of hearts has been very high (79%) and the patient survival rate at high (89% at 10 years). MC doctors may play a great role in increasing donor heart availability as well as in improving outcomes of cardiac recipients even from elderly donors or donors who died of post-resuscitation and anoxia in Japan. These strategies may be useful for maximizing heart transplant opportunities and improving post-transplant outcomes.

Author details

Norihide Fukushima
Department of Transplant Medicine, National Cerebral and Cardiovascular Center, Suita, Japan

*Address all correspondence to: nori@ncvc.go.jp

References

[1] Fukushima N. Revised organ transplant act and transplant surgeons. Japan Medical Association Journal. 2011;**54**(6):387-391

[2] Fukushima N, Ono M, Nakatani T, et al. Strategies for maximizing heart and lung transplantation opportunities in Japan. Transplantation Proceedings. 2009;**41**(1):273-276

[3] Novitzky D, Cooper DK, Rosendale JD, Kauffman HM. Hormonal therapy of the brain-dead organ donor: Experimental and clinical studies. Transplantation. 2006;**82**(11):1396-1401

[4] Mascia L, Mastromauro I, Viverti S, et al. Management of optimize organ procurement in brain dead donors. Minerva Anesthesiol. 2009;**75**:125-133

[5] Kaul DR, Vece G, Blumberg E, et al. Ten years of donor-derived disease: A report of the disease transmission advisory committee. American Journal of Transplantation. 2021;**21**:689-702. DOI: 10.1111/ajt.16178

[6] Audibert G, Charpentier C, Sequim-Devaux C, et al. Improvement of donor myocardial function after treatment of autonomic strom during brain death. Transplantation. 2006;**82**:1031-1036

[7] Ryan JB, Hicks M, Cropper JR, et al. Functional evidence of reversible ischemic injury immediately after the sympathetic storm associated with experimental brain death. The Journal of Heart and Lung Trasnplantation. 2003;**22**:922-928

[8] Boone M, Deen PM. Physiology and pathophysiology of the vasopressin-regulated renal water reabsorption. Pflügers Archives. 2008 Sep;**456**(6):1005-1024

[9] Pennefether SH, Bullock RE, Mantle D, Dark JH. Use of low dose arginine vasopressin to support brain-dead organ donors. Transplantation. 1995;**59**:58

[10] Kinoshita Y, Okamoto K, Yahata K, et al. Clinical and pathological changes of the heart in brain death maintained with vasopressin and epinephrine. Pathology, Research and Practice. 1990;**186**(1):173-179

[11] Iwai A, Sakano T, Uenishi M, et al. Effects of vasopressin and catecholamines on the maintena,nce of circulatory stability in brain-dead patients. Transplantation. 1989;**48**(4):613-617

[12] Fukushima N, Shirakura R, Nakata S, et al. Failure of rapid autonomic augmentation of cardiac performance in transplanted hearts. Transplantation Proceedings. 1998;**30**(7):3344-3346

[13] Huprikar S, Danziger-Isakov L, Ahn J, et al. Solid organ transplantation from hepatitis B virus-positive donors: Consensus guidelines for recipient management. American Journal of Transplantation. 2015;**15**(5):1162-1172. DOI: 10.1111/ajt.13187

[14] Ruiz I, Gavaldà J, Monforte V, Len O, Román A, et al. Donor-to-host transmission of bacterial and fungal infections in lung transplantation. American Journal of Transplantation. 2006;**6**:178-182

[15] Hynes CF, Ramakrishnan K, Alfares FA, et al. Risk of tumor transmission after thoracic allograft transplantation from adult donors with central nervous system neoplasm–A

UNOS database study. Clinical Transplantation. 2017;**31**(4):e12919. DOI: 10.1111/ctr.12919

[16] Desai R, Collett D, Watson CJE, Johnson P, Evans T, Neuberger J. Estimated risk of cancer transmission from organ donor to graft recipient in a national transplantation registry. BJS. 2014;**101**:768-774. DOI: 10.1002/bjs.946

[17] Grauhan O. Screening and assessment of the donor heart cardiopulmonary. Pathophysiology. 2011;**15**:191-197

[18] Laks H, Gates RN, Ardehali A, et al. Orthotopic heart transplantation and concurrent coronary bypass. The Journal of Heart and Lung Transplantation. 1993;**12**:810-815

[19] Marelli D, Laks H, Bresson S, et al. Results after transplantation using donor hearts with preexisting coronary artery disease. The Journal of Thoracic and Cardiovascular Surgery. 2003;**126**:821

[20] Kimura Y, Seguchi O, Iwasaki K, et al. Impact of coronary artery calcification in the donor heart on transmitted coronary artery disease in heart trnsplant recipients. Circulation Journal. 2018;**82**:3021-3028. DOI: 10.1253/circj.CJ-18-0107

[21] Bailey LL, Razzouk AJ, Hasaniya NW, Chinnock RE. Pediatric transplantation using hearts refused on the basis of donor quality. The Annals of Thoracic Surgery. 2009;**87**(6):1902-1908

[22] Khush KK, Potena L, Cherikh WS, et al. The international thoracic organ transplant registry of the International Society for Heart and Lung Transplantation: 37th adult heart transplantation report—2020; focus on deceased donor characteristics. The Journal of Heart and Lung Transplantation. 2020;**39**(10):1003-1015

[23] Sakagoshi N, Shirakura R, Nakano S, et al. Serial changes in myocardial beta-adrenergic receptor after experimental brain death in dogs. The Journal of Heart and Lung Transplantation. 1992;**11**:1054-1058

[24] Fukushima N, Sakagoshi N, Ohtake S, et al. Effects of exogenous adrenaline on the number of the beta-adrenergic receptors after brain death in humans. Transplantation Proceedings. 2002;**34**:2571-2574

[25] Fukushima N, Shirakura R, Nakata S, et al. Study of efficacies of leukocyte-depleted terminal blood cardioplegia in 24-hour preserved hearts. The Annals of Thoracic Surgery. 1994;**58**(6):1651-1656

[26] Russo MJ, Iribarne A, Hong KN, et al. Factors associated with primary graft failure after heart transplantation. Transplantation. 2010;**90**(4):444-450

[27] Fukushima N, Ono M, Saito S, et al. Japanese strategies to maximize heart and lung availabilities: Experience from 100 consecutive brain-dead donors. Transplantation Proceedings. 2013;**45**:2871-2874

[28] Hoshikawa Y, Okada Y, Ashikari J, et al. Medical consultant system for improving lung transplantation opportunities and outcomes in Japan. Transplantation Proceedings. 2015;**47**:746-750

Chapter 2

Primary Graft Dysfunction after Heart Transplantation

Soo Yong Lee

Abstract

The entire transplant journey that the donor heart experiences affect the donor heart function early after transplantation. The early graft dysfunction without discernible cause is primary graft dysfunction (PGD) and has been one of the critical complications and the cause of early mortality after orthotopic heart transplantation. Although, numerous researchers investigated the pathophysiology and the related biomarkers, the process is multifactorial and therefore no definite biomarker has been proposed. After the recent definition from the International Society of Heart and Lung Transplantation, the standard of management is still under investigation by each status. Here, the prevalence, pathophysiology, biomarkers, and recent progression of management of PGD will be reviewed.

Keywords: heart transplantation, primary graft dysfunction

1. Introduction

Heart transplantation (HTx) remains the most effective long-term treatment for eligible patients with advanced heart failure. Remarkable improvements in HTx outcomes over decades with advances in medicine and surgical techniques, Primary graft dysfunction (PGD) has been one of the critical complications after orthotopic heart transplantation and cause of early mortality [1, 2]. However, even the definition has formulated recently in 2014, by the International Society of Heart and Lung Transplantation (ISHLT) in the consensus statement and management guidelines are still absent [3]. The 30-day mortality of PGD had been reported with a wide range of 2.3-28.2% in the era before consensus definition. Although, applying new a definition, the early mortality with PGD patients showed no great difference, 6.06-18.4% [4–6].

2. Primary graft dysfunction

2.1 Definition, prevalence, diagnosis

2.1.1 Definition

PGD was defined as any graft dysfunction that occurs within 24 h after completion of transplant surgery (**Table 1**). This definition was established during the annual meeting of ISHLT in 2013. Primary means, not associated with a discernible cause, such as

PGD-left ventricle (PGD-LV)	Mild PGD-LV	One of the following criteria must be met: LVEF ≤40% by echocardiography, or Hemodynamics with RAP >15 mm Hg, PCWP >20 mm Hg, CI < 2.0 L/min/m^2 (lasting more than 1 h) requiring low-dose inotropes
	Moderate PGD-LV	Must meet one criterion from I and another criterion from II: I. Criteria LVEF ≤40%, or Hemodynamic compromise with RAP >15 mm Hg, PCWP >20 mm Hg, CI < 2.0 L/min/m2 Hypotension with MAP <70 mm Hg (> 1 h) II. Criteria. i. High-dose inotropes: Inotrope score > 10* or ii. Newly placed IABP (Regardless of inotropes)
	Severe PGD–LV	Dependence on left or biventricular mechanical support including ECMO, LVAD, BiVAD, or percutaneous LVAD. Excludes requirement for IABP.
PGD-right ventricle (PGD-RV)		Diagnosis requires either both i and ii, or iii alone: i. Hemodynamics with RAP >15 mmHg, PCWP <15 mmHg, CI < 2.0 L/min/m^2 ii. TPG <15 mmHg and/or sPAP <50 mm Hg, or iii. Need for RVAD

BiVAD, biventricular assist device; CI, cardiac index; ECMO, extracorporeal membrane oxygenation; IABP, intraaortic balloon pump; LVAD, left ventricular assist device; PCWP, pulmonary capillary wedge pressure; RAP, right atrial pressure; RVAD, right ventricular assist device; TPG, transpulmonary pressure gradient.
**Inotrope score = dopamine (×1) + dobutamine (×1) + amrinone (×1) + milrinone (×15) + epinephrine (×100) + norepinephrine (×100) with each drug dosed in μg/kg/min.*

Table 1.
Definition of severity scale for primary graft dysfunction [3].

hyperacute rejection, pulmonary hypertension, or uncontrolled intraoperative bleeding requiring massive blood product transfusions and prolonged graft ischemic time [3, 7].

2.1.2 Prevalence and outcomes

Primary graft dysfunction develops fairly common after HTx. A report from two Italian center studies described a 518-patient cohort with a 14% prevalence of PGD and a mortality of 54% in patients with severe PGD [8]. In addition, a UK National study evaluated medical records, PGD developed in 163 among 450 adult heart transplant cohort, and the overall incidence of PGD was 36.2%. The distribution of PGD according to severity was 4, 72, 81 and 6 for mild, moderate, severe LV PGD, and RV. A recently published data from South Korea showed 6.7% (38/570) of incidence, most of them were moderate to severe state (34/38). The early mortality rate in patients with moderate to severe PGD-LV (20.6%) differed significantly from that in patients without PGD (0.6%; $P < 0.001$). From the landmark analysis, the authors showed the strong effect of moderate to severe PGD-LV on early death, and no significant difference in late survival rates (>3mo) in patients with or without moderate to severe PGD-LV.

The outcomes of a different cohort of 191 patients found worse 30-day mortality of 25% in moderate to severe PGD group, the survival curves diverged during the first 3 months following transplantation but went parallel after this initial postoperative period [9]. That means, PGD mainly affects the early deaths, not the late deaths.

The detailed incidence and outcomes of each study is summarized in **Table 2**.

DOI: http://dx.doi.org/10.5772/intechopen.102506

References	Year of publish	Years of data obtained	PGD/Total patient number of cohort (%)	Mild LV PGD	Moderate LV PGD	Severe LV PGD	RV PGD	30-day mortality PGD vs no-PGD	Long-term outcome PGD vs no-PGD
Daronavalli et al.* UK [10]	2015	2007–2011	94/290 (32%)					37.2% versus 4.1%	1-year morality 41.5% versus 8.2%
Sabatino M., et al. [8] Italy	2017	1999–2013	72/518 (14%)	4/72 (5%)	33/72 (46%)	35/72 (49%)		27% versus 3% mild (0%), moderate (12%), severe (65%)	PGD no longer influenced mortality after hospital discharge
Squiers J., et al. [9] USA	2017	2012–2015	59/191 (31%)	35/59 (59%)	8/59 (14%)	16/59 (27%)		mild (0%), moderate (0%), severe (38%) versus 0%	1-year survival:mild (94%), moderate (75%), severe (44%)
Nicoara A. et al. [6] USA	2017	2009–2014	99/317 (31%)					1.7% without VAD 12.8% with VAD versus 0.9%	1-year mortality 15% without VAD 28% with VAD versus 4.1%
Foroutan F. et al. [11] Canada	2019	2004–2015	82/412 (20%)	15/82 (18%)	39/82 (48%)	19/82 (23%)	12/82 (15%)		
Singh S., et al. [5] UK	2019	2012–2015	163/450 (36%)	4/163 (3%)	72/163 (44%)	81/163 (50%)	6/163 (4%)	19% versus 4.5%	6 month mortality 31.9% versus 6.3%
Rhee Y., et al. [4] South Korea	2021	1992–2017	35/570 (6%)	1/35 (3%)	14/35 (40%)	20/35 (57%)	3/35 (8.6%)	mild (0%), moderate (14.3%), severe (25%) versus 0.6%	1-year survival: 72.5 ± 7.5% versus 95.1 ± 0.9%

Applied PGD criteria within 72 h after transplantation.

Table 2.
Incidences of PGD according to new ISHLT criteria showed in various reports.

2.1.3 Differential diagnosis with secondary graft dysfunction (SGD)

When it comes to the first facing of PGD, a novice in HTx could have difficulties in differentiating PGD from SGD. SGD has discernible causes such as pulmonary hypertension, surgical complications, or hyperacute rejection [3]. A significant improvement in the pretransplant management of both donors and recipients could contribute to reducing the incidence of SGD over a decade, from10 to 5.6% [8], although there are some differences in the reported incidences [2, 8]. For SGD and PGD share some risk factors and could develop concurrently. Therefore, the patient's condition is unacceptable for the satisfactory evaluation for differential diagnosis, treatment targeting both SGD and PGD is warranted. Several diagnostic pearls and pitfalls are summarized in **Table 3**.

2.2 Pathophysiology

The entire transplant journey that the donor heart experiences including brain death, storage of the organ in a hypothermic environment, potential exposure to warm ischemia, and reperfusion could affect the allograft dysfunction [15]. The surge of catecholamines following brain injury leads to myocardial ischemia, calcium overload, and alteration in the sensitivity of myocytes to calcium. This is further aggravated by exogenous catecholamines following cardiopulmonary bypass and reperfusion [16, 17].

In addition, the ischemia-reperfusion injury (IRI) has been thought to play another major role in the development of PGD. Once the aortic cross-clamp is applied, cold cardioplegia is infused via the aortic root at approximately 4°C. The retrieval process is completed with the heart placed in a cold storage container. The cold storage induces hypothermic arrest of metabolism and maintains viability during this reduced metabolic state, therefore minimizing cellular swelling and reperfusion injury [18]. At these temperatures, and with limited oxygenation, the heart switches from aerobic to anaerobic metabolism. Generally in the hypothermic state (0–4°C), there is a 12-fold decrease in metabolic rate and reduces the accumulation of mitochondrial byproducts of metabolism such as oxygen-free radicals. However, the duration at which the hearts are kept in cold storage matters in the formation of these free radicals. Cellular swelling and lactic acidosis occur in prolonged cold storage, causing an elevation of intracellular H^+ ions [19]. Then, the Na^+/H^+ exchanger is activated resulting in an increase in intracellular Na^+ which activates the Na^+/Ca^{2+} exchanger. The final pathway is the accumulation of cytosolic Ca^{2+} [20]. After releasing cross-clamp, Ca^{2+} overload results in hypercontraction of the myocardium, and a marked rise in end-diastolic pressure with increased ventricular wall stiffness. A greater myofibrillar shortening and cytoskeletal damage occur compared to the ischemic phase [21]. In cellular studies, re-perfused infarcts consist almost exclusively of contraction band necrosis. This process, known as hypercontracture-mediated sarcolemmal rupture (HMSR), impairs Na^+/Ca^{2+} exchanger pumps, and finally increases Na^+ influx into cardiomyocytes via gap junctions and may propagate to adjacent cells [22]. Clinically, the prolonged cold ischemic time of more than 4 h was reported as one of the most important predictors of PGD [23, 24].

2.3 Biomarkers

Several biomarkers have been suggested as potential predictors of PGD, however, the guidelines are absent, and none are in routine use currently.

DOI: http://dx.doi.org/10.5772/intechopen.102506

Secondary graft dysfunction	Incidence	Clinical characteristics	Diagnosis	Management	Prevention
RV failure by Pulmonary hypertension	The most common ~80% [8]	TPG >11 mmHg [12] PVR >2.8WU Young donor heart naïve to high PA pressure	Right heart catheterization RV failure detection by Echo	Inhaled NO (20–40 ppm) IV indicators Volume optimization High FiO_2 for limiting vasoconstriction MCS is needed in hemodynamic instability	Avoid HTx in the recipients with cpcPAH (rather apply LVAD first)
Surgical complications	Second most common	Occlusion of the coronary arteries (dissection, air embolism) Narrowed anastomosis Kinking of the pulmonary artery Significant adhesions >10 Units of packed RBCs	Imaging study (CT, Echo) Events in surgical field Markedly elevated EBL counts	Releasing the mechanical obstructive problems Careful fluid and electrolyte management	Thorough understanding of recipient anatomy and planning via imaging study before surgery
Hyperacute rejection	Very low 01–0.3% [8, 13, 14]	ABO mismatch High DSA with no desensitization	Graft failure within the first few minutes to hours	Inotropes, plasmapheresis, intense immunosuppression (IVIG, rituximab, eculizumab) MCS	Avoid ABO mismatch HTx Prospective cross-matching Desensitization

cpcPAH, combined pre and post pulmonary artery hypertension, CT, computed tomography, DSA, donor-specific antibody, EBL, estimated blood loss, Echo, echocardiography, FiO_2, the fraction of inspired oxygen, HTx, heart transplantation, IVIG, intravenous immunoglobulin, LVAD, left ventricular assisted devices, MCS, mechanical circulatory support, NO, nitric oxide, PA, pulmonary artery, PVR, pulmonary vascular resistance, RV, right ventricle, TPG, transpulmonary pressure gradient.

Table 3.
Brief characteristics of SGD for differential diagnosis with PGD.

2.3.1 Proinflammatory biomarkers in donors and recipients

The pathophysiology of PGD itself is deeply connected with the inflammatory processes after IRI, the related markers were investigated. Tumor necrosis factor-α (TNF-α) is a representative pro-inflammatory biomarker produced by lymphocytes and macrophages [25]. Venkateswaran et al. highlighted poorer biventricular function in donors with elevated levels of TNF-α using serum immunoassays. In the study, the authors also showed higher baseline donor procalcitonin (PCT) levels were related to worse cardiac index and RV and LVEF and demonstrated PCT level of more than 2 ng/mL might be a tool for the usability of donor heart [26]. Wagner et al. also suggested a PCT level of 2 ng/mL as a cut-off value for increasing 30-day mortality and early graft dysfunction after transplantation [27].

Birks and colleagues noted an increased expression of TNF-α in unused donor hearts due to poor function and compared them with donors with good ventricular function (used donors) and patients with advanced heart failure (HF). They also noted IL-6 mRNA expression was 2.4-fold higher in the unused donor hearts than in those used for HTx [28]. This was accompanied by similar changes in the serum and suggests those could be potential biomarkers for PGD.

Hypoxia-inducible factor (HIF)-1 is activated by various growth factors, cytokines, and vascular hormones, which are essential mediators of IRI. HIF-1 is a heterodimeric α, β transcription factor, and potentiates tissue responses to hypoxia [29]. HIF-1 along with the early growth response factor facilitates the transcription of inflammatory cytokines. Aharinejad et al. performed a prospective analysis in 200 heart donors over 7 years and identified HIF-1 as an independent predictor of PGD [30]. They demonstrated a significant increase in HIF-1 levels especially 10 min after reperfusion and were correlated with higher incidences of PGD.

Recently, the pro-inflammatory tendency of recipients rather than donors has been actively focused by investigators. Giangreco et al. reported KLKB1, a serine protease that controls the activation of both inflammation and coagulation in what is known as the kallikrein-kinin system (KKS), as a potential predictor for PGD using gene set enrichment analysis (GSEA) [31]. A classifier utilizing KLKB1 and inotrope therapy outperforms existing composite scores by more than 50%. In the inflammatory response, KLKB1 converts high molecular weight kininogen into bradykinin stimulating the release of nitric oxide and prostacyclin causing vasodilation and increased vascular permeability.

Truby et al. employed high-throughput proteomic profiling related to innate immune activation and inflammation in HTx recipients of pre-transplant serum from HTx recipients to identify relevant biomarkers [32]. Proteomic profiling revealed 9 out of 342 proteins showed statistical significance in the derivation set. When they were tested in the validation set, only CLEC4C (C-Type Lectin Domain Family 4 Member C, a protein marker of plasmacytoid dendritic cells (pDCs),) was significantly associated with PGD. The odd ratio (95% CI) for CLEC4C for PGD was 1.89 ([1.38, 2.64], $p = 1.3 \times 10^{-4}$) in sensitivity analysis combining the derivation and validation sets. Moreover, when the CLEC4C was added to the traditional risk stratification tool such as RADIAL score, they showed a better risk profile. The aforementioned studies identified not only the biomarkers but also the novel pathogenesis of PGD.

2.3.2 Biomarkers for damaged heart

The measurements of serum cardiac troponin I (cTnI) and cardiac troponin T (cTnT) have shown to be sensitive and specific markers of myocardial damage [33].

After SAH, sympathetic nervous system activation and release of norepinephrine from the myocardial sympathetic nerves could result in myocardial damage and troponin elevation [34]. Many systemic complications occur after brain death like myocardial dysfunction, neurogenic stunned myocardium, segmental wall motion abnormalities, stress cardiomyopathy, and these could affect the cardiac function after HTx. Deibert et al. assessed the clinical significance of elevated cTnI levels in patients with non-traumatic subarachnoid hemorrhage and found that an elevated cTnI (≥1.4 μg/l) was a good indicator of LV dysfunction in patients with subarachnoid hemorrhage [35]. However, the cardiac dysfunction in brain death donors was mostly reversible, and larger studies that investigated the association between donor serum troponin level and PGD showed no relevance [36, 37].

BNP and the BNP precursor N-terminal prohormone BNP (NT-proBNP) are released from myocardium in response to increased wall stress. These are the most useful markers utilized in the heart failure field, with significant predictive value on diagnosis and prognosis. The elevated levels of BNP have been identified in heart donors and high levels may distinguish those donors with severely impaired LV systolic function [38]. Elevated NT-proBNP levels (4125 pg/ml) have also been found to be a marker of poor hemodynamic function and echocardiographic data in potential donors after brain stem death [39].

2.3.3 Other biomarkers

Switch/sucrose non-fermentable, a matrix-associated, actin-dependent regulator of chromatin subfamily a-like 1(SMARCAL1) is an intracellular protein that acts as a DNA-dependent ATPase involved in transcription, DNA repair and chromatin dynamics [40]. In 2009, Ahrinejad et al. demonstrated in a cohort of 336 heart donors that SMARCAL1 levels were significant predictors of both short and long-term survival and PGD. Donor serum cutoff of ≥1.25 ng/ml showed 96% sensitivity and 88% specificity for predicting PGD, with corresponding positive predictive and negative predictive values of 83% and 97%, respectively [41]. It seemed SMARCAL1 could play as a potential biomarker before organ selection or donation, however, it has not been widely used in practice till recent days.

The potential biomarkers, related pathophysiology and clinical implications are summarized in **Table 4**.

2.4 Clinically identified risk factors

Numerous variables have been identified as risk factors for PGD. Broadly, they have been categorized in terms of donor, recipient, procurement, surgical procedural and post-operative factors (**Table 5**).

In general, PGD does not come from a single risk factor, rather from multiple or complex interplays of the risk factors. Therefore, a kind of scoring system for PGD would be reasonable to estimate the risk. In 2011, Segovia et al. suggested a risk scoring system called RADIAL for predicting PGD. 'RADIAL' represents 6 multivariate risk factors: Right atrial pressure ≥ 10 mm Hg, recipient Age ≥ 60 years, Diabetes mellitus, Inotrope dependence, Donor Age ≥ 30 years, Length of ischemic time ≥ 240. In a single-center cohort of 621 HTx recipients transplanted from 1984 to 2006, the percentages of PGD were 8.3%, 11.1%, 24% and, 44.4% in the score of 0–1, 2, 3, and ≥ 4 group. The validated score in an external multicenter cohort (698 HTx from 2006 to 2010) was acceptable for risk stratification [50, 52]. However, the transplanted patient

Biomarkers	Source of sample	Pathophysiology	Clinical implication	Clinical application
TNF-α [25–27]	Donor blood (serum)	Pro-inflammatory cytokine produced by lymphocytes and macrophages	High TNF-α levels are associated with donor heart dysfunction	Surrogate indices of donor heart function
Procalcitonin [26, 27]	Donor blood (serum)	Precursor of the hormone calcitonin Proinflammatory marker	PCT >2 ng/mL, worse cardiac index, RV, LV function, increasing 30-day mortality and early graft dysfunction	Donor heart usability
IL-6/IL-6R [28, 42]	Donor myocardium and serum	Proinflammatory cytokine Also exhibit anti-inflammatory effects	2.4-fold higher blood level in the unused donor hearts	Donor heart usability
HIF-1 [29, 30]	Recipient serum after reperfusion Donor myocardium	Heterodimeric α, β transcription factor mediates tissue responses to hypoxia	HIF-1α mRNA expression after ACC in donors and at 10 min following the release of the ACC in the recipient were significant predictors of PGD	PGD risk stratification?
KLKB1 [31]	Pretransplant recipient blood	A serine protease Down regulated in inactivated complement and immune response pathway	Pretransplant KLKB1 + inotrope enhances prediction of PGD	Recipient PGD risk stratification, selection of therapy?
CLEC4C [32]	Recipient serum	A surface marker of pDCs High pDCs may develop the higher risk of interferon and TNF mediated cardiotoxicity	Full clinical model + CLE4C best predicts the risk of PGD	Recipient PGD risk stratification, target therapy for PGD?
Troponin [43, 44]	Donor blood (serum)	Regulatory proteins that control the interaction between actin and myosin Marker of myocardial damage	Increased Troponin was associated with allograft dysfunction Incomplete myocardial preservation	Surrogate indices of donor heart function
BNP [45]	Donor blood (serum)	Increased wall stress of allograft	Donor serum BNP of >160 pg/mL had 89% accuracy to predict poor cardiac performance	Surrogate indices of donor heart function

BNP, brain natriuretic peptide, CLEC4C, C-Type Lectin Domain Family 4 Member C, HIF-1, hypoxia inducible factor-1, KLKB1, Kallikrein B1, PCT, procalcitonin, pDC, plasmacytoid dendritic cells, PGD, primary graft dysfunction, TNF-α, tumor necrosis factor.

Table 4.
Representative potential biomarkers, related pathophysiology and clinical implications.

Factors	Non-modifiable	Modifiable
Donor	• Age [46, 47] • Death from trauma [48] • Cardiac dysfunction • Cardiac resuscitation time • Substance abuse • Left ventricular hypertrophy [49] • Valvular disease • Coronary artery disease	• Sepsis • Inotropic support [50]
Procurement		• Procurement team experience • Cardioplegic solution
Recipient	• Age [50] • Mechanical support [5] • Congenital heart disease • Multiple thoracic operation [2] • Comorbidities (DM, CKD, Liver dysfunction) [5, 50] • Ventilator dependence • Pulmonary hypertension [8] • LVAD bridging [6]	• Amiodarone usage [51] • Infection
Surgery	• Non-cardiac organ donation • Center volume	• Ischemic time [4, 6] • Female to male recipient [5] • Undersized donor (≥30%) [9] • Blood transfusion requirement
Postop management		• Maintain optimal CO • Maintain optimal UO

DM, diabetes mellitus, CKD, chronic kidney disease, CO, cardiac output, UO, urine output.

Table 5.
Known risk factors for the development of primary graft dysfunction.

population bridged by LVAD was relatively low (16/621, 2.6%) in the study. In a recent single-center study, there was a trend toward increased PGD in pretransplant LVAD recipients (40.4% vs. 32.9%, $P = 0.0555$) [6]. The RADIAL score is the only validated scoring system for PGD thus far however, does not have a definitive role in donor selection or predicting PGD for its limited predictive power. The modifiable risk factors should be managed in every transplantation process. Female to male and undersized donors (≥30%) would have better been avoided. Possible infections should be controlled with antibiotics in both donor and recipient. Vasopressors such as vasopressin and terlipressin, are currently recommended as first-line treatment to reduce the noradrenaline requirement [53]. Insulin or thyroid hormone replacement would be helpful in some donors with hyperglycemia and hormone depletion [54, 55]. During procurement, the team should minimize allograft damage and try the best effort to reduce the ischemic time. Especially, donors with hypertrophied hearts should be kept to a minimum cold ischemic time due to susceptibility to ischemic injury [2].

2.5 Prevention

Patients with significant coronary artery disease, and/or LV hypertrophy, above 55 years are generally classified as marginal donors [56]. To resolve the severe donor shortage problem, many transplant centers accept extended use of marginal donor hearts [56]. Some authors recommend avoiding marginal donor hearts to reduce the risk of PGD [15]. However, for the absolute shortage of donor supply, and the absence of a groundbreaking alternative, utilization of marginal donors would be inevitable. Therefore, making efforts to minimize PGD after utilizing marginal donors seems more rational than just declining them unconditionally.

Proper donor management (hormone therapy, lower inotropes), better matching of the donor to recipient, improved procurement techniques, better organ preservation (Oran Care System, different additives in solutions), gradual wean of inotropes, utilization of nitric oxide, making efforts to decrease ischemic time and transfusion by improving surgical techniques and thorough planning are suggested as prevention [3]. Among them, the ex-vivo perfusion modifies many variables arising in the course of procurement and delivery of allograft. Ex-vivo perfusion may avoid the limitation of cold storage by providing warm blood perfusion to the donor heart [57]. The Harefield Hospital team reported favorable results in their experience using marginal donors with mild LVH with normothermic ex vivo perfusion [58]. In the prospective, multicenter, randomized, clinical investigation of TransMedics Organ Care System (OCS) for Cardiac Use II trial, 130 patients were randomized to ex-vivo donor heart perfusion or standard cold storage and demonstrated no difference in 30-day patient and graft survival rates or serious adverse events.

The development of more effective donor management and donor heart preservation strategies may reduce the incidence of PGD. Each effort to reduce the risk of PGD could make better results when they gather.

2.6 Management

The current definition for PGD is including the treatment options for each status.

By far the treatment of PGD is still primarily supportive care. PGD is initially managed by using inotropic support using catecholamines and phosphodiesterase inhibitors.

2.6.1 Mild to moderate LV PGD

Mild to moderate PGD cases could be treated medically first with inotropes, vasopressors, nitric oxide, and inhaled prostaglandins. If hemodynamics is not able to be improved to a level of adequate organ perfusion, mechanical support is implemented. IABPs may be a first-line device that gives counter pulsation that reduces afterload and improves coronary perfusion pressure, and it can be placed quickly at the bedside. However, it has limited utilization for partial hemodynamic support (maximum 30% increase in cardiac output) in severe graft dysfunction [15].

2.6.2 Severe LV PGD

In patients experiencing severe PGD early after transplantation, mechanical circulatory support other than IABP (by definition) is required to maintain adequate end-organ perfusion. This involves veno-arterial extracorporeal membrane oxygenator (VA-ECMO) support or implantation of a temporary ventricular assist device (VAD) without oxygenators such as Centrimag (Thoratec Corporation, Pleasanton, CA), TandemHeart (Tandem Life, Pittsburgh, PA), or Impella (Abiomed, Danvers, MA). Choice of the device, the timing of insertion, device configuration, and management differ even among high-volume transplant centers [3].

The incidence differs from report to report, a significant proportion of PGDs develop as biventricular involvement. Therefore, when it comes to severe PGD, MCS that supports both ventricles could be a better choice than a single ventricular support system. Takeda et al. demonstrated improved outcomes with the use of ECMO compared with temporary surgically implanted VAD for severe PGD with retrospective analysis of data collected in Columbia University Medical Center [59].

In general, it is thought that ECMO leads to better results when applied in early cardiogenic shock before multi-organ failure progresses. The forementioned institution adopted an aggressive ECMO approach for patients with evidence of severe PGD in 2015. VA-ECMO support was initiated early in the assessment of graft dysfunction in the immediate perioperative period, often during or immediately after weaning from cardiopulmonary bypass. In-hospital mortality improved from 28% (conservative) to 5% (prompt, $P = 0.083$). Post-transplant survival at 1 year was 67% in the conservative ECMO cohort and 90% in the prompt ECMO cohort ($P = 0.117$). Although, there was no statistical difference in survival rate for 3 yrs., they concluded that a possible mortality reduction in the prompt ECMO after severe PGD could be expected [60]. Regardless of modality, early intervention and short-term mechanical support seem to be associated with improved survival in severe LV PGD.

2.6.3 RV PGD

Currently, available treatment options for postoperative RV failure are optimization of acid-base status, fluid management, intravenous inotropes and vasodilators, and right-sided mechanical support. Inhaled vasodilators are often preferred because of their more direct effect on the pulmonary vasculature [61]. However, treatment options tend to be dependent on physicians or institutional preferences due to the lack of guidelines. Pulmonary vasodilators have been indicated only for the mild form of PGD-RV, with mechanical circulatory support indicated at an early stage for signs of severe PGD-RV [3].

3. Conclusions

PGD is the leading cause of early morbidity following heart transplantation. It is thought to be multifactorial in origin and several risk factors implicated. Researchers for potential biomarkers have been reporting novel predictors and are still ongoing. Prevention with adjusting modifiable risk factors is needed. Treatment options remain supportive with no definitive pharmacological agents identified yet, however, in terms of severe PGDs, timely mechanical circulatory support could reverse the fatal clinical outcome.

Acknowledgements

This work was supported by the National Research Foundation of Korea (NRF) grant funded by the Korea government (MSIT) (No. 2020R1F1A106657312).

Author details

Soo Yong Lee
Division of Cardiology, Department of Internal Medicine and Research Institute for Convergence of Biomedical Science and Technology, Pusan National University School of Medicine, Pusan National University Yangsan Hospital, South Korea

*Address all correspondence to: shonge0906@gmail.com

References

[1] Iyer A, Kumarasinghe G, Hicks M, Watson A, Gao L, Doyle A, et al. Primary graft failure after heart transplantation. Journal of Transplantation. 2011;**2011**: 175768

[2] Singh SSA, Dalzell JR, Berry C, Al-Attar N. Primary graft dysfunction after heart transplantation: A thorn amongst the roses. Heart Failure Reviews. 2019;**24**(5):805-820

[3] Kobashigawa J, Zuckermann A, Macdonald P, Leprince P, Esmailian F, Luu M, et al. Report from a consensus conference on primary graft dysfunction after cardiac transplantation. The Journal of Heart and Lung Transplantation. 2014;**33**(4):327-340

[4] Rhee Y, Kim HJ, Kim JJ, Kim MS, Lee SE, Yun TJ, et al. Primary graft dysfunction after isolated heart transplantation-incidence, risk factors, and clinical implications based on a single-center experience. Circulation Journal. 2021;**85**(9):1451-1459

[5] Avtaar Singh SS, Banner NR, Rushton S, Simon AR, Berry C, Al-Attar N. ISHLT primary graft dysfunction incidence, risk factors, and outcome: A UK National Study. Transplantation. 2019;**103**(2):336-343

[6] Nicoara A, Ruffin D, Cooter M, Patel CB, Thompson A, Schroder JN, et al. Primary graft dysfunction after heart transplantation: Incidence, trends, and associated risk factors. American Journal of Transplantation. 2018;**18**(6):1461-1470

[7] Kim IC, Youn JC, Kobashigawa JA. The past, present and future of heart transplantation. Korean Circulation Journal. 2018;**48**(7):565-590

[8] Sabatino M, Vitale G, Manfredini V, Masetti M, Borgese L, Maria Raffa G, et al. Clinical relevance of the International Society for Heart and Lung Transplantation consensus classification of primary graft dysfunction after heart transplantation: Epidemiology, risk factors, and outcomes. The Journal of Heart and Lung Transplantation. 2017;**36**(11):1217-1225

[9] Squiers JJ, Saracino G, Chamogeorgakis T, MacHannaford JC, Rafael AE, Gonzalez-Stawinski GV, et al. Application of the International Society for Heart and Lung Transplantation (ISHLT) criteria for primary graft dysfunction after cardiac transplantation: Outcomes from a high-volume centredagger. European Journal of Cardio-Thoracic Surgery. 2017;**51**(2):263-270

[10] Dronavalli VB, Rogers CA, Banner NR. Primary cardiac allograft dysfunction-validation of a clinical definition. Transplantation. 2015;**99**(9):1919-1925

[11] Foroutan F, Alba AC, Stein M, Krakovsky J, Chien KGW, Chih S, et al. Validation of the International Society for Heart and Lung Transplantation primary graft dysfunction instrument in heart transplantation. The Journal of Heart and Lung Transplantation. 2019;**38**(3):260-266

[12] Gorlitzer M, Ankersmit J, Fiegl N, Meinhart J, Lanzenberger M, Unal K, et al. Is the transpulmonary pressure gradient a predictor for mortality after orthotopic cardiac transplantation? Transplant International. 2005;**18**(4):390-395

[13] Bourge RC, Naftel DC, Costanzo-Nordin MR, Kirklin JK, Young JB, Kubo SH, et al. Pretransplantation risk factors for death after heart

transplantation: A multiinstitutional study. The transplant cardiologists research database group. The Journal of Heart and Lung Transplantation. 1993;**12**(4):549-562

[14] Murali S, Kormos RL, Uretsky BF, Schechter D, Reddy PS, Denys BG, et al. Preoperative pulmonary hemodynamics and early mortality after orthotopic cardiac transplantation: The Pittsburgh experience. American Heart Journal. 1993;**126**(4):896-904

[15] Subramani S, Aldrich A, Dwarakanath S, Sugawara A, Hanada S. Early graft dysfunction following heart transplant: Prevention and management. Seminars in Cardiothoracic and Vascular Anesthesia. 2020;**24**(1):24-33

[16] Pratschke J, Wilhelm MJ, Kusaka M, Basker M, Cooper DK, Hancock WW, et al. Brain death and its influence on donor organ quality and outcome after transplantation. Transplantation. 1999;**67**(3):343-348

[17] D'Amico TA, Meyers CH, Koutlas TC, Peterseim DS, Sabiston DC Jr, Van Trigt P, et al. Desensitization of myocardial beta-adrenergic receptors and deterioration of left ventricular function after brain death. The Journal of Thoracic and Cardiovascular Surgery. 1995;**110**(3):746-751

[18] Schipper DA, Marsh KM, Ferng AS, Duncker DJ, Laman JD, Khalpey Z. The critical role of bioenergetics in donor cardiac allograft preservation. Journal of Cardiovascular Translational Research. 2016;**9**(3):176-183

[19] Anaya-Prado R, Delgado-Vazquez JA. Scientific basis of organ preservation. Current Opinion in Organ Transplantation. 2008;**13**(2):129-134

[20] Karmazyn M, Gan XT, Humphreys RA, Yoshida H, Kusumoto K. The myocardial Na(+)-H(+) exchange: Structure, regulation, and its role in heart disease. Circulation Research. 1999;**85**(9):777-786

[21] Piper HM, Abdallah Y, Schafer C. The first minutes of reperfusion: A window of opportunity for cardioprotection. Cardiovascular Research. 2004;**61**(3): 365-371

[22] Garcia-Dorado D, Rodriguez-Sinovas A, Ruiz-Meana M. Gap junction-mediated spread of cell injury and death during myocardial ischemia-reperfusion. Cardiovascular Research. 2004;**61**(3):386-401

[23] Russo MJ, Iribarne A, Hong KN, Ramlawi B, Chen JM, Takayama H, et al. Factors associated with primary graft failure after heart transplantation. Transplantation. 2010;**90**(4):444-450

[24] Jahania MS, Sanchez JA, Narayan P, Lasley RD, Mentzer RM Jr. Heart preservation for transplantation: Principles and strategies. The Annals of Thoracic Surgery. 1999;**68**(5):1983-1987

[25] Locksley RM, Killeen N, Lenardo MJ. The TNF and TNF receptor superfamilies: Integrating mammalian biology. Cell. 2001;**104**(4):487-501

[26] Venkateswaran RV, Dronavalli V, Lambert PA, Steeds RP, Wilson IC, Thompson RD, et al. The proinflammatory environment in potential heart and lung donors: Prevalence and impact of donor management and hormonal therapy. Transplantation. 2009;**88**(4):582-588

[27] Wagner FD, Jonitz B, Potapov EV, Qedra N, Wegscheider K, Abraham K, et al. Procalcitonin, a donor-specific predictor of early graft failure-related mortality after heart transplantation. Circulation. 2001;**104**(12 Suppl 1): I192-I196

[28] Birks EJ, Burton PB, Owen V, Mullen AJ, Hunt D, Banner NR, et al. Elevated tumor necrosis factor-alpha and interleukin-6 in myocardium and serum of malfunctioning donor hearts. Circulation. 2000;**102**(19 Suppl. 3):III352-III358

[29] Jiang BH, Rue E, Wang GL, Roe R, Semenza GL. Dimerization, DNA binding, and transactivation properties of hypoxia-inducible factor 1. The Journal of Biological Chemistry. 1996;**271**(30):17771-17778

[30] Aharinejad S, Schafer R, Krenn K, Zuckermann A, Schneider B, Neumann F, et al. Donor myocardial HIF-1alpha is an independent predictor of cardiac allograft dysfunction: A 7-year prospective, exploratory study. American Journal of Transplantation. 2007;**7**(8):2012-2019

[31] Giangreco NP, Lebreton G, Restaino S, Jane Farr M, Zorn E, Colombo PC, et al. Plasma kallikrein predicts primary graft dysfunction after heart transplant. The Journal of Heart and Lung Transplantation. 2021;**40**(10):1199-1211

[32] Truby LK, Kwee LC, Agarwal R, Grass E, DeVore AD, Patel CB, et al. Proteomic profiling identifies CLEC4C expression as a novel biomarker of primary graft dysfunction after heart transplantation. The Journal of Heart and Lung Transplantation. 2021;**40**(12):1589-1598

[33] Sharma S, Jackson PG, Makan J. Cardiac troponins. Journal of Clinical Pathology. 2004;**57**(10):1025-1026

[34] Zahid T, Eskander N, Emamy M, Ryad R, Jahan N. Cardiac troponin elevation and outcome in subarachnoid hemorrhage. Cureus. 2020;**12**(8):e9792

[35] Deibert E, Barzilai B, Braverman AC, Edwards DF, Aiyagari V, Dacey R, et al. Clinical significance of elevated troponin I levels in patients with nontraumatic subarachnoid hemorrhage. Journal of Neurosurgery. 2003;**98**(4):741-746

[36] Khush KK, Menza RL, Babcock WD, Zaroff JG. Donor cardiac troponin I levels do not predict recipient survival after cardiac transplantation. The Journal of Heart and Lung Transplantation. 2007;**26**(10):1048-1053

[37] Madan S, Saeed O, Shin J, Sims D, Goldstein D, Pina I, et al. Donor troponin and survival after cardiac transplantation: An analysis of the United Network of Organ Sharing Registry. Circulation: Heart Failure. 2016;**9**(6):e002909

[38] Nicolas-Robin A, Salvi N, Medimagh S, Amour J, Le Manach Y, Coriat P, et al. Combined measurements of N-terminal pro-brain natriuretic peptide and cardiac troponins in potential organ donors. Intensive Care Medicine. 2007;**33**(6):986-992

[39] Dronavalli VB, Ranasinghe AM, Venkateswaran RJ, James SR, McCabe CJ, Wilson IC, et al. N-terminal pro-brain-type natriuretic peptide: A biochemical surrogate of cardiac function in the potential heart donor. European Journal of Cardio-Thoracic Surgery. 2010;**38**(2):181-186

[40] Dronavalli VB, Banner NR, Bonser RS. Assessment of the potential heart donor: A role for biomarkers? Journal of the American College of Cardiology. 2010;**56**(5):352-361

[41] Aharinejad S, Andrukhova O, Gmeiner M, Thomas A, Aliabadi A, Zuckermann A, et al. Donor serum SMARCAL1 concentrations predict primary graft dysfunction in cardiac transplantation. Circulation. 2009;**120**(11 Suppl):S198-S205

[42] Plenz G, Eschert H, Erren M, Wichter T, Bohm M, Flesch M, et al. The interleukin-6/interleukin-6-receptor system is activated in donor hearts. Journal of the American College of Cardiology. 2002;**39**(9):1508-1512

[43] Potapov EV, Wagner FD, Loebe M, Ivanitskaia EA, Muller C, Sodian R, et al. Elevated donor cardiac troponin T and procalcitonin indicate two independent mechanisms of early graft failure after heart transplantation. International Journal of Cardiology. 2003;**92**(2-3):163-167

[44] Riou B, Dreux S, Roche S, Arthaud M, Goarin JP, Leger P, et al. Circulating cardiac troponin T in potential heart transplant donors. Circulation. 1995;**92**(3):409-414

[45] Vorlat A, Conraads VM, Jorens PG, Aerts S, Van Gorp S, Vermeulen T, et al. Donor B-type natriuretic peptide predicts early cardiac performance after heart transplantation. The Journal of Heart and Lung Transplantation. 2012;**31**(6):579-584

[46] Russo MJ, Chen JM, Sorabella RA, Martens TP, Garrido M, Davies RR, et al. The effect of ischemic time on survival after heart transplantation varies by donor age: An analysis of the United Network for Organ Sharing database. The Journal of Thoracic and Cardiovascular Surgery. 2007;**133**(2):554-559

[47] Marasco SF, Esmore DS, Negri J, Rowland M, Newcomb A, Rosenfeldt FL, et al. Early institution of mechanical support improves outcomes in primary cardiac allograft failure. The Journal of Heart and Lung Transplantation. 2005;**24**(12):2037-2042

[48] D'Alessandro C, Golmard JL, Barreda E, Laali M, Makris R, Luyt CE, et al. Predictive risk factors for primary graft failure requiring temporary extra-corporeal membrane oxygenation support after cardiac transplantation in adults. European Journal of Cardio-Thoracic Surgery. 2011;**40**(4):962-969

[49] Stehlik J, Edwards LB, Kucheryavaya AY, Aurora P, Christie JD, Kirk R, et al. The registry of the International Society for Heart and Lung Transplantation: Twenty-seventh official adult heart transplant report--2010. The Journal of Heart and Lung Transplantation. 2010;**29**(10):1089-1103

[50] Segovia J, Cosio MD, Barcelo JM, Bueno MG, Pavia PG, Burgos R, et al. RADIAL: A novel primary graft failure risk score in heart transplantation. The Journal of Heart and Lung Transplantation. 2011;**30**(6):644-651

[51] Wright M, Takeda K, Mauro C, Jennings D, Kurlansky P, Han J, et al. Dose-dependent association between amiodarone and severe primary graft dysfunction in orthotopic heart transplantation. The Journal of Heart and Lung Transplantation. 2017;**36**(11):1226-1233

[52] Cosio Carmena MD, Gomez Bueno M, Almenar L, Delgado JF, Arizon JM, Gonzalez Vilchez F, et al. Primary graft failure after heart transplantation: Characteristics in a contemporary cohort and performance of the RADIAL risk score. The Journal of Heart and Lung Transplantation. 2013;**32**(12):1187-1195

[53] McKeown DW, Bonser RS, Kellum JA. Management of the heartbeating brain-dead organ donor. British Journal of Anaesthesia. 2012;**108**(Suppl. 1):i96-i107

[54] Novitzky D, Mi Z, Collins JF, Cooper DK. Increased procurement of thoracic donor organs after thyroid hormone therapy. Seminars in Thoracic and Cardiovascular Surgery. 2015;**27**(2):123-132

[55] Wood KE, Becker BN, McCartney JG, D'Alessandro AM, Coursin DB. Care of the potential organ donor. The New England Journal of Medicine. 2004;**351**(26):2730-2739

[56] Khush KK. Donor selection in the modern era. Annals of Cardiothoracic Surgery. 2018;**7**(1):126-134

[57] DePasquale EC, Ardehali A. Primary graft dysfunction in heart transplantation. Current Opinion in Organ Transplantation. 2018;**23**(3):286-294

[58] Garcia Saez D, Zych B, Sabashnikov A, Bowles CT, De Robertis F, Mohite PN, et al. Evaluation of the organ care system in heart transplantation with an adverse donor/recipient profile. The Annals of Thoracic Surgery. 2014;**98**(6):2099-2105. discussion 105-6

[59] Takeda K, Li B, Garan AR, Topkara VK, Han J, Colombo PC, et al. Improved outcomes from extracorporeal membrane oxygenation versus ventricular assist device temporary support of primary graft dysfunction in heart transplant. The Journal of Heart and Lung Transplantation. 2017;**36**(6):650-656

[60] DeRoo SC, Takayama H, Nemeth S, Garan AR, Kurlansky P, Restaino S, et al. Extracorporeal membrane oxygenation for primary graft dysfunction after heart transplant. The Journal of Thoracic and Cardiovascular Surgery. 2019;**158**(6):1576-1584 e3

[61] Khan TA, Schnickel G, Ross D, Bastani S, Laks H, Esmailian F, et al. A prospective, randomized, crossover pilot study of inhaled nitric oxide versus inhaled prostacyclin in heart transplant and lung transplant recipients. The Journal of Thoracic and Cardiovascular Surgery. 2009;**138**(6):1417-1424

Chapter 3

Hepatic and Endocrine Aspects of Heart Transplantation

Andrea Székely, András Szabó and Balázs Szécsi

Abstract

End-organ dysfunction is a progression that can often develop in patients with end-stage heart failure. Hepatic abnormalities in advanced systolic heart failure may affect several aspects of the liver function. Hepatic function is dependent on age, nutrition, previous hepatic diseases, and drugs. The hepatic dysfunction can have metabolic, synthetic, and vascular consequences, which strongly influence the short- and long-term results of the transplantation. In this chapter, the diagnostic and treatment modalities of the transplanted patient will be discussed. On the other hand, endocrine abnormalities, particularly thyroid dysfunction, are also frequently detected in patients on the waiting list. Endocrine supplementation during donor management after brain death is crucial. Inappropriate management of central diabetes insipidus, hyperglycemia, or adrenal insufficiency can lead to circulatory failure and graft dysfunction during procurement. Thyroid dysfunction in donors and recipients is conversely discussed.

Keywords: hepatic dysfunction, heart transplant, MELD score, thyroid function, donor management, endocrine dysfunction

1. Introduction

The increased need for transplantation cannot be met because of the shortage of the available grafts. In the last decades, the number of heart transplantation has not increased. As a consequence, the patients will be longer on the waiting list, becoming older and having more severe end organ dysfunction, or even they lose their candidacy for transplantation because of the irreversible hepatic or liver failure. Bridging techniques, such as temporary extracorporeal circulation or implantable mechanical assist devices, may improve and reverse the end-organ failure and transplantation can be done. The physician of the transplantation team must be familiar with the diagnosis and possible treatment of these organ dysfunctions. Recently, recognition and extended investigation of the end-stage heart-failure-related hepatic failure have been highlighted, since the liver dysfunction can worsen in the posttransplantation period through hypoxic hepatitis or by the immunsuppressive medications, which should be taken lifelong.

Besides the liver, another important system, the endocrine hormones, must be strictly followed in the perioperative period. End-stage heart failure can cause thyroid dysfunction, and it can lead to circulatory failure or hemodynamic instability.

Amiodarone, a frequently applied antiarrhythmic drug, can cause severe hypo- or hyperthyreosis. In the postoperative period, the physicians must distinguish the nonthyroidal illness syndrome from the chronic illness-related thyroid dysfunction. Endocrine replacement must be also initiated during the donor procurement to decrease the graft loss or the graft dysfunction in the posttransplant period.

In this chapter, we aimed to describe briefly the basic liver function, the diagnostic modalities in the preoperative evaluation, and the special considerations related to transplantation care. The endocrine part will overview the thyroid dysfunction, the treatment of central diabetes insipidus, and the posttransplantation endocrine management.

2. Hepatic aspects of heart transplantation

2.1 Basic anatomy and physiology of the liver

The human liver is wedge-shaped with two lobes, and it weighs cca 1.5 kg [1, 2]. The hepatic artery via the celiac trunk and the portal vein are the main blood supply of the liver. The liver receives approximately one-fourth of the cardiac output, which secures one-third of the blood supply, and the rest will be supplied by the portal system. These blood vessels divide into small capillaries, called hepatic sinusoids, which then build the lobules. Lobules are the functional units of the liver. Each lobule is made up of hepatocytes. The lobules are held together by fibroelastic connective tissue that extends from a fibrous capsule covering the entire liver [3]. The function of the liver is very complex and diversified. Liver has excretion function, including synthesis and excretion of biliary acids. Furthermore, liver also plays a key role in endocrine homeostasis in the metabolism of various hormones. To understand the potential perioperative issues, it is necessary to review the complex role of the liver in the human body. Oxidative capacity decreases with the age and congestive disorders, which may cause delayed drug metabolism [4].

2.2 Congestive heart-failure-related hepatic dysfunction

Heart failure with reduced ejection fraction can alter many pathways in the liver. As a forward failure due to (the) low cardiac output syndrome, reduced systolic function leads to hypoperfusion, while backward failure caused by biventricular or isolated right ventricular dysfunction will result in venous congestion. As a response for the constantly elevated high pressure in the inferior caval and hepatic veins, the perivenular space of the lobule will be dilated, and fibrotic transformation will be initiated. As the congestive state persists, perivenular-perivenular bridging develops, which has less effect on centrally located portal tracks. This pattern is the reverse lobulation. As the circulatory failure progresses, the portal part also undergoes fibrotic transformation and complete congestive hepatopathy may develop. The collagen is deposited in the subendothelial region and in the Disse space. The elevated right ventricular pressure can now affect the portal circulation, causing cirrhotic portal hypertension. The well-known symptoms of cirrhosis, such as ascites and development of the varices of esophageal veins, are often present. Laboratory parameters remain unchanged or minimally elevated in the early phase of the congestion. Only elevation of aspartate aminotransferase (AST) and alanine transaminase (ALT) may be abnormal, an increase in bilirubin or obstructive enzyme (alkaline phosphatase, ALP) levels is frequently seen. Highly elevated transaminase levels and increased bilirubin levels are more common in advanced or end-stage liver failure, usually associated with acute on chronic heart failure.

2.3 Preoperative evaluation algorithms

Routine laboratory tests, including hepatic function tests, are good but rough indicators of hepatic dysfunction in the pre-transplant period. It should be stressed that normal transaminase and serum bilirubin levels are not suitable for early detection of hepatic problems. As shown in the scores presented, elevated serum bilirubin levels and spontaneous prolonged coagulation are strong predictors of a negative outcome. Nonalcoholic fatty liver disease is a sign that the congestion has reached a distinct stage caused by heart failure with or without reduced ejection fraction. Transient elastography is a good and reliable method to measure fibrotic transformation of the liver. In the decompensated period of advanced heart failure, fibroelastography shows higher than real fibrotic results.

Liver biopsy is the most accurate way to assess fibrotic transformation of liver tissue. In some advanced cases, a liver biopsy can be used to rule out candidates for a heart transplantation or to determine the need for combined heart and liver transplantation [4]. Existing gallstone should be removed before surgery as it is potential infectious focus.

2.4 Laboratory tests

The classic laboratory tests for estimating hepatic function are serum bilirubin, transaminases (ALT, AST), alkaline phosphatase, lactate dehydrogenase, total serum protein and albumin, serum bilirubin, and coagulation parameters, especially prothrombin time. Most patients with advanced heart failure were found to have moderately elevated levels of transaminase in random blood samples. Chronic anticoagulation can influence the prothrombin levels and must be considered in the calculation of model for end-stage liver disease (MELD) scores.

In acute hypoxic hepatitis, transaminases (AST, ALT) can rise more than 100-fold above normal ranges. This increase reflects the severity of centrolobular hepatic necrosis. Peak transaminase is usually expected within 12–24 hours, and normalization take 2 weeks with treatment. Abnormalities in alkaline phosphates and serum bilirubin levels are less common. Prolonged prothrombin time has important prognostic value. Thrombocytopenia, if present, occurs simultaneously with prolonged prothrombin time. Renal failure is often associated with global hypoperfusion.

2.5 Hepatic vein flow Doppler measurement

Nowadays, hepatic vein flow measurement using duplex Doppler technic is an arising increasingly common method of assessing changes caused in heart failure. It may also be useful and feasible for noninvasive hemodynamic monitoring in acute conditions. Accurate interpretation of spectral Doppler tracing from hepatic veins is valuable, because they reflect important cardiac and hepatic physiology. There are usually four phases: A, S, V, and D; the S and D waves indicate the antegrade flow toward the heart. In hepatic and cardiac disease, these normal waves may be absent, indicating non-physiological flow in the hepatic circulation. In addition, transient patient factors, such as phase of the respiratory cycle, may can affect the appearance of the spectral trace. Knowledge of the normal and abnormal spectral Doppler waveforms of the hepatic veins and the corresponding physiology and pathophysiology provide valuable insights. Systematic analysis of the direction, regularity, and phasing of the spectral trace and the ratio of S- and D-wave amplitudes allows in most cases a correct differential diagnosis [5].

Under abnormal conditions, the normal triphasic pattern is altered, and the original waves may not exist or be distinguishable. The biphasic pattern may indicate severe tricuspid valve regurgitation and/or acute right ventricular overload. Normally, the hepatic vein spectrum shows the normal S-wave to D-wave ratio, where the S-wave is larger than the D-wave. According to Scheinfeld, there are three types of right-sided heart failure. (According to its classification, in mild tricuspid regurgitation, the relationship between the S-wave and the D-wave changes, with the S-wave being smaller than the D-wave.) Type 1 tricuspid regurgitation is classified as a change in the relationship between the S-wave and the D-wave, with the S-wave being smaller than the D-wave. However, there is still antegrade flow during the ventricular systole. In type 2 tricuspid regurgitation, there is no systolic flow during the ventricular systole. In type 3 tricuspid regurgitation, there is retrograde flow during the ventricular systole [5].

In the early state of fibrotic hepatic transformation or nonalcoholic fatty liver disease (NAFLD). the hepatic vein waveform may be remarkably damped due to stiffness of hepatic tissue and vessel walls. Flow pattern changes, such as monophasicity or blunt waveform, are also often observed in these conditions. Hepatic vein flow patterns also suitable for follow-up of the right ventricular function, the severity of tricuspidal regurgitation, and the venous congestion during the perioperative period. On the pictures 1 and 2, hepatic vein flow patterns are shown (**Figure 1**).

2.6 Transient elastography

Transient elastography (TE) is a noninvasive, simple, fast, and highly accurate clinical examination method. During TE, a special probe is used to measure the liver stiffness, which correlates well with the fibrotic hepatic remodeling [6]. However, the test has high reliability and may overestimate the level of liver fibrosis depending on the severity of decompensation. Thus, the examination should be planned in an elective setting with relatively well-compensated patient [7, 8].

In the literature reports could be seen with examination of the relationship between chronic coronary syndrome and nonalcoholic fatty liver disease (NAFLD). Reports have appeared in the literature examining the association between chronic coronary syndrome and nonalcoholic fatty liver disease (NAFLD). These findings are noteworthy because the liver structure transformation begins before the presence of a notable reduction in global cardiac function or congestive right heart failure [9].

2.7 Risk stratification system

Precise multidisciplinary risk assessment in the pre-transplant period is a key factor. The possible contraindicating coexisting diseases and states should be ruled out. The risk estimation can be helpful in planning, preparing, and managing the intraoperative and postoperative period. For preoperative hepatic dysfunction, two scores are mostly used. The Child-Pugh score is a traditional risk estimation method.

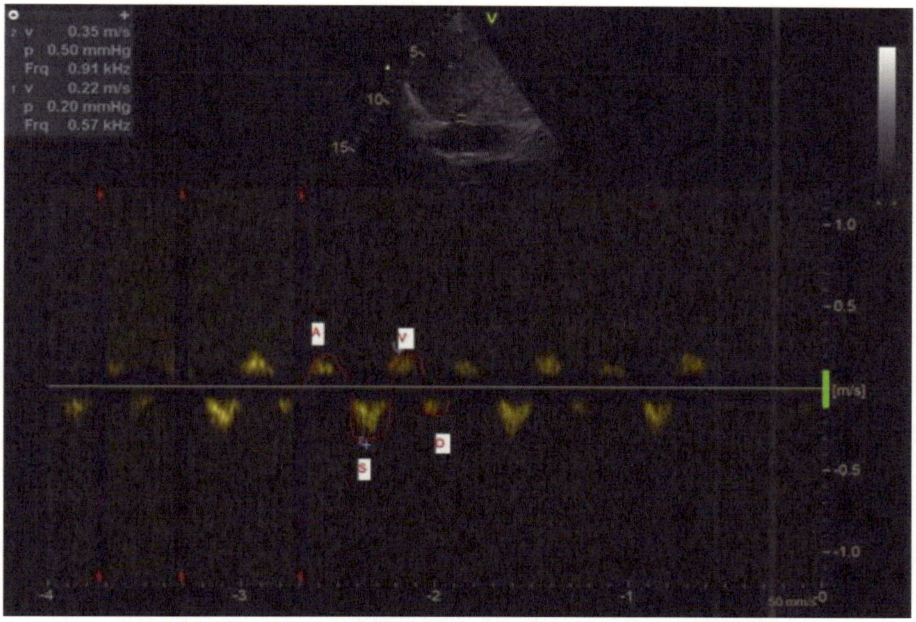

Figure 1.
Hepativ vein flow pattern.

The Child-Pugh score was based on serum bilirubin and albumin levels, international normalized ratio (INR), and the presence of ascites and encephalopathy. While the Child-Pugh score is useful for risk stratification in the clinical practice, MELD score(s) are more feasible for patients admitted to intensive care unit (ICU) due to their better prognostic value and lower negative likelihood ratio [10].

2.7.1 Model for end-stage liver disease (MELD) score

MELD score was originally developed to predict mortality in patients with hepatopathy and/or cirrhosis after porto-jugular shunt placement. The baseline MELD score gives an estimate of 3-month mortality as a function of the need for dialysis, INR, serum bilirubin, and creatinine (**Table 1**) [11].

$$MELD\ score\ calculation = \left(0.957\times\ln(seCreat)+0.378\times\ln(seBilirubin)+1.120\times\ln(INR)+0.643\right)\times 10 \quad (1)$$

The MELD score has several modifications according to the patients' comorbidities. MELD XI score excludes INR from the equation. MELD XI is promoted for use in patients receiving anticoagulant therapy. Frequent anticoagulant therapy in end-stage heart failure emphasizes the INR-independent MELD score.

Since UNOS (United Network for Organ Sharing) started using the MELD score, its importance for estimating the risk of liver complications and mortality before heart transplantation is unquestioned. Use of Na-corrected or XI (INR excluded) MELD scores in patients with end-stage heart failure in the pre-transplant period is the basics for liver failure risk estimation [12].

Parameter, factor	Range
Dialysis twice at the last week (or continuous veno-venosus hemodialysis ≥24 hours at last week)	yes/no
Creatinine	normal range: 62–115 μmol/L (0.7–1.3 mg/dL)
Bilirubin	normal range: 5.13–32.49 μmol/L
INR	0.8–1.2
Sodium	normal range: 136–145 μmol/L (mEq/L)

Table 1.
The components of updated MELD score (used for 12 years and older patients after 2016).

3. Perioperative considerations

3.1 Synthetic dysfunctions in perioperative period

Decreased serum albumin levels are present in 30–50% of patients, but the serum level is usually not less than 25 g/L. Low albumin levels do not correlate with hepatic injury, but are associated with nutritional impairment and protein wasting. The serum albumin level is an independent risk factor for mortality after heart transplantation [13]. Multiple studies suggest that serum albumin level under 35 g/L is related with worse mortality. Intravenous albumin substitution was not proven useful in the perioperative period.

Mild increase of the prothrombin time (PT) indicates a secondary impairment of the coagulation factor synthesis. In case of portal hypertension, the protein content of the ascites is usually more than 25 g/L and the ratio higher than 1:1 (serum albumin to ascites albumin). Some studies have reported a significant relationship between central venous pressure, low cardiac index, and elevated total bilirubin, AST, or ALT levels [14]. Increased transaminase levels correlate with the severity of hepatocellular injury caused by hypoperfusion. Increased direct bilirubin and ALP with ALT/ALP levels are markers of cholestatic injury and increased venous congestion. Increased bilirubin levels have been reported to be associated with high inotropic requirement, low cardiac output states, early readmission, in patients with advanced heart failure [15].

3.2 Hepatic dysfunction in patients during mechanical circulatory support (MCS)

End-stage heart failure patients with significantly impaired end-organ dysfunction often need a bridging method to become candidates for heart transplantation. For these patients, more frequent use of various mechanical circulatory supports may be a solution. However, even short to medium periods of support for planned pathophysiological changes caused by devices should be of concern. Short-term devices (veno-arterial extracorporeal membrane oxygenation, VA-ECMO) and various mid-term ventricular assist devices, such as left ventricular assist device (LVAD) or biventrular assist devices (BIVAD), also have a major impact on complex physiological processes. In case of LVAD implantation—similar than in heart transplantation cases—the low serum albumin level (≤35 g/L) is related to worse survival (**Figures 2** and **3**) [16].

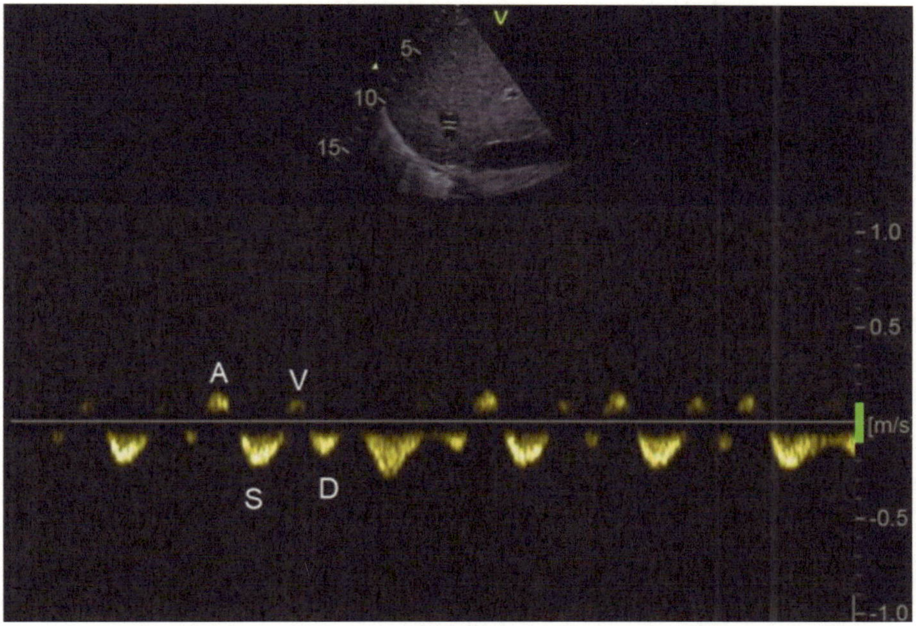

Figure 2.
Normalization of hepatic vein flow pattern in a patient with end-stage heart failure on BiVAD treatment for 85 days. The flow pattern is normal with minimal retrograde flow in venticular systole.

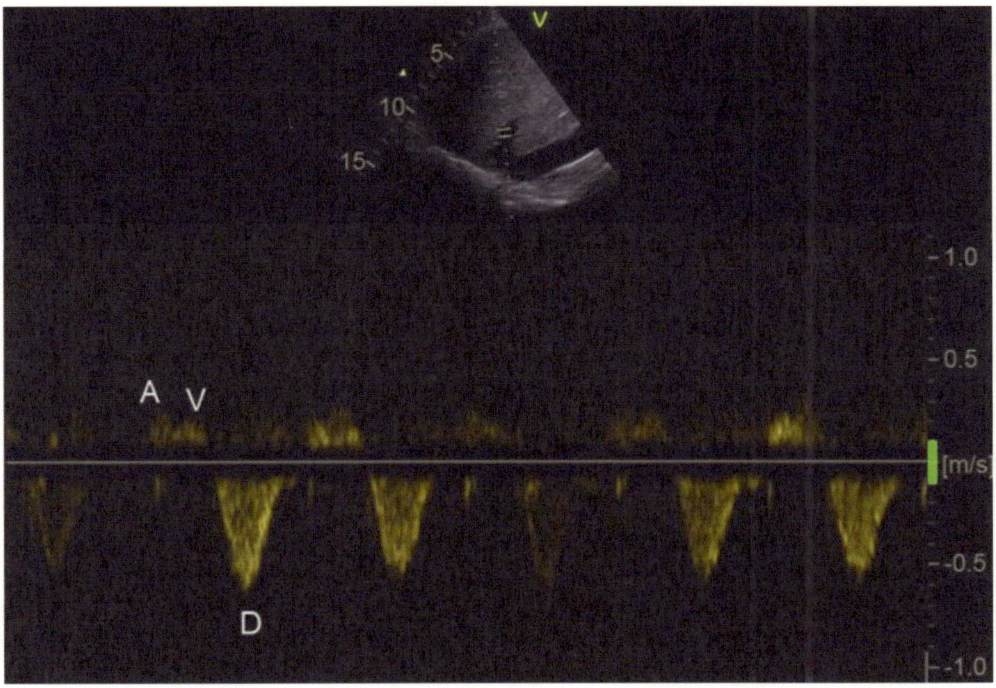

Figure 3.
Hepatic vein flow in a patient with end-stage heart failure treated with implantable LVAD for 22 days. Regarding grade 3 tricuspidal regurgitation, prominent V wave could be seen. Often the A, S, and V waves are fusional and indicate severe retrograde flow during the global systole.

3.3 Lactic acidosis, decreased lactate clearance

The liver is 60% responsible for the elimination of lactate via the Cori cycle, (lactate is therefore a glycogen precursor molecule). Renal lactate excretion is meaningful as serum lactate levels above 6–8 mM. In cirrhosis patients, lactate clearance is decreased, which can lead to type B lactic acidosis caused by reduced activity of lactate dehydrogenase. A parallel problem is the dysregulated carbohydrate balance. Without a well-functioning hepatic enzyme system, accumulated substrate levels slowly return to normal.

3.4 Coagulation disorders

In intraoperative settings, hepatic impairment is often associated with hemostatic disorders. The liver plays a crucial role in hemostasis through the synthesis of procoagulants, anticoagulants, and components of the fibrinolytic system, as well as the clearance of activated clotting factors. In hepatic dysfunction, these synthetic functions are insufficient, and hemostatic changes within and between procoagulant, anticoagulant, and fibrinolytic systems result in a new balance, defined as a rebalanced hemostatic state. This conception is defined as a) dysfunction in thrombin generation/disturbance in thrombus production and b) instability in the face of relatively small disturbances that commonly lead to a disruption of the balance between bleeding or thrombotic events [17].

The most sensitive laboratory parameters are prothrombin time (PT) and partial thromboplastin time (PTT), which are sensitive to reduced levels of procoagulants but not to anticoagulants; this has led to the erroneous assumption in the past that patients with liver disease are auto-anticoagulated and are protected against thrombosis. Nevertheless, PT and INR are not reliable risk factors for bleeding after surgery or invasive procedures [17, 18].

Under VA-ECMO support, patients with preexisting hepatic dysfunction have increased morbidity and mortality, with obviously serious implications for the planning and further bridging [19]. According to the current recommendations for the implantable LVAD devices, the candidacy for implantation must fulfill strong criteria in their hepatic function. Mid-term and especially long-term LVADs are associated with serious side effects by altering the molecular mass spectrum of von Willebrand factor (vWf). A kind of degradation (more precisely multimerization into smaller molecules) of von Willebrand factor caused by shear stress associated with mechanical circulatory devices can lead to device specific coagulopathy and unexpected and defective angiogenesis—smaller multimers of vWf may act as vascular endothelial growth factor. The clinical context is often driven by unexplained bleeding from interstitial angiodysplasias. The acquired von Willebrand factor dysfunction type of hemostatic dysfunction is diagnosed mostly by viscoelastic tests [20].

Furthermore, coagulopathy based on hepatic dysfunction is often accompanied by thrombocytopenia. Platelet function seems to be normal in patients with cirrhosis, but intrinsic dysfunction has not yet been confirmed [21].

4. Immunosuppressive therapy and the liver

A major function of the liver is drug metabolism. Drugs given in the perioperative period, lifelong immunosuppressive therapy often interact with the liver. In the perioperative period, special attention should be paid to hepatic function problems caused by immunosuppressive therapy. The impaired liver condition before surgery makes these interactions more complex and difficult.

In heart transplant patients, the drugs that induce immunosuppression are mostly anti-thymocyte globulin (ATG). ATG is safe to use in liver failure; however, some case reports have reported extremely elevated transaminase levels within a few hours of infusion. Liver damage associated with ATG therapy is usually mild and asymptomatic, self-limited [22].

Calcineurin inhibitors are metabolized by the liver's P450 enzyme system (CYP 3A4). The most commonly used calcineurin inhibitors are cyclosporin and tacrolimus. Initiation of cyclosporine therapy may sometimes be associated with a slight increase in serum bilirubin levels, often without a considerable increase in serum ALT or alkaline phosphatase. Tacrolimus therapy is associated with a mild to moderate increase in serum aminotransferase levels in 5–10% of patients. Rises in serum aminotransferase levels are usually mild, asymptomatic, and self-limiting, but occasionally persistent and may require a dose modification. Tacrolimus has also been implicated in the development of cholestatic hepatitis, but clinically apparent liver damage is rare [22].

Corticosteroids are the basis of the immunosuppressive therapy, particularly in the early period and in case of rejection. Corticosteroids also have major effects on the liver, particularly when given in long term and in higher doses. Glucocorticoid usage may result in liver enlargement, steatosis, or glycogenosis. Hepatomegaly and moderate elevation of serum aminotransferase levels are common in glycogenosis. There is little or no change in alkaline phosphatase and serum bilirubin levels. Furthermore, steroids can aggravate nonalcoholic fatty liver disease. Long-term therapy can also worsen chronic viral hepatitis. Thus, hepatic complications of corticosteroids are mostly associated with high intravenous dosing and usually represent the worsening or triggering of an underlying liver disease, and rarely are the result of drug

Modality	Information	Pathology	Optimal timing
Laboratory tests	Transaminase levels	Hepatocellular injury caused by congestion Excessively increased levels often seen in hypoperfusion NB: viral hepatitis, medical therapy	Routinely preoperative examination and heart failure care (monthly)
	Serum bilirubin level	Indicator of severe hepatic (conjugation) function loss	
	Albumin, Total protein	Related to the hepatic synthetic function and nutritional state (NB: adsorption problems, protein loss in enteropathy)	
	INR, PT	Indicator of hemostatic disorders regarding synthesis of coagulation system factors	
Transient elastography		Classification of hepatic fibrotic transformation	Before transplantation in well compensated state
Biopsy	Microscopic structure of liver tissue	Classification of fibrotic transformation/cirrhosis	Before transplantation in case of serious indication

Table 2.
The preoperative examination modalities, their focus and optimal timing before the heart transplantation.

hepatotoxicity. High doses of intravenous corticosteroids, such as those used in anti-rejection shot therapy, are rarely associated with fatal acute liver injury [22].

Among antiproliferative agents, azathioprine and mycophenolate-mofetil (MMF) are commonly used in heart transplant patients. Azathioprine has a worse side effect profile, including severe hepatic problems, so MMF is usually preferred. In mild cases, azathioprine has been associated with a transient and asymptomatic rise in serum aminotransferase levels, which is associated with acute cholestatic damage in the first year after initiation of therapy. Chronic damage to the liver characterized by peliosis hepatis, veno-occlusive disease or nodular regeneration is typical with long-term use. Hepatocellular carcinomas have also been reported with long-term azathioprine use. In contrast, MMF use is safe, with side effects mostly nausea and digestive problems that respond well to dose reduction (**Table 2**) [22].

5. Thyroid function and transplantation

Nonthyroidal illness (NTI) is a syndrome that is observed in critically ill patients. As the name suggests, it is not a primary endocrine disease, but a result of severe systemic stress. Many conditions can lead to a generalized stress, such as severe infection, sepsis, prolonged starvation, bone marrow transplantation, extensive myocardial infarction, end-stage heart failure, heart transplantation, or any potentially life-threatening condition [23]. As for the changes in hormone levels, plasma T3 levels decrease, followed by a decrease in plasma T4 levels, while rT3 levels show an increasing trend. This is due to both altered protein binding and altered deiodinase enzyme activity. However, in the vast majority of cases, plasma TSH levels remain unchanged or decrease slightly [24]. In the international literature, several synonyms for nonthyroidal illness are common, such as euthyroid sick syndrome or low T3 syndrome (**Table 3**) [23].

The course of nonthyroidal illness can be divided into two basic phases, an acute phase and a chronic phase. The first acute phase is observed during a sudden change in critical condition. The main laboratory parameters in the acute phase are characterized by decreased peripheral free T3 levels and elevated rT3 concentrations. This is due to mechanisms such as reduced binding of plasma proteins to thyroid hormones and altered activity of certain deiodinase enzymes (D1, D3). In fact, the acute phase of NTI is an adaptive response to a reduced nutrient supply to the body due to a critical condition. Consequently, this phase of NTI, whose primary purpose is to reduce the catabolism of the body, has a positive effect on the body [24]. Other research has also observed that during starvation, the catabolism of peripheral skeletal muscle slows down as T3 levels decrease, while thyroid hormone administration increases its breakdown again [25, 26]. However, some research is in stark contrast to this view, as there is no correlation between a decrease in T3 levels during starvation and a concomitant decrease in peripheral skeletal muscle breakdown [27].

In the event that the acute phase is prolonged, the adaptive response that initially seems beneficial is replaced by a phase that is already less beneficial to the body. This is the chronic phase of NTI. In terms of thyroid laboratory parameters, not only the T3 but also the T4 levels start to decrease, while the plasma TSH levels fall below the lower limit of the normal range [24]. According to one study, these changes are due to a decrease in hypothalamic TRH secretion for an as yet unknown reason. This is because the research team found an association between TRH gene expression and plasma T3 and TSH levels [28]. During the chronic phase, adaptive mechanisms are developed in the peripherical located tissues to maximize the utilization of reduced thyroid hormones: increased

Nonthyroidal illness syndrome		
	Acute phase	**Chronic phase**
other names	"Low T_3 syndrome"	"Central hypothyroidism"
CAUSE	Starvation, stress, inflammation	Endo–/exogen dopamine, cortisol
T_3	↓	↓↓
T_4	↑	↓
rT_3	↑↑	↑
TSH	↑/normal (no peak)	norm./↓ (no pulsatility)
TRH	Normal	↓
TBG, albumin	↓	↓
D_1 ($T_4 \rightarrow T_3$)	↓	↓
D_3 ($T_4 \rightarrow rT_3$)	↑	↑
D_2 ($T_4 \rightarrow T_3$)	Normal	↑ (feedback)
Receptor sensitivity	Normal	↑
Result	Adaptive, useful	Maladaptive
Hormonal replacement	Not recommended	Considerable

Table 3.
Hormonal changes in NTI.

transcription and activity of the D2 enzyme, increased localization of certain transporters, and increased activity of active isoforms of TRs' expression [24].

A clear, definite pathomechanism for the nonthyroidal illness syndrome has not been established. Samples of muscle and liver tissue from several patients who died in intensive care units (ICU) were collected. Biopsies from liver and muscle tissue from died patients were found to be increased in the expression of type 3 deiodinase enzymes and decreased in the expression of type 1 deiodinase enzymes. Blood collected from died patients showed decreased total T3, T4, TSH levels, while rT3 levels were higher than normal. In this study, a correlation was found that the plasma T3/rT3 ratio was positively correlated with the expression of type 1 deiodinase enzyme [29]. rT3 level, T3/rT3 ratio and D3 enzyme expression measured on the very first day of ICU admission may have prognostic value for mortality [30].

In the chronic phase of NTI, decreased TRH gene expression may be strongly influenced by increased D2 enzyme activity mediated by inflammatory mediators, transcription factor NFκB (nuclear factor κB), and corticosterone [31, 32]. Certain drugs, such as dopamine can keep plasma T3, T4, and TSH levels, are low [33]. The role of different drugs in the suppression of the hypothalamic–pituitary-thyroid axis is conversely discussed [34, 35]. This association could not be demonstrated by another study group that used dopexamine and dobutamine simultaneously in high-risk surgical patients (**Figure 4**) [35].

5.1 Amiodarone

Amiodarone is a commonly used antiarrhythmic drug in patients with end-stage heart failure. Moreover, antiarrhythmic treatment of atrial or ventricular arrhythmias with amiodarone is an effective and widely known phenomenon in clinical practice. Amiodarone maintains normal sinus rhythm in patients with atrial fibrillation (AF)

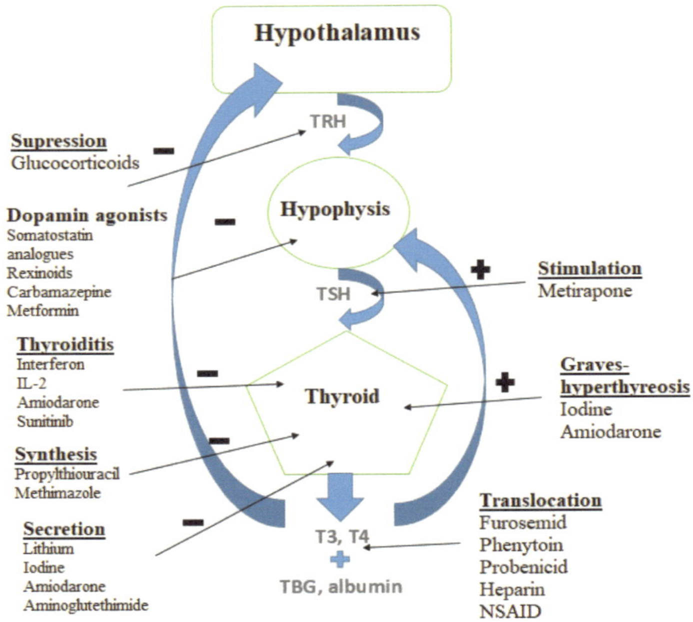

Figure 4.
Regulation of hypothalamic–pituitary-thyroid axis.

and also reduces the recurrence rate of ventricular tachycardia. Amiodarone remains the preferred treatment, particularly for patients awaiting heart transplantation (HTX). Due to its slow distribution in body's tissue, amiodarone may take several months to reach steady-state tissue concentrations and to exert a sufficient antiarrhythmic effect. In addition, the registered half-life of amiodarone is highly variable. Because of this phenomenon, the administration of amiodarone before transplantation has been controversially discussed in the literature, and different results have been reported for morbidity and mortality after heart transplantation [36, 37].

The administration of this antiarrhythmic medication may increase the probability of one-year mortality, graft failure, transplantation, and permanent pacemaker implantation [38]. Amiodarone-induced hypothyroidism (AIH) and amiodarone-induced thyrotoxicosis (AIT) can also occur during chronic administration. In addition, there is a mixed/indefinite form to which both pathogenic mechanisms mentioned above contribute. Type 1 AIT develops in patients with preexisting thyroid disorders, while type 2 AIT occurs in substantially normal thyroid gland. On the one hand, the rate of serious adverse cardiovascular events was three times higher in AIT compared with euthyroid patients [39]. On the other side, several studies demonstrated the safety of amiodarone in end-stage heart failure and in early postoperative atrial fibrillation [36, 37].

6. Donor management

Endocrine dysfunction is common in severe brain injury. Traumatic brain injury is usually associated with increased intracranial pressure, which can be followed by a brainstem herniation, resulting in brainstem infarction [40]. Ischemic lesions can cause dysfunction in the hypothalamic–pituitary axis. One of the most frequent complications is the posterior pituitary deficiency, characterized by central diabetes insipidus (CDI). Arginine vasopressin (AVP) deficiency can cause inadequate diuresis with hypovolemia, hyperosmolality, and hypernatremia [41]. Anterior pituitary gland dysfunction has also been detected with hypothyroidism and hypocortisolemia. Lack of these hormones may lead to hemodynamic instability, with reduced myocardial function, hypovolemia, inadequate stress response, increased proinflammatory condition. Each of them can impair graft function [42, 43]. Endogenous catecholamine release is enhanced in both neurological death and acute critical illness. Although it causes increased systemic vascular resistance, cardiac output is compromised by myocardial suppression induced by neurological death and by a reduced thyroid hormone release due to pituitary gland deficiency. Therefore, a theoretical advantage exists for exogenous thyroid hormone supplementation [44].

6.1 Arginine-vasopressin

Arginine-vasopressin should be considered if hypotension persists despite adequate volume resuscitation or if central diabetes insipidus (CDI) occurs. Damage of the posterior lobe of the pituitary gland, hypothalamic paraventricular nuclei, and supraoptic nuclei results in undetectable or low levels of AVP. The deficiency of AVP can lead to inadequate diuresis and is associated with hyperosmolality, hypovolemia, and hypernatremia, which is consistent with DI. In addition, even in patients who do not meet the criteria for DI, baroreflex-mediated secretion of AVP can be impaired in response to decreased hypotension and decreased circulatory volume. Appropriate therapy with early intervention can restore hemodynamic stability and prevent end-organ damage. A recent analysis of the OPTN database has shown that the administration of AVP in organ donors is independently associated with an increased rate of organ recovery. The study did not recommend indications for AVP use (such as DI and hypotension). Prolonged hypernatremia ($Na+ > 155$ mmol/L) due to untreated DI has been associated with postoperative graft dysfunction in several retrospective studies and one prospective study; however, this association was not generally reported. Maintaining normal sodium levels remains a reasonable goal of the appropriate treatment. Hypernatremia, excessive diuresis, and volume depletion can occur for reasons other than DI (e.g., osmotic diuresis due to hyperglycemia or mannitol administration) and should be investigated [45]. Treatment of AVP deficiency could be considered if hypotension persists despite adequate resuscitation or in the presence of DI, which is likely to occur if one or more of the following criteria are identified, unless there is another cause of the disorder: polyuria (urinary output>3–4 l/d or 2.5–3.0 ml/kg/h); normal or increased serum motility; inadequately diluted urine (specific gravity <1.005, urinary osmolality <200 mOsm/kg H_2O); hypernatremia ($Na+ > 145$ mmol/L) [45].

6.2 The use of corticosteroids

The use of corticosteroids can reduce the inflammation caused by brain death and modulating immune functions can improve the quality of donor organs (e.g., lungs) and posttransplant graft function. Corticosteroid administration for brain-dead organ donors is highly recommended for two reasons. The first reason is the treatment of hypothalamic–pituitary–adrenal (HPA) axis failure, which could potentially lead to hemodynamic instability. However, like the axis of the thyroid gland, the HPA axis is generally not deficient after brain death. Additionally, in observational studies, the donor's hemodynamic instability was not associated with hypocortisolemia or lack of adrenal corticotropin sensitivity. Nevertheless, corticosteroids may improve hemodynamics through their vasopressor effects. The second possible reason for the administration of corticosteroids is reduced inflammation, which can have a negative effect on graft function. Observational studies highlight the increased organ procurement and improved graft and survival of the recipient by administration of corticosteroids. However, good-quality RCT evidence is lacking. With high heterogeneity of the study design and concomitant therapies, as well as poor quality, most RCTs rule out a strong conclusion. Several studies analyzed the effect of high-dose methylprednisolone. Theoretically, corticosteroid-induced hyperglycemia may outweigh all possible benefits. Recently, lower doses of hydrocortisone have been studied. Improved blood glucose was improved by a small observational study control by such strategy without any benefit on patient-centered outcomes. In summary, the indications of corticosteroid use in possible organ donors remain controversial, but can be considered in hemodynamic instability. It is important that it could be administered only after sampling for tissue typing, as it can reduce the expression of human leukocyte antigen [43]. Administration of high-dose corticosteroids (methylprednisone 1000 mg IV, 15 mg/kg IV, or 250 mg IV bolus followed by an infusion at a rate of 100 mg/h) reduces the potential adverse effects of the inflammatory cascade on donor organ function after brain death. Ideally, it should be administered after taking blood for tissue typing as it is able to suppress human leukocyte antigen expression [45].

6.3 The use of thyroid hormone

Changes in the axis of the thyroid are common after brain death, and levels of biologically active T3 are generally low. However, several studies with brain-dead organ donors have shown that the majority of patients have maintained pituitary function with normal or elevated thyroid-stimulating hormone levels due to internal carotid supply. T4 levels generally remain in the normal range and inactive reverse T3 levels are normal or elevated. This constellation points to non-thyroid disease rather than central hypothyroidism in the presence of thyroid gland with increased peripheral inactivation of thyroid hormone, as is the case in patients in the general intensive care unit. Because prolonged and severe hypothyroidism can lead to myocardial dysfunction, low T3 levels are thought to induce hemodynamic instability in the potential donor.

The changes in the neuroendocrine axes have a biphasic manner. During the acute phase of critical illness, it seems to be evolutionarily selective and is likely to be beneficial for survival. Therefore, exogenous intervention may not be required at this stage of critical illness. If these profound changes last longer, a maladaptive phase begins. Although treatment with exogenous active hormones in the chronic phase seems to be a reasonable option, experimental studies have highlighted the difficulties of optimal dosing and posology [46]. In addition, a large study has highlighted the fact that thyroid hormone supplementation may be associated with an increased risk of early graft loss (EGL) and early graft dysfunction (EGD) [47, 48]. However, reliable data have shown that thyroid hormone supplementation in combination with methylprednisolone may reduce the likelihood of developing of primer graft dysfunction (PGD). In addition, thyroxine administration may also have a beneficial effect on long-term survival after HTX [49].

However, it remains unclear whether non-thyroid disease following cerebral death should be treated. An extensive observational study that included data from 63,593 brain-dead organ donors independently linked thyroid hormone replacement to an increased number of procured organs. The apparent benefits of thyroid hormone replacement were not confirmed by another RCT. However, the relatively low number of patients with hemodynamic stability in RCTs can preclude a conclusion in this subset of patients. Consensus guidelines have suggested that thyroid hormone replacement should be considered in hemodynamically unstable donors. Both T4 and T3 substitutions have been used for this purpose, although T4 is increasingly degraded to inactive reverse T3(46). One commonly utilized protocol is the following: T4 IV administration with a 20 μg bolus, followed by an infusion at 10 μg/h, or administer T3 IV with a 4.0 μg bolus, followed by an infusion at 3 μg/h [45].

Although target glucose levels for intensive insulin therapy in critically ill patients are still a matter of debate, hyperglycemic organ donors should be treated in the same way as other critically ill patients [45].

7. Hormone replacement therapy in recipients during transplantation

Although donor organ replacement therapies are still a matter of debate, there are some reliable data on HRT for cardiac recipients [50]. The use of triiodothyronine (T3) and thyroxine (T4) should be considered in patients with hemodynamic instability or potential cardiac donors with reduced ejection fraction [45]. The perioperative l-thyroxine treatment supplementation of cardiac recipients revealed that thyroid hormone administration initiated preoperatively was associated with a significantly

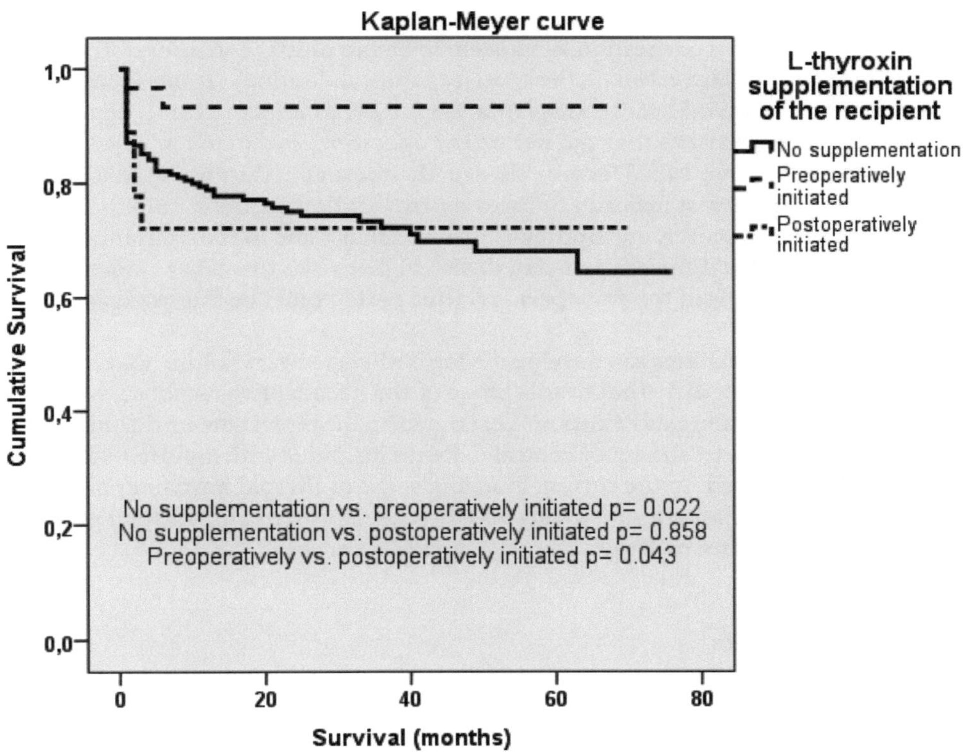

Figure 5.
Kaplan–Meier curve. Survival function according to the initiation of l-thyroxine supplementation in recipients. Preoperatively initiated supplementation was associated with significantly better survival function than no or postoperatively initiated supplementation.

better survival than either no thyroid hormone substitution or postoperative thyroid hormone substitution [50]. According to our institutional practice, thyroid hormone levels should be measured before the transplantation and thereafter weekly. While T3 levels are usually low and considered as a consequence of a natural response for huge stress, T4 levels should be closely monitored and values lower than the normal range must be treated. TSH levels in the perioperative period have also become interest of recent research (**Figure 5**).

8. Conclusions

Detection of hepatic dysfunction during preoperative evaluation, even in subclinical form, is the cornerstone of postoperative mortality estimation. As discussed above, hepatic dysfunction can affect both the intraoperative and postoperative period. In early-stage liver fibrosis, higher transaminase levels after surgery were associated with worse survival [51]. Moderate and elevated MELD XI scores predict increased short- and mid-term mortality after heart transplantation [52]. A remarkable increased MELD XI score is also associated with higher rates of postoperative stroke, need of dialysis, infection, and rejection [53].

Hepatic vein flow patterns are an intensively researched topic. Results suggest that pathological changes in flow patterns, such as damped, reduced, and reversed flow, may be an early predictor of hepatic tissue fibrotic transformation. Therefore, it can be an important marker of adverse outcome after adult heart transplantation. Moreover, hepatic vein congestion signs seem to be not only the marker of the right heart failure but can also estimate the severity of the abdominal venous insufficiency. After a successful heart transplantation [or LVAD implantation], congestive problems no longer exist as they did before the operation. In a manner, hepatic functions may improve. MELD scores are usually improving during the first postoperative year. In the vast majority of cases, normalization occurs within the first two months [54]. However, our findings indicated that a rise in the transaminase levels after transplantation was associated with higher risk of two-year mortality [19]. Hypoxic hepatitis in the early perioperative period must be followed, as it can worsen survival.

Endocrine abnormalities can develop during end-stage heart failure, and it should be monitored to detect early the chronic phase of the maladaptive response, which requires thyroid hormone substitution. Certain hormone replacements during donor procurement, such as treatment of central diabetes insipidus with arginine-vasopressin, are well established. In the current guidelines, use of thyroid hormones has been debated. After transplantation, the steroids can cause impaired glucose tolerance or diabetes. Thyroid hormone levels should be regularly checked.

Acknowledgements

We would like to thank you Veronika Rajki RN, PhD, for English editing.

Conflict of interest

The authors declare no conflict of interest related to this chapter.

DOI: http://dx.doi.org/10.5772/intechopen.102418

Abbreviations

AF	atrial fibrillation
AIH	amiodarone-induced hypothyroidis
AIT	amiodarone-induced thyrotoxicosis
ALP	alkaline phosphatase
ALT	alanine aminotransferase
AST	aspartate aminotransferase
ATG	anti-thymocyte globulin
AVP	arginine vasopressin
BIVAD	biventricular assist device
CDI	central diabetes insipidus
CYP	cytochrome P450 enzymes
D1	type 1 iodothyronine deiodinase
D2	type 2 iodothyronine deiodinase
D3	type 3 iodothyronine deiodinase
EGD	early graft dysfunction
EGL	early graft loss
HRT	hormone replacement therapy
HTX	heart transplantation
ICU	intensive care unit
IL-1	interleukin-1
IL-6	interleukin-6
INR	international normalized ratio
LVAD	left ventricular assist device
MCS	mechanical circulatory support
MELD	model for end-stage liver disease
MMF	mycophenolate-mofetil
NAFLD	nonalcoholic fatty liver disease
NFκB	nuclear factor κB
NTI	nonthyroidal illness
PGD	primer graft dysfunction
PT	prothrombin time
PTT	partial thromboplastin time
RAAS	renin-angiotensin-aldosterone system
rT3	reverse triiodothyronine
SERCA	sarcoplasmic reticulum calcium adenosine triphosphatase
SVR	systemic vascular resistance
T3	triiodothyronine
T4	thyroxine
TE	transient elastography
TNF-α	tumor necrosis factor
TRH	thyrotropin-releasing hormone
TRα1	thyroid hormone receptor alfa-1
TSH	thyroid-stimulating hormone
UNOS	United Network for Organ Sharing
VA-ECMO	veno-arterial extracorporeal membrane oxygenation
vWF	von Willebrand factor

Author details

Andrea Székely[1]*, András Szabó[1] and Balázs Szécsi[2]

1 Department of Anesthesiology and Intensive Therapy, Semmelweis University, Budapest, Hungary

2 Doctoral School of Theoretical and Translational Medicine, Semmelweis University, Budapest, Hungary

*Address all correspondence to: andi_szekely@yahoo.com

References

[1] Molina DK, DiMaio VJM. Normal organ weights in women: Part II—The brain, lungs, liver, spleen, and kidneys. The American Journal of Forensic Medicine and Pathology. 2015;**36**(3):182-187

[2] Molina DK, DiMaio VJM. Normal organ weights in men: Part II—The brain, lungs, liver, spleen, and kidneys. The American Journal of Forensic Medicine and Pathology. 2012;**33**(4):368-372

[3] Yen T-C, Chen Y-S, King K-L, Yeh S-H, Wei Y-H. Liver mitochondrial respiratory functions decline with age. Biochemical and Biophysical Research Communications. 1989;**165**(3): 994-1003

[4] Louie CY, Pham MX, Daugherty TJ, Kambham N, Higgins JPT. The liver in heart failure: A biopsy and explant series of the histopathologic and laboratory findings with a particular focus on pre-cardiac transplant evaluation. Modern Pathology. 2015;**28**(7):932-943

[5] Scheinfeld MH, Bilali A, Koenigsberg M. Understanding the spectral Doppler waveform of the hepatic veins in health and disease. Radiographics. 2009;**29**(7):2081-2098

[6] Fraquelli M, Rigamonti C, Casazza G, Conte D, Donato MF, Ronchi G, et al. Reproducibility of transient elastography in the evaluation of liver fibrosis in patients with chronic liver disease. Gut. 2007;**56**(7):968-973

[7] Castéra L, Foucher J, Bernard PH, Carvalho F, Allaix D, Merrouche W, et al. Pitfalls of liver stiffness measurement: A 5-year prospective study of 13,369 examinations. Hepatology. 2010;**51**(3):828-835

[8] Castera L, Forns X, Alberti A. Non-invasive evaluation of liver fibrosis using transient elastography. Journal of Hepatology. 2008;**48**(5):835-847

[9] Friedrich-Rust M, Schoelzel F, Maier S, Seeger F, Rey J, Fichtlscherer S, et al. Severity of coronary artery disease is associated with non-alcoholic fatty liver dis-ease: A single-blinded prospective mono-center study. PLoS One. 2017;**12**(10):e0186720

[10] Peng Y, Qi X, Guo X. Child-Pugh versus MELD score for the assessment of prognosis in liver cirrhosis: A systematic review and Meta-analysis of observational studies. Medicine. 2016;**95**(8):e2877

[11] Kamath PS, Wiesner RH, Malinchoc M, Kremers W, Therneau TM, Kosberg CL, et al. A model to predict survival in patients with end-stage liver disease. Hepatology. 2001;**33**(2):464-470

[12] Kim MS, Kato TS, Farr M, Wu C, Givens RC, Collado E, et al. Hepatic dysfunction in ambulatory patients with heart failure: Application of the MELD scoring system for outcome prediction. Journal of the American College of Cardiology. 2013;**61**(22):2253-2261

[13] Kato TS, Cheema FH, Yang J, Kawano Y, Takayama H, Naka Y, et al. Preoperative serum albumin levels predict 1-year postoperative survival of patients undergoing heart transplantation. Circulation. Heart Failure. 2013;**6**(4):785-791

[14] Anand IS, Ferrari R, Kalra GS, Wahi PL, Poole-Wilson PA, Harris PC. Edema of cardiac origin. Studies of body water and sodium, renal function,

hemodynamic indexes, and plasma hormones in untreated congestive cardiac failure. Circulation. 1989;**80**(2): 299-305

[15] Maleki M, Vakilian F, Amin A. Liver diseases in heart failure. Heart Asia. 2011;**3**(1):143-149

[16] Kato TS, Kitada S, Yang J, Wu C, Takayama H, Naka Y, et al. Relation of preoperative serum albumin levels to survival in patients undergoing left ventricular assist device implantation. The American Journal of Cardiology. 2013;**112**(9):1484-1488

[17] Caldwell S, Intagliata N. Dismantling the myth of "autoanticoagulation" in cirrhosis: An old dogma dies hard. Hepatology. 2012;**55**(5):1634-1637

[18] Tripodi A, Primignani M, Mannucci PM, Caldwell SH. Changing concepts of cirrhotic coagulopathy. The American Journal of Gastroenterology. 2017;**112**(2):274-281

[19] Nagy Á, Holndonner-Kirst E, Eke C, Kertai MD, Fazekas L, Benke K, et al. Model for end-stage liver disease scores in veno-arterial extracorporeal membrane oxygenation. The International Journal of Artificial Organs. 2020;**43**(10):684-691

[20] Nascimbene A, Neelamegham S, Frazier OH, Moake JL, Dong JF. Acquired von Willebrand syndrome associated with left ventricular assist device. Blood. 2016;**127**(25):3133-3141

[21] Lisman T, Porte RJ. Platelet function in patients with cirrhosis. Journal of Hepatology. 2012;**56**(4):993-994

[22] Hoofnagle JH, Serrano J, Knoben JE, Navarro VJ. LiverTox: A website on druginduced liver injury. Hepatology. 2013;**57**:873-874. DOI: 10.1002/HEP.26175

[23] De Groot LJ. Dangerous dogmas in medicine: The nonthyroidal illness syndrome. The Journal of Clinical Endocrinology and Metabolism. 1999;**84**(1):151-164

[24] Van den Berghe G. Non-thyroidal illness in the ICU: A syndrome with different faces. Thyroid. 2014;**24**(10):1456-1465

[25] Burman KD, Wartofsky L, Dinterman RE, Kesler P, Wannemacher RWJ. The effect of T3 and reverse T3 administration on muscle protein catabolism during fasting as measured by 3-methylhistidine excretion. Metabolism. 1979;**28**(8): 805-813

[26] Gardner DF, Kaplan MM, Stanley CA, Utiger RD. Effect of tri-iodothyronine replacement on the metabolic and pituitary responses to starvation. The New England Journal of Medicine. 1979;**300**(11): 579-584

[27] Byerley LO, Heber D. Metabolic effects of triiodothyronine replacement during fasting in obese subjects. The Journal of Clinical Endocrinology and Metabolism. 1996;**81**(3):968-976

[28] Fliers E, Guldenaar SE, Wiersinga WM, Swaab DF. Decreased hypothalamic thyrotropin-releasing hormone gene expression in patients with nonthyroidal illness. The Journal of Clinical Endocrinology and Metabolism. 1997;**82**(12):4032-4036

[29] Peeters RP, Wouters PJ, Kaptein E, van Toor H, Visser TJ, Van den Berghe G. Reduced activation and increased inactivation of thyroid hormone in tissues of critically ill patients. The Journal of Clinical Endocrinology and Metabolism. 2003; **88**(7):3202-3211

[30] Peeters RP, Wouters PJ, van Toor H, Kaptein E, Visser TJ, Van den Berghe G. Serum 3,3′,5′-triiodothyronine (rT3) and 3,5,3′-triiodothyronine/rT3 are prognostic markers in critically ill patients and are associated with postmortem tissue deiodinase activities. The Journal of Clinical Endocrinology and Metabolism. 2005;**90**(8):4559-4565

[31] de Vries EM, Fliers E, Boelen A. The molecular basis of the non-thyroidal illness syndrome. The Journal of Endocrinology. 2015;**225**(3):R67-R81

[32] de Vries EM, Kwakkel J, Eggels L, Kalsbeek A, Barrett P, Fliers E, et al. NFkappaB signaling is essential for the lipopolysaccharide-induced increase of type 2 deiodinase in tanycytes. Endocrinology. 2014;**155**(5): 2000-2008

[33] Van den Berghe G, de Zegher F, Lauwers P. Dopamine and the sick euthyroid syndrome in critical illness. Clinical Endocrinology. 1994;**41**(6):731-737

[34] Lee E, Chen P, Rao H, Lee J, Burmeister LA. Effect of acute high dose dobutamine administration on serum thyrotrophin (TSH). Clinical Endocrinology. 1999;**50**(4):487-492

[35] Schilling T, Gründling M, Strang C, Möritz K-U, Siegmund W, Hachenberg T. Effects of dopexamine, dobutamine or dopamine on prolactin and thyreotropin serum concentrations in high-risk surgical patients. Intensive Care Medicine. 2004;**30**:1127-1133

[36] Rivinius R, Helmschrott M, Ruhparwar A, Schmack B, Erbel C, Gleissner CA, et al. Long-term use of amiodarone before heart transplantation significantly reduces early post-transplant atrial fibrillation and is not associated with increased mortality after heart transplantation. Drug Design, Development and Therapy. 2016;**10**:677

[37] Rivinius R, Helmschrott M, Ruhparwar A, Darche FF, Thomas D, Bruckner T, et al. Comparison of posttransplant outcomes in patients with no, acute, or chronic amiodarone use before heart transplantation. Drug Design, Development and Therapy. 2017;**11**:1827

[38] Cooper LB, Mentz RJ, Edwards LB, Wilk AR, Rogers JG, Patel CB, et al. Amiodarone use in patients listed for heart transplant is associated with increased 1-year post-transplant mortality. The Journal of Heart and Lung Transplantation. 2017;**36**(2):202-210

[39] Jabrocka-Hybel A, Bednarczuk T, Bartalena L, Pach D, Ruchała M, Kamiński G, et al. Amiodarone and the thyroid. Endokrynologia Polska. 2015;**66**(2):176-196

[40] Smith M. Physiologic changes during brain stem death - Lessons for management of the organ donor. Journal of Heart and Lung Transplantation. 2004;**23**(9):217-222

[41] Loh JA, Verbalis JG. Disorders of water and salt metabolism associated with pituitary disease. Endocrinology and Metabolism Clinics of North America. 2008;**37**:213-234

[42] Dimopoulou I, Tsagarakis S, Anthi A, Milou E, Ilias I, Stavrakaki K, et al. High prevalence of decreased cortisol reserve in brain-dead potential organ donors. Critical Care Medicine. 2003;**31**(4):1113-1117

[43] Meyfroidt G, Gunst J, Martin-Loeches I, Smith M, Robba C, Taccone FS, et al. Management of the brain-dead donor in the ICU: General

and specific therapy to improve transplantable organ quality. Intensive Care Medicine. 2019;**45**:343-353

[44] Ball IM, Hornby L, Rochwerg B, Weiss MJ, Gillrie C, Chassé M, et al. Management of the neurologically deceased organ donor: A Canadian clinical practice guideline. CMAJ. 2020;**192**(14):E361-E369

[45] Kotloff RM, Blosser S, Fulda GJ, Malinoski D, Ahya VN, Angel L, et al. Management of the potential organ donor in the ICU: Society of Critical Care Medicine/American College of Chest Physicians/Association of Organ Procurement Organizations Consensus Statement. Critical Care Medicine. 2015;**43**(6):1291-1325

[46] Teblick A, Langouche L, Van den Berghe G. Anterior pituitary function in critical illness. Endocrine Connections. 2019;**8**(8):R131-R143

[47] Peled Y, Ram E, Klempfner R, Lavee J, Cherikh WS, Stehlik J. Donor thyroid hormone therapy and heart transplantation outcomes: ISHLT transplant registry analysis. The Journal of Heart and Lung Transplantation. 2020;**39**(10):1070-1078

[48] Lander MM. Thyroid hormone in cardiac transplantation: Cat chasing its tail? Journal of Heart and Lung Transplantation. 2020;**39**:1079-1080

[49] Nagy Á, Szécsi B, Eke C, Szabó A, Mihály S, Fazekas L, et al. Endocrine management and hormone replacement therapy in cardiac donor management: A retrospective observational study. Transplantation Proceedings. 2021;**53**(10):2807-2815

[50] Holndonner–Kirst E, Nagy A, Czobor NR, Fazekas L, Dohan O, Kertai MD, et al. The impact of l-thyroxine treatment of donors and recipients on postoperative outcomes after heart transplantation. Journal of Cardiothoracic and Vascular Anesthesia. 2019;**33**(6):1629-1635

[51] Holndonner-Kirst E, Nagy A, Czobor NR, Fazekas L, Lex DJ, Sax B, et al. Higher transaminase levels in the postoperative period after Orthotopic heart transplantation are associated with worse survival. Journal of Cardiothoracic and Vascular Anesthesia. 2018;**32**(4):1711-1718

[52] Grimm JC, Shah AS, Magruder JT, Kilic A, Valero V 3rd, Dungan SP, et al. MELD-XI score predicts early mortality in patients after heart transplantation. The Annals of Thoracic Surgery. 2015;**100**(5):1737-1743

[53] Deo SV, Al-Kindi SG, Altarabsheh SE, Hang D, Kumar S, Ginwalla MB, et al. Model for end-stage liver disease excluding international normalized ratio (MELD-XI) score predicts heart transplant outcomes: Evidence from the registry of the united network for organ sharing. The Journal of Heart and Lung Transplantation. 2016;**35**(2):222-227

[54] Chokshi A, Cheema FH, Schaefle KJ, Jiang J, Collado E, Shahzad K, et al. Hepatic dysfunction and survival after orthotopic heart transplantation: Application of the MELD scoring system for outcome prediction. The Journal of Heart and Lung Transplantation. 2012;**31**(6):591-600

Section 2

Mechanical Circulatory Support

Chapter 4

Durable Ventricular Assist Device for Bridge to Transplantation

Minoru Ono

Abstract

A durable ventricular assist device (VAD) is a key mechanical circulatory support to safely bridge a heart transplant candidate to transplantation over a long waiting period. Recent UNOS policy change has a great impact on the role of continuous-flow VAD as a bridging device. The rest of the majority of countries still rely on a cf-VAD as a safe and effective support device. A sole durable VAD for bridge to transplantation in pediatric patients is Berlin Heart EXCOR, for which there is a growing demand through the improvement of a long-term result. In this chapter, I will overview the history and the present status of durable VAD for bridge to transplantation in both adult and pediatric patients.

Keywords: heart transplantation, ventricular assist device, bridge to transplantation

1. Introduction

The first bridge to transplantation strategy was started in the 1980s, but a patient needed to stay in hospital due to a huge driving console, even if the device was implantable. First-generation of implantable ventricular assist device (VAD) was not widely implanted due to its huge size and a limited reliable support period. Development and introduction to the clinical arena of a rotary blood pump in the early 2000 completely changed the landscape. The smaller pump size enabled easier implantation in smaller body size patients and an operation of the device by portable batteries paved a way to outpatient management. A so-called second-generation device is driven in the presence of contact bearings, which were found to lead to several tough complications, such as pump thrombosis and gastrointestinal bleeding. Advent of the third-generation device, in which an impeller is rotated without contact to an inner housing by magnetic and/or hydrodynamic levitation systems. Most updated devices are manufactured by incorporating a magnetic levitation system. Thanks to these technological refinements and improvements of continuous-flow VAD (cf-VAD) support patients, the survival of patients on a VAD has been steadily prolonging. In this chapter, the current status and survival of cf-VAD patients for bridge to transplantation (BTT) in Japan and the United States (US) are reviewed.

2. Bridge to transplantation in Japan: analysis of J-MACS report

Two Japan-made cf-LVAD (EVAHEART, Sun Medical Research Corp., Nagano, Japan and DuraHeart, Terumo Heart Inc., Ann Arbor, MI) were approved for health insurance coverage as a BTT in April 2010. Subsequently, HeartMate II (Abbott, Chicago, IL) in April 2013, Jarvik 2000 (Jarvik Heart Inc., New York, NY) in January 2014, HVAD (Medtronic, Minneapolis, MN) in February 2019 and HeartMate 3 (Abbott, Chicago, IL) in July 2019 were approved for a BTT. Similar to Interagency Registry for Mechanically Assisted Circulatory Support (INTERMACS) in the US, we have the Japanese Registry for Mechanically Assisted Circulatory Support (J-MACS) as a mandatory registry system of cf-LVAD. J-MACS was established in 2009 with an intention of harmonization by doing with Food and Drug Administration (FDA) in the US [1].

Registry summary report is published every year, and the most recent one was published online in March 2021 [2]. HeartMate 3 was approved as the first DT device in May 2021, so the most recent J-MACS registry report included solely data regarding a BTT strategy. This report analyzed data of cf-LVADs which were implanted by October 31, 2020. The total number of implantation was 1353, among which primary implantation was in 956 (70.7%), bridge to bridge (BTB, conversion from paracorporeal device to cf-LVAD) in 218 (16.1%) and device exchange from cf-LVAD in 179 (13.2%). The total number of patients was 1174 (primary VAD + BTB). There were 871 male patients (74.2%) with an average age of 43.5 years. The distribution of the age in decade is shown in **Table 1**. The height, weight, body mass index (BMI) and body surface area (BSA) were 167.0 +/− 8.7 cm, 57.6 +/− 11.8 kg, 20.5 +/− 3.3 kg/m^2 and 1.64 +/− 0.19 m^2, respectively (**Table 2**). The majority of the patients were implanted for non-ischemic dilated cardiomyopathy (DCM; 64.8%), followed by ischemic heart disease (12.2%) and dilated-phase of hypertrophic cardiomyopathy (10.6%) (**Table 3**). The severity INTERMACS/J-MACS profile of the patients before cf-LVAD implantation was shown in **Table 4**. Almost half of the patients were implanted at profile 3 (46.7%), and only 9.1% belonged to profile 1. Kaplan–Meier survival curve showed that 1- and 2-year survival rates were 92% and 89% (**Figure 1**). The longest support exceeded 5 years.

		N	%
Total number		1174	
Gender	Male	871	74.2
	Female	303	25.8
Age distribution	< 10	1	0.1
	10–19	66	5.6
	20–29	129	11.0
	30–39	227	19.3
	40–49	307	26.1
	50–59	304	25.9
	60–69	139	11.8
	> 70	1	0.1

Table 1.
Gender and age distribution.

	Mean ± SD
Age (years)	43.5 ± 13.4
Height (cm)	167.0 ± 8.7
Weight (kg)	57.6 ± 11.8
BMI (kg/m^2)	20.5 ± 3.3
BSA (m^2)	1.64 ± 0.19

Table 2.
Patient demographics. BMI: Body mass index, BSA: Body surface area.

	N	%
CHD	22	1.9
IHD	143	12.2
HCM (dilated phase)	125	10.6
HCM (no dilated phase)	5	0.4
VHD	10	0.9
DCM	761	64.8
RCM	5	0.4
Others	102	8.7
Unknown	1	0.1
Total	1174	

CHD: congenital heart disease, IHD: ischemic heart disease, HCM: hypertrophic cardiomyopathy, VHD: valvular heart disease, DCM: idiopathic dilated cardiomyopathy, RCM: restrictive cardiomyopathy.

Table 3.
Causative diseases.

INTERMACS/J-MACS profile	N	%
Profile 1	107	9.1
Profile 2	453	38.6
Profile 3	548	46.7
Profile 4	52	4.4
Profile 5–7	14	1.2
Total	1174	

Table 4.
Preimplant INTERMACS/J-MACS profile.

Figure 2 shows Kaplan–Meier survival stratified by the age group by decade. Patients with age in 50s and over 60 years had significantly worse survival ($p < 0.0001$). **Figure 3** shows the survivals divided by preoperative J-MACS profiles, demonstrating a significantly worse survival in profile 1 ($p = 0.032$). **Figure 4** shows the competing

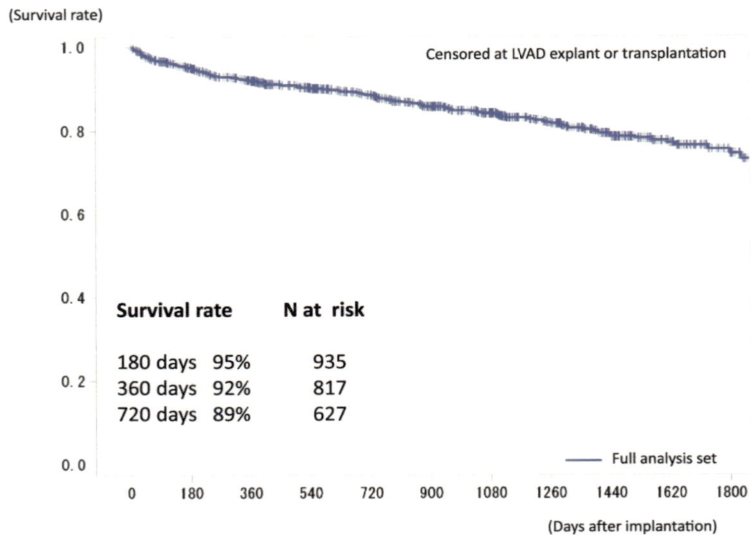

Figure 1.
Actuarial survival after BTT cf-LVAD implantation.

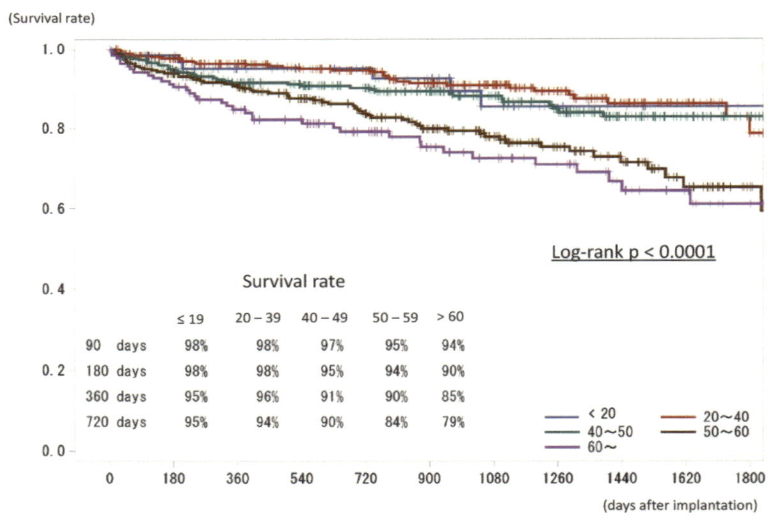

Figure 2.
Actuarial survival after BTT cf-LVAD implantation stratified by age group.

outcomes. Waiting time for heart transplantation is more than 4 years recently, so the curve of survival on the device crosses that of transplantation around 1500 days.

Pump thrombosis-free curve is shown in **Figure 5** with 1- and 2-year event-free rates of 97% and 97% for the primary implant, which is much less compared to an INTERMACS report. Driveline infection-free curve is shown in **Figure 6**, demonstrating that 1- and 2-year event-free rates are 78% and 67% for a primary implant.

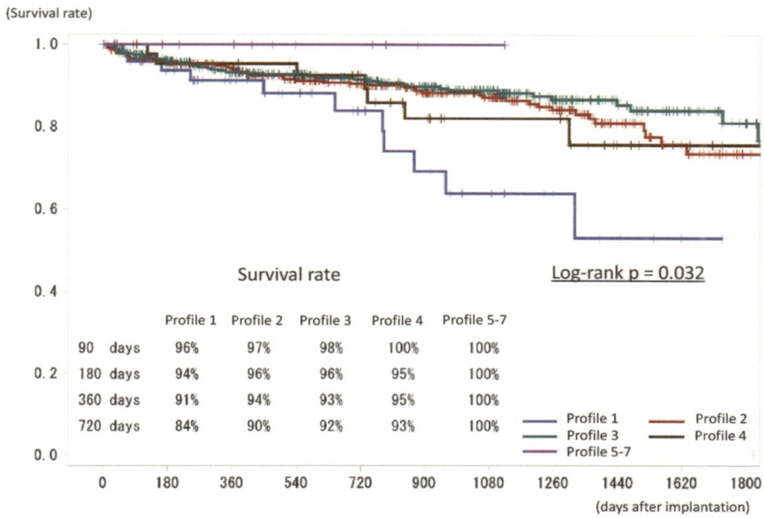

Figure 3.
Actuarial survival after BTT cf-LVAD implantation stratified by preimplant profiles.

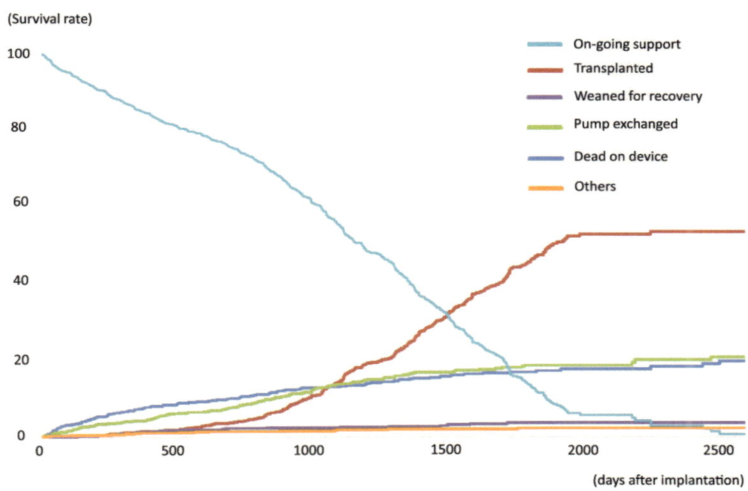

Figure 4.
Competing outcomes.

Figure 7 shows stroke-free curve including all stroke events of any grade. The gastrointestinal bleeding-free curve is shown in **Figure 8**, demonstrating 1- and 2-year event-free rate of 95% and 93% for primary implantation, which is much more infrequent compared to the US. **Figure 9** shows the readmission-free rate. Almost two-thirds of the patients were readmitted within 1 year and three-quarters in 2 years, which is still an important issue to be solved. **Figure 10** shows a pump exchange free rate with a 1- and 2-year event-free rate of 96% and 92% for primary implantation.

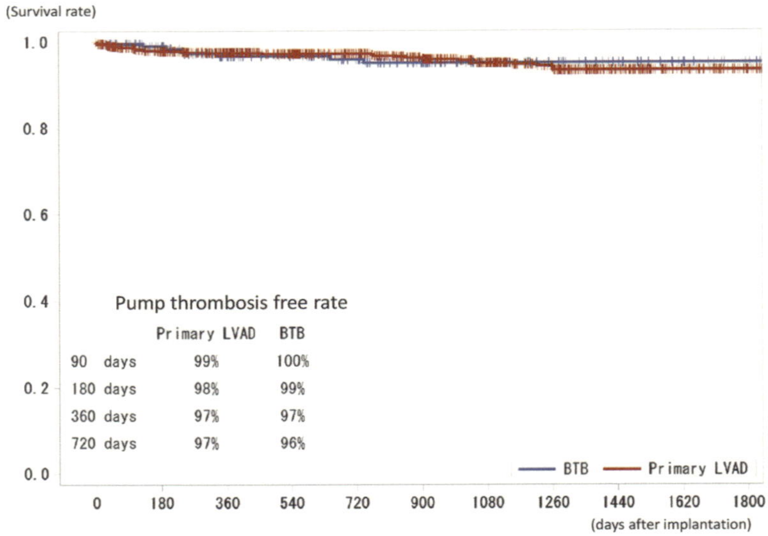

Figure 5.
Pump thrombosis-free rate divided by primary VAD and BTB.

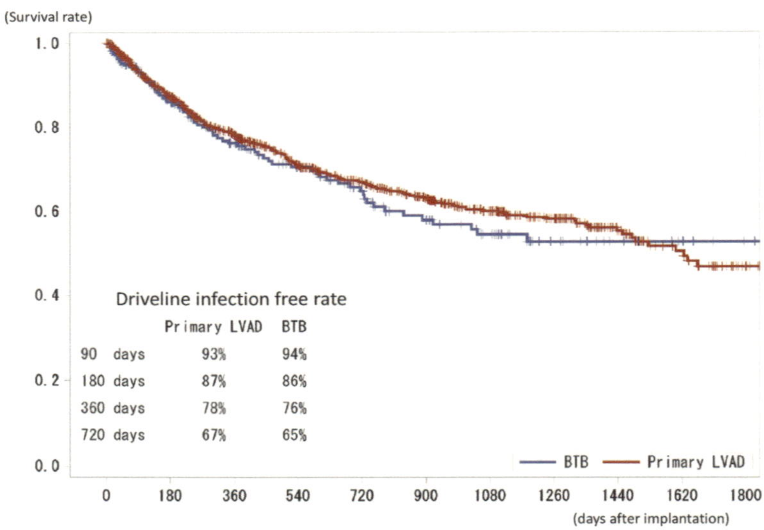

Figure 6.
Driveline infection-free rate divided by primary VAD and BTB.

3. Heart transplantation in Japan: analysis of heart transplantation registry

Five hundred sixty-six heart transplantations (512 adult and 54 pediatric HTx) were performed by December 2020 in Japan since the Organ Transplantation Act came into force in October 1997 [3]. **Figure 11** shows the number and the type of circulatory support device on which the recipient was placed at the time of HTx [4]. There were only three recipients who were not on any circulatory support including inotropes. All these

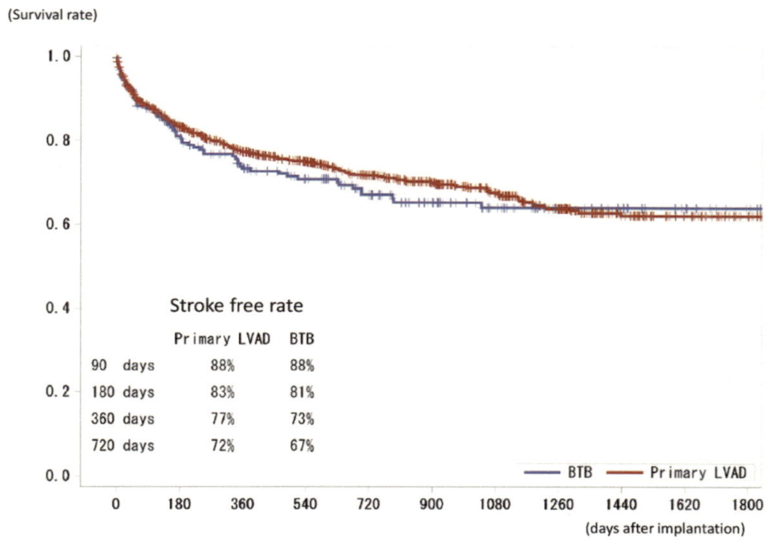

Figure 7.
Stroke (any grade)-free rate divided by primary VAD and BTB.

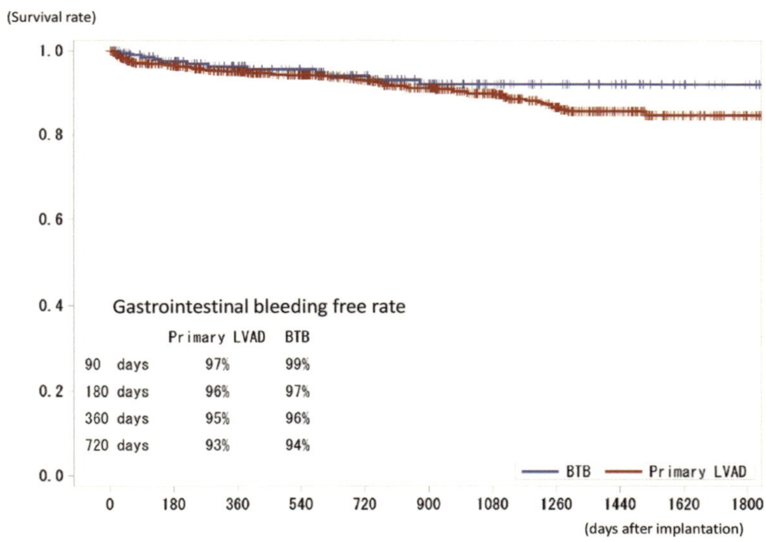

Figure 8.
Gastrointestinal bleeding-free rate divided by primary VAD and BTB.

three were pediatric patients. Thirty-two recipients (5.7%) were on continuous inotropic support. Thus, the majority of the recipients (93.8%) were on any type of mechanical circulatory support. Paracorporeal air-driven LVAD was used in 126 patients (22.3%), including 110 Nipro VAD (Nipro, Osaka, Japan) and 16 Berlin Heart Excor pediatric VADs (Berlin Heart GmbH, Berlin, Germany). Implantable LVAD was used in 393 recipients (69.4%) and 12 patients (2.1%) were on biventricular VAD (BIVAD) support. Most frequently implanted cf-LVAD device was HeartMate II in 166, followed by EVAHEART in 86, Jarvik 2000 in 61, DuraHeart in 56 and so on. A small number of first-generation implantable pulsatile devices were used in the early years (n = 11).

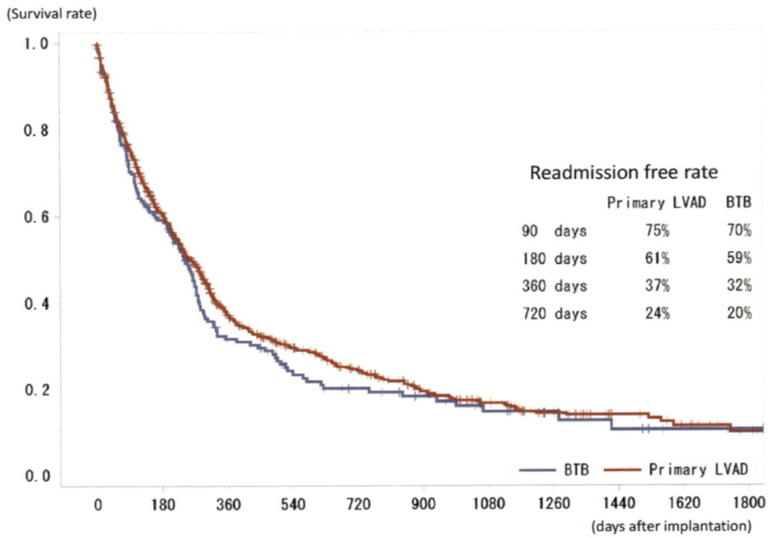

Figure 9.
Readmission-free rate divided by primary VAD and BTB.

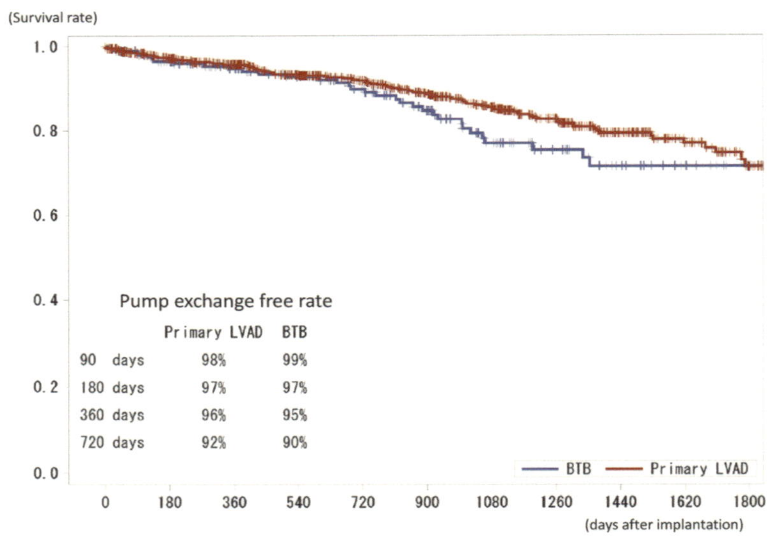

Figure 10.
Pump exchange-free rate divided by primary VAD and BTB.

Figure 12 shows a yearly trend of the type of circulatory support [4]. Paracorporeal VADs were mainly used for a BTT before the year 2011 when two Japan-made cf-LVAD were approved for health insurance coverage. Berlin Heart Excor pediatric was started to be covered by health insurance in 2015. **Figure 13** shows a yearly trend of waiting time for HTx divided by adult and pediatric recipients [4]. Since a shortage of brain-dead donations is extreme in Japan, a waiting time has continuously prolonged and reached 1625 days in adult recipients in 2020. A waiting time was variable year by year in pediatric recipients, but in general longer than that of Western countries.

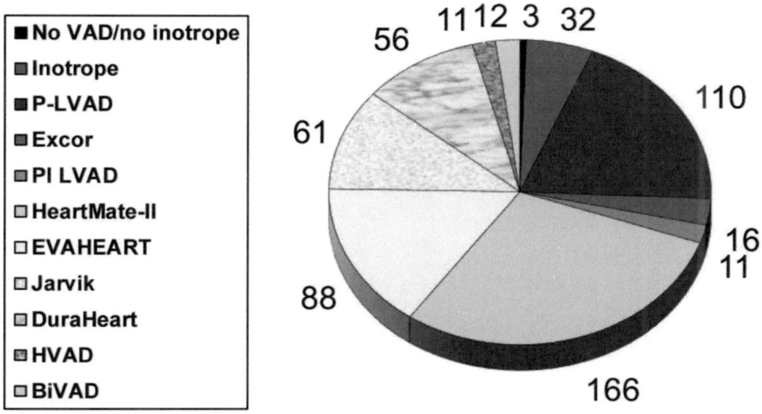

Figure 11.
The number and the type of circulatory support at HTx(n = 566). Cf-VAD: continuous-flow left ventricular assist device, PI VAD: pulsatile implantable left ventricular assist device, P-LVAD: paracorporeal left ventricular assist device.

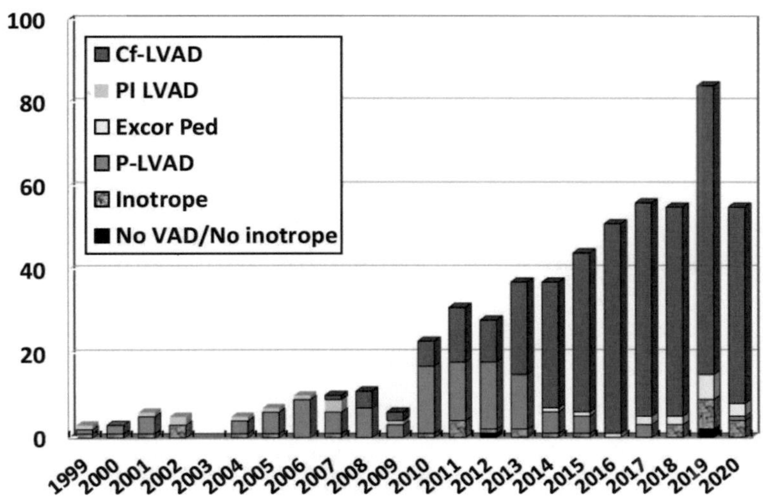

Figure 12.
The number and the type of circulatory support at HTxin each year. Cf-VAD: continuous-flow left ventricular assist device, PI VAD: pulsatile implantable left ventricular assist device, P-LVAD: paracorporeal left ventricular assist device.

4. Impact of bridge to transplantation on the results of heart transplantation: from ISHLT registry report

A cf-VAD has been widely used for a BTT in these two decades due to improvement of long-term safe support, less complications and size miniaturization. **Figure 14** is from ISHLT (International Society for Heart and Lung Transplantation) 2019 Annual Report Slides [5], showing an annual trend of a ratio of adult patients who were bridged to HTx with mechanical circulatory support devices. Including LVAD, BIVAD, VAD + ECMO and isolated RVAD, 52.5% and 49.6% of the recipients were bridged to HTx in 2016 and 2017, respectively. An isolated LVAD support was the

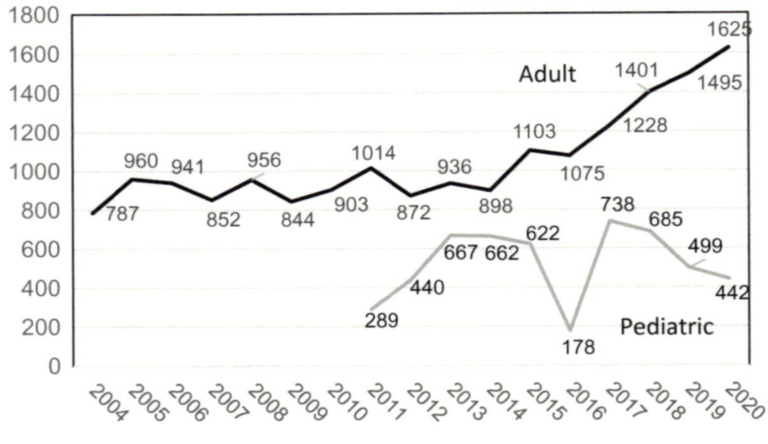

Figure 13.
Waiting time for heart transplantation in both adult and pediatric recipients.

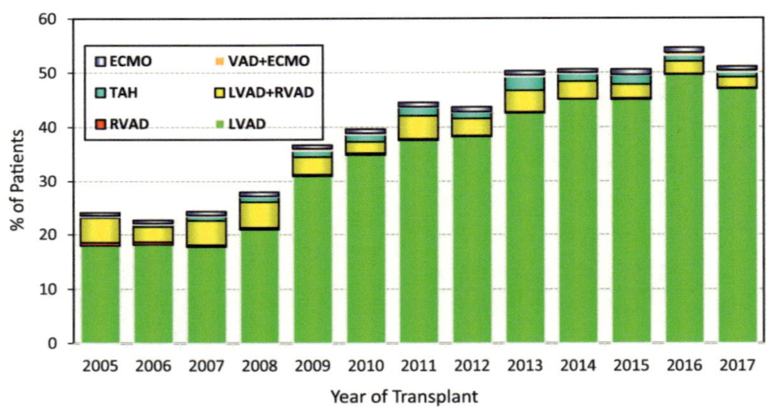

Figure 14.
Adult heart transplants. The ratio of patients bridged with mechanical circulatory support by year and device type.

majority like 49.6% and 47.0% in 2016 and 2017, respectively. **Figure 15** from ISHLT 2019 Report demonstrates that survival (89.9% and 77.6% at 1 and 5 years) in patients with cf-LVAD support is identical with that of no LVAD/no inotrope group (90.0% and 79.0%) or no LVAD/Inotrope group (91.9% and 78.7%) [5]. Cox-hazard analysis of risk factors for 1-year mortality among adult heart transplants between 2012 and June 2017 showed that VAD support was a significant risk factor ($p < 0.01$; HR 1.241, 95% CI 1.082–1.424). However, VAD bridge was not a significant risk factor for cardiac allograft vasculopathy (CAV) or severe renal dysfunction within 5 years by Cox-hazard analysis of adult heart transplants conditional on survival to discharge between 2008 and June 2013 [5].

Figure 16 from ISHLT Pediatric HTx 2019 Annual Report shows an annual trend of a ratio of patients who were bridged with mechanical circulatory support [6]. Different from adult recipients, an increasing trend of the MCS bridge ratio was not steady, but there was a trend for increase with 31.8% in VAD or TAH and 1.5% in VAD + ECMO. **Figure 17** demonstrates that about a quarter of pediatric

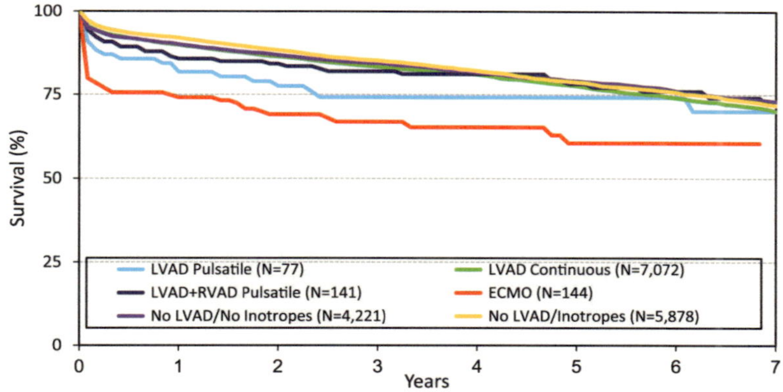

Figure 15.
Adult heart transplants. Kaplan–Meier survival by pre-transplant mechanical circulatory support use (transplants: Jan 2010 –June 2017).

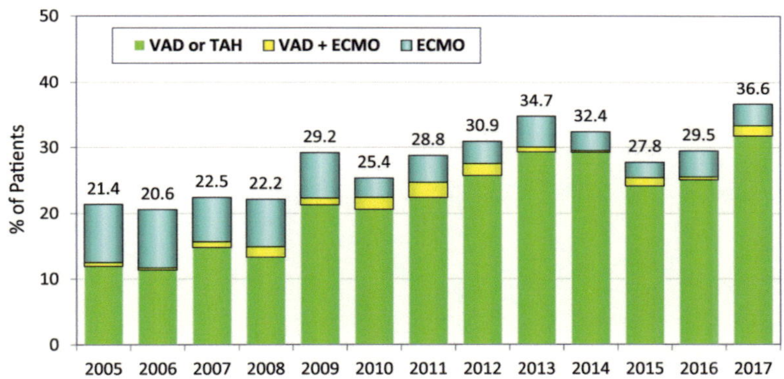

Figure 16.
Pediatric heart transplants. Ratio of patients bridged with mechanical circulatory support by year (transplants: Jan 2005 –Dec 2017).

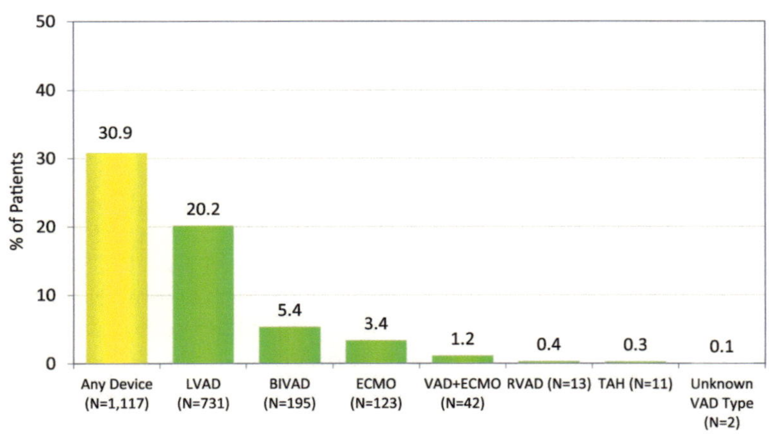

Figure 17.
Pediatric heart transplants. The ratio of patients bridged with mechanical circulatory support by the device (transplants: Jan 2010 –June 2018).

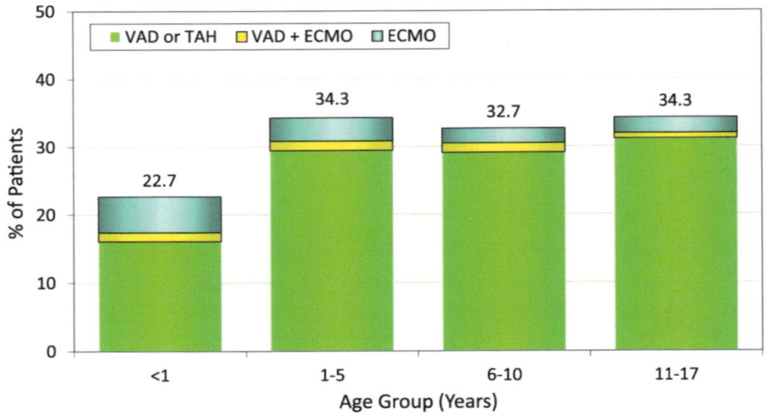

Figure 18.
Pediatric heart transplants. The ratio of patients bridged with mechanical circulatory support by age group (transplants: Jan 2010 –June 2018).

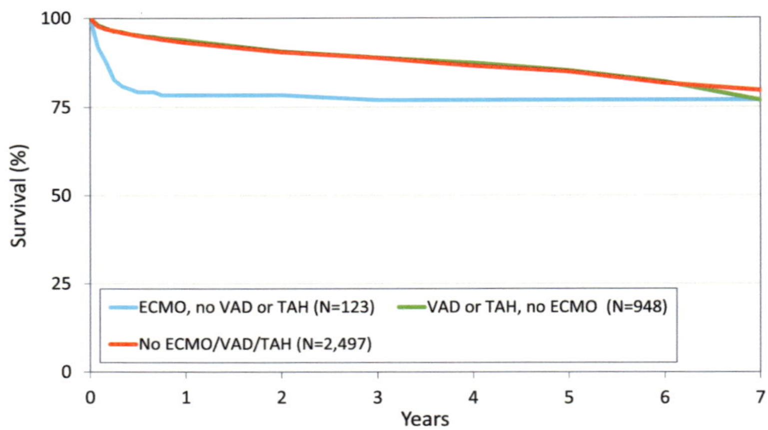

Figure 19.
Pediatric heart transplants. Kaplan–Meier survival by mechanical circulatory support usage (transplants: Jan 2010 –June 2017).

recipients were bridged with LVAD (20.2%) or BIVAD (5.4%) between 2010 and June 2018 [6]. Notably, almost a half of the recipients were bridged with LVAD (39.8%) or BIVAD (8.7%) in DCM among transplants between 2010 and June 2018 [6]. **Figure 18** shows a ratio of patients who were bridged with MCS divided by age group [6]. A total of 30% patients with age of 1 to 17 years were bridged with VAD or TAH, or VAD + ECMO [6]. **Figure 19** is a Kaplan–Meier survival curve stratified by device strategies, demonstrating that survivals of the VAD or TAH group (93.7% and 85.2% at 1 and 5 years) are not different from those of no support group (93.1% and 84.8%) [6]. The VAD support was a risk factor for 1-year mortality by Cox-hazard analysis (p = 0.02; HR 1.396, 95% CI 1.047–1.860). However, as in adult HTx, pretransplant VAD use was not associated with CAV progression or renal dysfunction within 5 years conditional on survival to discharge.

5. Most recent publications on bridge to transplantation

In addition to BTT, a cf-VAD has been implanted for bridge to candidacy or destination therapy. A recent trend of survival after cf-VAD implantation for each strategy was reported in The Society of Thoracic Surgeons (STS) INTERMACS 2020 annual Report [7]. Survival of cf-LVAD patients by a device strategy is shown in **Figure 20**. Patients with a BTT strategy enjoyed better survival than those with other strategies. The absolute difference of survival at each year between BTT and DT strategies ranged from 6.7% to 10.3%. Steady improvement of survival after HTx with cf-VAD support was clearly demonstrated in the ISHLT adult heart transplantation 2021 report [8]. As shown in **Figure 21**, a significant improvement in survival is achieved as years elapsed. A similar finding was also confirmed in pediatric recipients with a BTT strategy [9].

A new heart allocation policy was introduced in October 2018 with an intention to: 1. decrease a wait-list death, and 2. equalize a chance to be transplanted for a severely ill recipient. This policy change made the new donor heart allocation system to prioritize candidates supported by temporary devices. However, waitlist and post-transplant outcomes in candidates with durable LVAD remain to be elucidated. Mullan et al. analyzed the United Network for Organ Sharing (UNOS) database of adults with cf-LVAD at listing or implanted while listed between April 2017 and April 2020, and elucidated that the number of patients listed with LVAD decreased nationally over time from 102 in April 2017 to 12 in April 2020 ($p < 0.001$). The proportion of patients with LVAD at the time of transplant decreased from 47% to 14% (**Figure 22**) [10]. They also showed that transplantation rates were not different before and after the allocation policy change (85.4% vs. 83.6%; $p = 0.225$), but waitlist time decreased in the post-period (82 vs. 65 days; $p = 0.004$). Waitlist survival did not change, but post-transplantation survival was worse in patients with BTT post-change ($p < 0.001$) [10]. Abrupt decrease of a BTT strategy among cf-LVAD implantation was endorsed by the STS INTERMACS 2020 annual Report (**Figure 23**) [7].

Edelson et al. conducted an ISHLT data analysis to seek the influence of mechanical circulatory support on post-transplant outcomes in pediatric patients [11]. Among

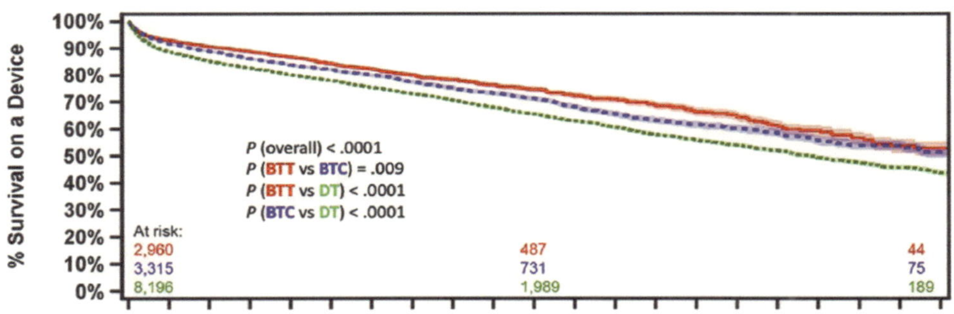

Months after Implant	Survival by Strategy BTT	BTC	DT
12	86.8%	83.8%	80.1%
24	78.3%	75.2%	70.6%
36	70.9%	65.5%	60.6%
48	61.3%	58.6%	52.1%
60	52.7%	51.4%	43.6%

Figure 20.
Kaplan–Meier survival curves for primary cf-LVAD for 2015–2019 by implant strategy. BTC: Bridge to candidacy, BTT: Bridge to transplant, Cf-LVAD, continuous-flow left ventricular assist device, DT: Destination therapy.

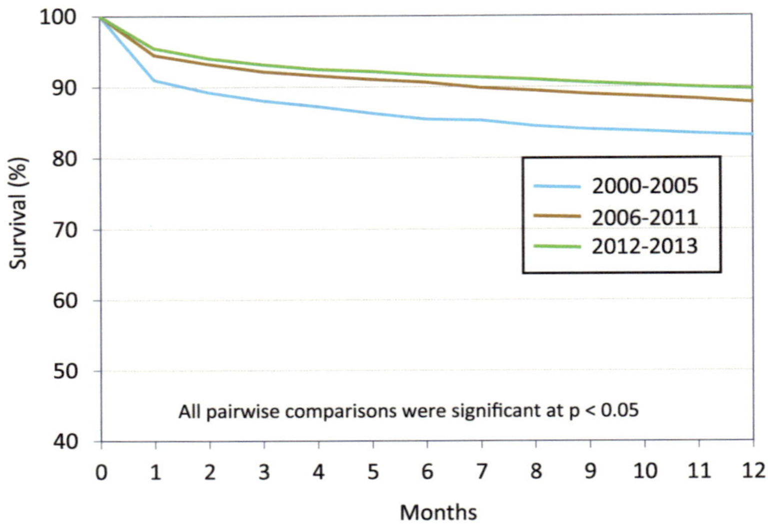

Figure 21.
Adult heart transplants with cf-VAD BTT. Kaplan–Meier survival within 12 months by recipient era (transplants: Jan 2000 -Jun 2017).

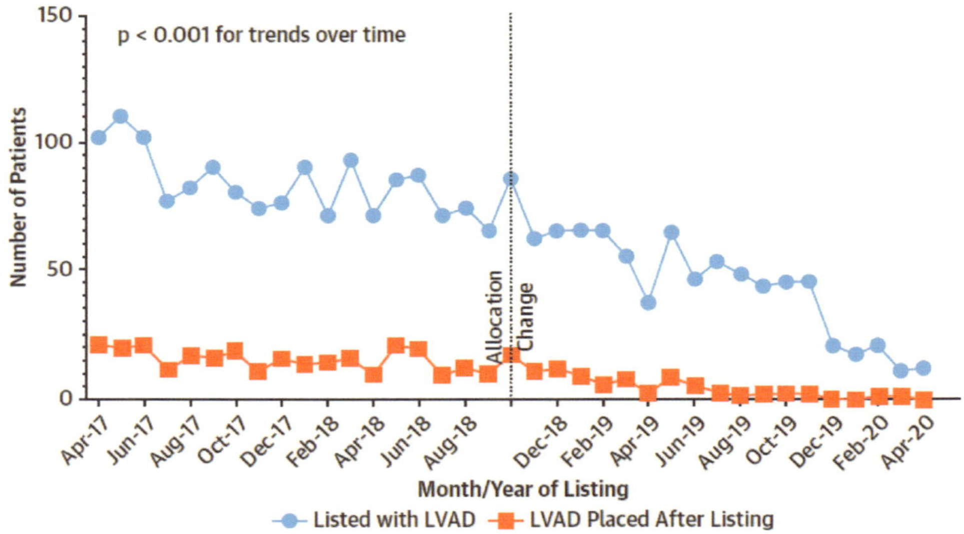

Figure 22.
Trends in LVAD utilization in patients listed for heart transplantation.

5095 patients between 2005 and 2017, 26% of patients received MCS prior to transplant: 240 (4.7%) on extracorporeal membrane oxygenation (ECMO), 1030 (20.2%) on VAD, and 54 both. They found that survival in congenital heart disease (CHD) and DCM was similar in patients with no MCS or those with VAD, while pretransplant ECMO use is strongly associated with death after transplant particularly in children with CHD. HTx in patients with Fontan operation has been challenging, and a durable LVAD has been used to bridge a post-Fontan patient anecdotally. The first collective study of durable VAD support in Fontan patients was reported in 2021. Cedars

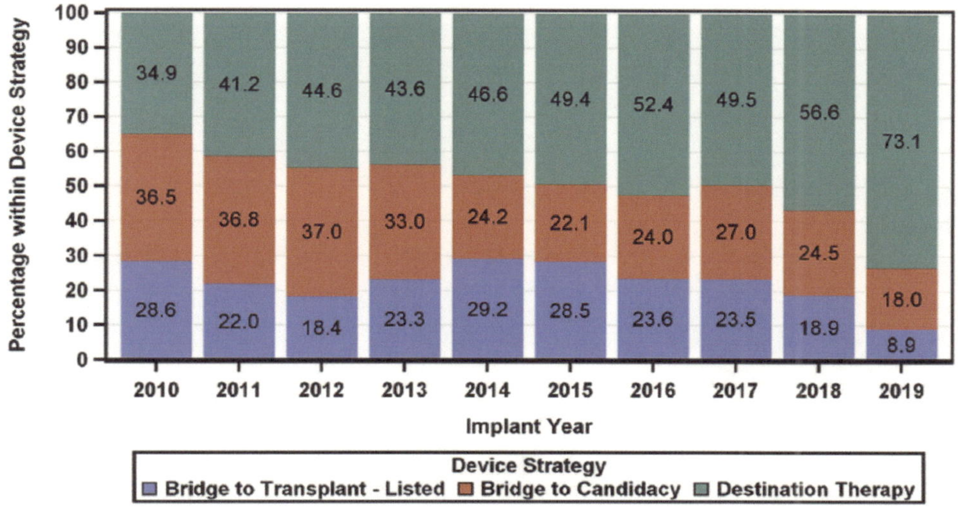

Figure 23.
Implant strategy by implant year for primary continuous-flow LVADs.

et al. conducted a retrospective analysis of data collected in the Advanced Cardiac Therapies Improving Outcomes Network (ACTION) registry, a multicenter learning network of pediatric hospitals actively involved in the implantation and management of VADs in children and adults with CHD [12]. They identified 45 Fontan patients implanted with a VAD. The average age of patients was 10 years (interquartile range: 4.5–18). The majority of patients were INTERMACS Profile 2 (56%). The most commonly employed device was the Medtronic HVAD (56%). A total of 13 patients were discharged on device support, and 67% of patients experienced adverse events, the most common of which were neurologic (25%). At 1 year after device implantation, the rate of transplantation was 69.5%, 9.2% of patients continued to be VAD supported, and 21.3% of patients had died.

6. Conclusions

In this chapter, the author reviews durable VAD used for a BTT. BTT strategy both in adult HTx by cf-LVAD and in pediatric HTx by Berlin Heart Excor or cf-LVAD is mandatory in Japan because a waiting time is over 4 years in adults and over 2 years in children due to a severe donor shortage. A total of 95% of adult HTx and 80% of pediatric HTx were bridged with a durable LVAD as of December 2020. As shown by J-MACS registry data, the survival of cf-LVAD patients was favorable. In the majority of European countries and the US cf-VAD use for a BTT was steadily increasing. VAD support was employed successfully in about 50% in adult and about 30% in pediatric HTx recipients. Survival after HTx with durable VAD support has been improving, and no survival difference is observed compared to that of recipients without VAD support. Recent heart allocation policy change in the US had a great impact on a judgment to choose a durable LVAD for a BTT. A chance to choose BTT strategy by using cf-LVAD will be declining undoubtedly, but nobody still knows what will be a future outcome.

Author details

Minoru Ono
Department of Cardiovascular Surgery, The University of Tokyo, Tokyo, Japan

*Address all correspondence to: ono-tho@h.u-tokyo.ac.jp

References

[1] Nakatani T, Sase K, Oshiyama H, Akiyama M, Horie M, Nawata K, et al. J-MACS investigators. Japanese registry for Mechanically Assisted Circulatory Support: First report. The Journal of Heart and Lung Transplantation. 2017;**36**(10):1087-1096

[2] J-MACS statistical report. Available from: https://www.jpats.org/society/jmacs/report.html [Accessed: December 3, 2021]

[3] Numbers of donated and transplanted organs in Japan. Available from: https://www.jotnw.or.jp/data/offer03.php [Accessed: December 10, 2021]

[4] The number and the type of circulatory support at heart transplantation in Japan. Available from: http://www.jsht.jp/2021/04/17/registry/japan/20201231%E3%83%AC%E3%82%B8%E3%82%B9%E3%83%88%E3%83%AA2.pdf [Accessed: December 11, 2021]

[5] ISHLT adult heart transplantation statistics in 2019. Available from: https://ishltregistries.org/registries/slides.asp?yearToDisplay=2019 [Accessed: December 11, 2021]

[6] ISHLT pediatric heart transplantation statistics in 2019. Available from: https://ishltregistries.org/registries/slides.asp?yearToDisplay=2019 [Accessed: December 11, 2021]

[7] Molina EJ, Shah P, Kiernan MS, Cornwell WK 3rd, Copeland H, Takeda K, et al. The Society of Thoracic Surgeons Intermacs 2020 Annual Report. The Annals of Thoracic Surgery. 2021;**111**(3): 778-792

[8] Khush KK, Hsich E, Potena L, Cherikh WS, Chambers DC, Harhay MO, et al. Stehlik J; International Society for Heart and Lung Transplantation. The International Thoracic Organ Transplant Registry of the International Society for Heart and Lung Transplantation: Thirty-eighth adult heart transplantation report - 2021; Focus on recipient characteristics. The Journal of Heart and Lung Transplantation. 2021;**40**(10):1035-1049

[9] Singh TP, Cherikh WS, Hsich E, Chambers DC, Harhay MO, Hayes D, et al. International Society for Heart and Lung Transplantation. The International Thoracic Organ Transplant Registry of the International Society for Heart and Lung Transplantation: Twenty-fourth pediatric heart transplantation report - 2021; Focus on recipient characteristics. The Journal of Heart and Lung Transplantation. 2021;**40**(10):1050-1059

[10] Mullan CW, Chouairi F, Sen S, Mori M, Clark KAA, Reinhardt SW, et al. Changes in Use of Left Ventricular Assist Devices as Bridge to Transplantation With New Heart Allocation Policy. JACC Heart Fail. 2021;**9**(6):420-429

[11] Edelson JB, Huang Y, Griffis H, Huang J, Mascio CE, Chen JM, et al. The influence of mechanical Circulatory support on post-transplant outcomes in pediatric patients: A multicenter study from the International Society for Heart and Lung Transplantation (ISHLT) Registry. The Journal of Heart and Lung Transplantation. 2021;**40**(11):1443-1453

[12] Cedars A, Kutty S, Danford D, Schumacher K, Learning Network Investigators ACTION, Auerbach SR, et al. Systemic ventricular assist device support in Fontan patients: A report by ACTION. The Journal of Heart and Lung Transplantation. 2021;**40**(5):368-376 Erratum in: J Heart Lung Transplant. 2021 Dec;40(12):1685

Chapter 5

Heart Transplant after Mechanical Circulatory Support

Elena Sandoval and Daniel Pereda

Abstract

Heart transplant is the gold-standard treatment for end-stage heart failure. However, the aging of the population, increase in the prevalence of heart failure and the shortage of available donors have led to a significant increase in the wait-list times. This increase in waiting time may cause some patients clinically deteriorate while on the list. Several bridging strategies have been developed to help patients reach heart transplant. It is mandatory to know the current results of these techniques and the specific tips and tricks these different devices may have. Survival results would also be presented to help us decide the best strategy for each of our patients.

Keywords: heart transplant, short-term mechanical circulatory support, ECMO, long-term mechanical circulatory support, survival

1. Introduction

Heart transplant is the gold-standard treatment for end-stage heart failure since the first case, performed by Christiaan Barnard, on December 3, 1967 in Cape Town [1]. This first case was the results of previous works led mainly by Norman Shumway at Stanford. After an initial spread of the technique and the development of different transplant programs, the actual number of heart transplants declined due to impaired outcomes, mostly due to infections and rejection [2]. Only a few groups, mainly Stanford in the USA and the Pitié-Salpêtrière in Europe, continued investigating and working on trying to improve their patients' outcomes. It was not until the introduction of cyclosporine as an immunosuppressor, that solid organ transplant outcomes significantly improved [3]. This significant change in patient management led to the final expansion of the technique and the development of multiple programs across the world.

Technical and medical developments have caused previously lethal conditions that evolve into chronic ones, increasing the prevalence of end-stage heart failure. This increase, in addition to the aging of the population, has led to a disbalance in the number of donors available, which has remained stable over the last years according to ISHLT data [4]. This disbalance has caused an increase in the waiting time period, leading to the development of different strategies to sustain patients.

This abovementioned shortage of donors, which is common to most countries, forced the transplant programs to expand their acceptance criteria with the such called "extended-criteria donors." This means that older donors with longer ischemic times were now accepted. Despite the initial concerns, results have been acceptable, with similar survivals at 1-year, 89% vs. 86% in the published reports [5, 6]. The increase achieved in the donor pool was still insufficient, so additional donors were evaluated. The pediatric groups developed the ABO group non-compatible heart transplant [7], while adult groups developed strategies for accepting HCV+ donors [8], treating recipients with the new antiviral in the immediate postoperative period, or started programs of donation after circulatory death (DCD donors) [9, 10]. It is important to remark that these different strategies to expand the donor pool have accomplished similar survival, both short (96% vs. 89% at 1-year) and medium-term (94% vs. 82% at 5 years) results, as the conventional donors [11].

As mentioned, the shortage in the donor pool leads to prolonged times on the waiting list. Some patients, however, would deteriorate during this waiting time. Different support strategies have been developed to sustain declining patients to allow for organ recovery and patient rehabilitation before the transplant. These bridging strategies can be classified into two main groups—short-term support and long-term support. Both of them have particularities that will be further developed.

2. Short-term mechanical circulatory support (ST-MCS)

Short-term support devices are the first line of support in patients who need emergent support, such as INTERMACS 1 patients, as they provide immediate hemodynamic support with an almost immediate deployment time, in some of them, such as ECMO or Impella®. In addition to those, there are other devices, such as Levitronix-Centrimag®, that need a surgical implant. It is worth mentioning that whereas ECMO provides complete circulatory support with one device, the other ones would need two pumps to provide full biventricular support.

Recently, several allocation systems changed their distribution policies aiming at providing a fair allocation of donors. These modifications meant that patients under ST-MCS achieve the highest priority on the waiting list [12].

2.1 Indications

All ST-MCS devices share common indications, the most common ones are as follows [13]:

- Postcardiotomy shock
- Primary graft failure after transplant
- Cardiogenic shock due to acute coronary syndrome
- Myocarditis
- Peripartum cardiomyopathy
- Arrhythmic storm
- Cardiac arrest.

The choice of the device would depend mostly on availability and patient factors. The different devices provide variable degrees of support and have inherent implantation requirements; there is general agreement that ECMO would be the device of choice in cases with cardiac arrest as it can be implanted percutaneously at the bedside. It would also be the preferred option in cases of respiratory compromise and biventricular failure.

Impella® support is most commonly used for cardiogenic shock secondary to myocardial infarction; the smaller (2,5 and CP) devices can be inserted percutaneously but the bigger ones (5,0 and 5,5) require insertion through a prosthesis.

Levitronix Centrimag® requires a surgical implant. It is commonly used in postcardiotomy shock, primary graft failure, or isolated right ventricular failure after a long-term ventricular assist device. It allows for the longest support; so, it is the preferable device in cases of the bridge to recovery.

2.2 General management

During the recovery period or the waiting time, it is recommended to extubate patients if possible. If this can be accomplished, oral nutrition is the preferred option. If the patient cannot be extubated, tube feedings would be the best option, above parenteral nutrition; this should be reserved for patients with significant instability and the need for high-dose pressors.

Volume status should be maintained as neutral as possible, initially with diuretics, but it is not uncommon that patients under ST-MCS develop acute kidney injury and need renal replacement therapies (RRT). In our group, we promote early use of RRT to help to manage the volume status and avoid hypervolemia at the time of the transplant.

In addition to recovering the organ, it is important to keep the muscular tone with daily physical therapy, even with static bicycle or ambulation within the unit, whenever possible.

Simultaneously to recovering the patient, special attention should be paid to the management of the device. It should provide enough support to allow for organ recovery minimizing the potential complications. To prevent them, it is recommended to perform daily echocardiograms and keep close monitoring of central venous pressure and pulmonary pressure. Blood pressure control is mandatory to reduce the risk of neurological complications but also to reduce afterload that may interfere with the device function; the higher the afterload, the lower the left ventricular unloading. We would suggest avoiding medications with a long half-life to minimize the risk of vasoplegia during the transplant.

2.3 Specialized management

2.3.1 Anticoagulation

All devices require systemic anticoagulation; unfractionated heparin is the most common anticoagulant used. A single bolus, normally 1 mg/kg, is administered at the time of ECMO or Levitronix implant. Systemic infusion is not started until the coagulation parameters have been normalized and there are no signs of bleeding. For example, in cases of central cannulation, anticoagulation would be started once the chest tube output is less than 50–80 ml/h for 6 hours.

ECMO is a device that requires a higher dose as it has an oxygenator. The patient receives a bolus of heparin at the time of the implant and after that ACT is kept around 180–200 seconds and/or aPTT around 60–80 seconds [14].

Impella systems ® require a heparinized dextrose-based purge solution and systemic heparinization with ACT around 160–160 seconds for its proper functioning. A recent publication by Beavers [15] proposes variations of the purge solution that can be modified depending on the patients' status.

Levitronix-Centrimag ® also requires systemic anticoagulation; the usual aPTT goal is 50–70 seconds. In all cases, systemic anticoagulation is maintained until the time of the transplant.

During the time on support, careful attention should be paid to the platelet count; in case, a sudden drop is noticed we would recommend to test for heparin-induced thrombocytopenia. Type 2 HITT may be a terrible complication that limits a patient's options. If suspected, heparin should be immediately replaced by bivalirudin or argatroban.

2.3.2 Infections

There is no general consensus regarding antibiotic prophylaxis while on short-term support. However, most groups administer it, especially if the implant has been performed in emergent circumstances. Regarding the duration of the therapy, the ELSO ID Taskforce [16] does not recommend using antibiotic prophylaxis for more than 48 hours. In cases of central cannulation when the chest is left open, most groups would maintain the prophylaxis while the sternum is open.

Patients on short-term support are highly instrumentalized, with increased transfusion requirements and a higher incidence of renal failure compared to the general intensive care unit population; all these factors increase the risk of systemic infections. Biffi et al. reported bacteriemia rates around 20% and lower respiratory tract infections that oscillated between 4 and 55% [17].

Due to the higher instrumentalization, the most common pathogens are coagulase-negative *staphylococci*, followed by *Candida spp* and *Pseudomonas pp*. The use of parenteral nutrition in these patients increases the risk of fungal infections.

Infections while on support can significantly impact the patients' treatment options. A recent publication by the Spanish transplant group proved that infections while of support reduced the options of reaching a heart transplant [18].

2.4 Pretransplant assessment

At the time of the transplant, specific considerations should be taken into account depending on the device the patient is being bridged with:

2.4.1 ECMO or extracorporeal membrane oxygenator

ECMO has increased its use as a bridging device, as it provides immediate support for rapidly declining patients and those unstable or in cardiogenic shock. When using ECMO as a bridging strategy, several aspects should be taken into account. From the technical perspective, there are two key points. The first one is venous cannulation; careful attention must be paid to reduce the ECMO flows at the time of venous cannulation to avoid air entry. If this occurs, the device may stop or the patient may suffer systemic emboli. Secondly, ECMO support has the risk of developing left-sided intracavitary stasis with its inherent risk of systemic emboli. Unnecessary cardiac manipulation should be avoided before applying the aortic clamp.

From the medical standpoint, the team must be aware that ECMO support may cause lung congestion, which may be not evident while on support, but that may appear when trying to abandon cardiopulmonary bypass. This pulmonary impairment may cause hypoxemia or right ventricular failure.

2.4.2 IMPELLA®

This percutaneous axial pump is normally placed through the femoral artery or the axillary artery, inside the left ventricle. When used as a bridge-to-transplant, the axillary artery insertion is preferable as it allows the patient to ambulate and facilitates the patient's rehabilitation.

At the time of the transplant, as the device crosses the aortic valve, surgeons should remove it into the aorta before applying the aortic clamp. After the implant is performed, attention should be paid to repairing the arterial entry site.

2.4.3 Levitronix-centrimag®

This magnetically levitated device provides up to 8 l/min of support and it is approved for 30 days support. It requires surgical intervention for its implant, in general, through a median sternotomy. However, some minimally invasive strategies have been proposed [19].

Its surgical implant should be performed considering the current patients' clinical status but also the future transplant. For instance, when tunneling the cannulas, it is recommended to keep the exit site far away from the sternotomy, to avoid any potential cross-contamination. In addition, surgeons should also keep in mind the future transplant; to ease that, it is our preferred approach to place the arterial cannula low in the aortic root; so, the entry site is removed at the time of the implant and we have enough ascending aorta to cannulate and perform the aortic anastomosis. If the patient has some residual ventricular function and the surgical team decides to cannulate the left atrium as an inflow cannula, our suggestion would be to cannulate the left atrial roof. This structure would be removed while doing the cardiectomy and avoid manipulation of the pulmonary veins.

At the time of the transplant, the surgical team must take into account the time needed for surgical dissection; if the patient has been supported for more than 10 days, some extra time might be necessary to isolate the different cardiac structures. In addition, some technical details should also be considered; special attention should be placed to avoid unnecessary manipulation of the cardiac structures before applying the aortic clamp. Some small clots might have formed in the cardiac chambers and there is the risk of systemic emboli in cases of aggressive manipulation.

Cannulation is also an important step, particularly at the time of the double venous cannulation in the patient under biventricular support. In these cases, special attention must be paid to ensure the right-side device flow reduction at the time of the cannula insertion to avoid air entry. Both cannulas should be placed already clamped to prevent air entry.

As mentioned, we prefer to place the outflow cannula low in the aortic root, but if the cannula is placed in the ascending aorta, the surgical team would have to decide if the left side device is interrupted and the arterial cannula reused for the cardiopulmonary bypass (CPB) machine or if a second arterial cannula is necessary.

At the end of the procedure, it is mandatory to achieve careful hemostasis to minimize postoperative bleeding; some groups propose to leave the chest open to reduce the risk of tamponade and bleeding.

2.5 Surgical considerations

Short-term mechanical support is normally implanted in patients under cardiogenic shock. This extremely acute situation, with patients that are usually under mechanical ventilation and who can barely move due to a peripheral device, makes it difficult to complete the detailed transplant evaluation that would be performed in an ambulatory situation. Despite the urgency of the situation, we would encourage to follow a so-called "parallel pathway," while recovering the patient like in **Figure 1**, an evaluation as complete as possible is performed, even more, if the patient has not been previously managed by the team. Our group has diagnosed end-stage neoplasm during these preoperative studies (**Figures 2** and **3**).

2.6 Results

Despite the systemic recovery achieved with these devices, several groups have shown their concerns regarding the outcomes of transplants with this ST-MCS bridging strategy. In 2018, the Spanish Transplant working group published a manuscript showing a 33% mortality when patients were bridged with ECMO and 11.9% when bridged with short-term left-sided devices [20]. Other reports have also shown reduced initial survival results when patients are bridged with ST-MCS [21, 22]. In previous publications, ECMO reveals as the bridging strategy with the shortest waiting times but also the worst post-transplant survival results. These

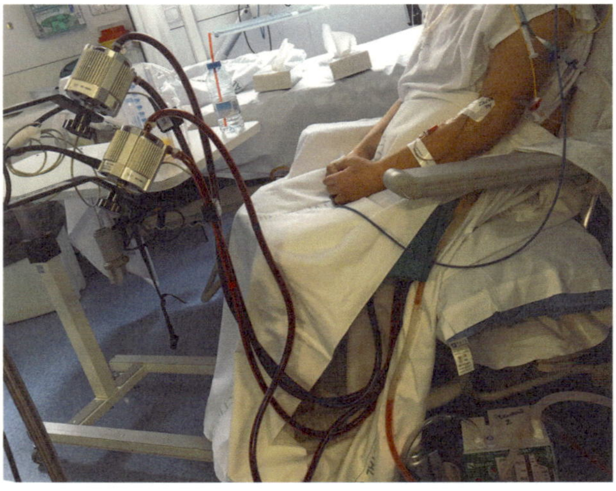

Figure 1.
Shows a patient, who is under biventricular temporary support, sitting on a chair during his/her intensive care unit stay. The patient was able to eat by himself/herself and do some physical therapy.

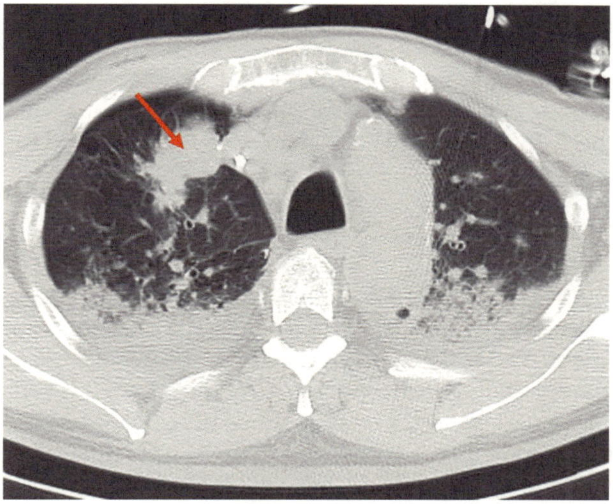

Figure 2.
Shows a lung tumor found in the pre-transplant assessment of patient support with peripheral ECMO.

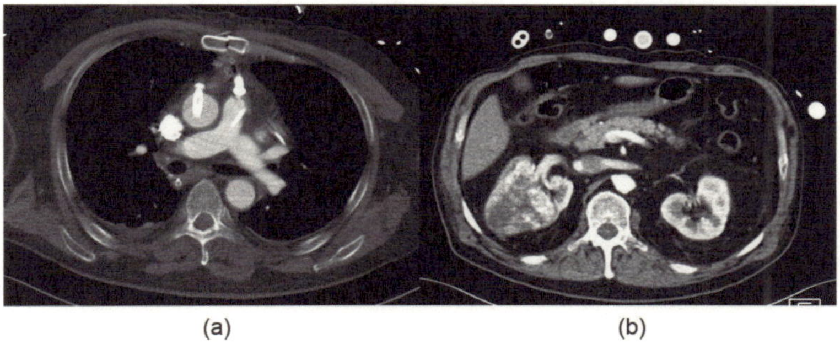

Figure 3.
(a) shows the entry site of the arterial cannulas from a biventricular Levitronix-Centrimag®. (b) displays the abdominal study of the same patient, where a right renal tumor can be observed.

worst results may be due to an early transplant with incomplete recovery of the organs in addition to pulmonary impairment due to insufficient left ventricular unloading.

In addition to this increased early mortality, different publications show a higher rate of postoperative transfusions and longer hospital length of stay compared to direct heart transplant or even, transplant with long-term devices [23].

3. Long-term mechanical circulatory support (LT-MCS)

As stated before, the increase in waiting list times may cause the clinical deterioration of patients awaiting a suitable organ. Long-term mechanical circulatory support offers these patients clinical stability and avoidance of multiorgan deterioration during this waiting time. Several devices have been developed, such as the Heartmate XVE®, the Heartmate II®, Heartware-HVAD®, Jarvik®, Syncardia®, and the HeartMate 3®. The last one is the most commonly used nowadays.

Most of them provide only univentricular support, mostly to the left ventricle. In cases where biventricular support is needed, a second device can be used "of-label' to provide right ventricular support. Syncardia® and Carmart® are also known as "total artificial hearts" providing biventricular support with a single device. The major drawback of all these devices is the need for an additional surgical intervention before the heart transplant.

3.1 Indications

The primary indication of LT-MCS devices is end-stage chronic heart failure. Most left ventricular assist devices require a minimal end-diastolic left ventricular diameter for their implant, which is easily accomplished in cases of ischemic or dilated cardiomyopathy. In cases of restrictive cardiomyopathy, with small left ventricular cavities or cases with biventricular failure, a total artificial heart would be indicated.

The hemodynamic indications according to ISHLT guidelines [13, 24] are as follows:

- Stage D refractory heart failure
- Systemic hypotension with systolic blood pressure below 90 mm Hg
- Cardiac index below 1,8 l/min/m2
- Pulmonary capillary wedge pressure above 15 mm Hg
- Evidence of end-organ perfusion
- Peak oxygen consumption <12–14 ml/kg2.

3.2 Specialized management

3.2.1 Anticoagulation

LT-MCS requires antithrombotic treatment since the early postoperative period to prevent thrombotic events [25, 26]. Each manufacturer has its own specific recommendations; however, in general, most centers follow the below strategy:

- Low-dose heparin in the first 12–24 hours if there are no signs of bleeding (chest tube output below 50 ml/h during >4 hours).
- Heparin infusion is gradually titrated to achieve full anticoagulation after 48 hours.
- Aspirin is started on the second postoperative day.
- Vitamin K antagonists are started on the third postoperative day once the patient is stable and tolerates oral intake.

The target INR is 2.0–3.0. The antithrombotic treatment should be tailored to the patient's clinical status.

In cases of heparin-induced thrombocytopenia, intravenous direct thrombin inhibitors, such as bivalirudin or argatroban, can be used. New oral anticoagulants have not been validated for the treatment of long-term MCS devices.

3.2.2 Infection

Infections will occur in nearly 60% of the implanted patients and the rate increases with the duration of support [27, 28]. The most common pathogens are gram-positive bacteria that colonize the skin and adhere to the implanted material creating biofilms; *staphylococci spp* account for more than 50% of infections followed by *enterococci spp.* Between the gram-negative rods, *Pseudomonas spp* is the most frequent, being responsible for 22–28% of infections [28].

Before a scheduled implant, it is recommended to remove all unnecessary lines and ensure there are no active infections. In cases of active infection, in special if bacteriemia, it is recommended to delay the implant until clearance of the infection, whenever possible.

A few years ago, antibiotic prophylaxis included gram-positive cocci, gram-negative rods, and fungi and it was maintained for days. The most current recommendations moved to the general cardiac surgery prophylaxis, using a cephalosporin that is maintained for 24–48 hours. In addition, MRSA should be discarded with a preoperative nasal swab and nasal mupirocine is applied [25].

Once the device has been implanted if an infection develops, it can be classified as [26, 27]:

- Device-specific infections
- Device-related infections (result of the surgery, for example, bloodstream infection).
- Non-device-related infections (pneumonia, urinary tract infections, etc.).

Device-specific infections are the ones that actually involve the device and they vary from driveline infection to pump infection with mediastinitis. The most important aspect is prevention. For example, during the surgical implant, it is recommended to keep all the velour parts of the driveline covered and ensure proper fixation of the driveline to avoid excessive movements.

It is of extreme importance that both the patient and the caregiver learn how to perform the sterile dressing changes of the driveline; patients also need to recognize signs of alarm, such as erythema or purulent discharge. Keeping a photographic diary might be helpful. It is also important that the wound is periodically evaluated during the clinic visits.

Driveline infections should be individually addressed; if the patient has no general symptoms, treatment can start with increased dressing changes and culture-directed antibiotics. On the other hand, in case of systemic symptoms, intravenous antibiotics should be started. In these cases, a PET-CT scan might be performed to assess the extension of the infection. If image tests reveal the presence of collections, re-routing of the driveline might be necessary. If the infection has affected the actual device, pump exchange or transplant might be the only curative option and it is recommended that blood cultures are negative at the time of the surgery.

When transplanting a patient with an infected device, the surgical must minimize deeper contaminations; for example, in cases of driveline infection, the exit site must be sealed from the rest of the surgical fields avoiding contact between infected and non-infected fields. In cases of device-specific infections involving blood contact surfaces, surgeons should minimize the embolic risk by early initiation of cardiopulmonary bypass, stoppage of the pump, and application of the aortic clamp. If active mediastinal infection is found, extensive debridement and antibiotic irrigation are recommended. After that, all surgical materials should be changed. In these circumstances, some groups would leave the chest open with antibiotic irrigation. After the surgery, antibiotic treatment should be targeted to prior cultures.

It may seem controversial to transplant patients with a current infection. However, several reports have shown no differences in survival compared with patients transplanted on LT-MCS support without infection [29].

3.2.3 Blood pressure control

Blood pressure control is mandatory while on long-term support. Hypertension leads to increase afterload, thus reducing the device flows and the left ventricular unloading. In addition, there is a significant relationship between high blood pressure and adverse events, such as stroke or aortic regurgitation [30, 31].

As the devices are continuous flow, it is possible that patients have no pulse; in an intensive care unit, it is recommended to use invasive lines to monitor the blood pressure; whereas if the patient is ambulatory, a doppler measurement of the blood pressure is the preferred system [25]. The doppler reading is equivalent to the mean blood pressure.

For blood pressure control, the current recommendations include the use of renin-angiotensin-aldosterone system antagonists as first-line; beta-blockers are recommended in cases of arrhythmias but should be carefully used if the right ventricular function is poor. Calcium channel blockers would be the third option for blood pressure control [24, 25].

3.3 Surgical implant

When a bridge-to-transplant strategy is considered in a patient who is going to receive an LT-MCS device, the surgical implant must be carefully planned to ease the future heart transplant.

The device could be divided into different components, the inlet cannula and the pump, the outflow graft, and the driveline.

The inlet cannula is placed inside the left ventricle and secured with a sewing ring. Some groups reinforce this ring with surgical glues, which may lead to increased adhesions.

Careful attention should be paid to the length and layout of the outflow graft, in special at the time of the chest closure. It should run smoothly along with the right-side cavities. A short graft would lay immediately under the sternum (**Figure 4A**), increasing the risk of damaging it during the reesternotomy. An excessively long graft is at risk of twisting, impairing the pump function. Its anastomotic site in the ascending aorta should be performed, taking into account that it should be removed at the time of the transplant and that enough ascending aorta should be left to perform the anastomosis.

The driveline should also be carefully placed. Our group does a double route; we exteriorize the driveline into the subcutaneous tissue at the left upper quadrant and

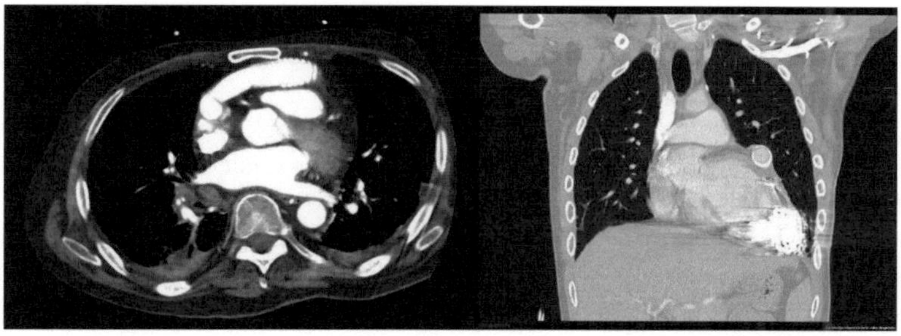

Figure 4.
A shows an outflow tract running immediately below the sternum. In this case, the implant was performed minimally invasive, so the risk of injury at the time of the transplant was lower. B shows non-conventional outflow tract layouts; this patient had the outflow anastomosis placed at the descending aorta. This risk of injury was lower at the reesternotomy but achieving control of it might be more difficult.

then tunnel it to the right upper quadrant, leaving a short intrapericardial portion away from the sternum, to avoid damaging it during the mediastinal reentry at the transplant time.

Reinterventions in patients with long-term devices are challenging due to extensive adhesion formation [32]. Several strategies have been developed to facilitate these reinterventions. The most extended one is covering the device and the outflow tract with PTFE sheets that would reduce the adhesions and, at the same time, might protect the pump components during the dissection [33, 34]. A different approach would be pursuing a less-invasive approach, either with two thoracotomies or a left thoracotomy and a mini-sternotomy. In these less invasive approaches, the avoidance of an extended pericardial opening and limited cardiac manipulation reduces the development of adhesions [35].

3.4 Transplant surgery

Despite the careful surgical implant, we would suggest that every patient with an LT-MCS who is a transplant candidate should have a postimplant computed tomography to know the final position of the different device components (**Figure 4A** and **B**).

At the time of the implant, the surgical team must carefully plan the times as surgical dissection may be more difficult and time-consuming than conventional reinterventions. Once we accept the organ, it is our preferred approach to reverse anticoagulation with prothrombin complex to avoid volume overload and start the anesthetic process. Our advice would be to start the reintervention enough in advance to be able to perform an extremely careful dissection in order to minimize intraoperative and postoperative bleeding.

We suggest that both the abdomen and the groins should be prepped; the abdomen should be accessible to remove the driveline and femoral vessel cannulation may be necessary in some cases.

Once the reesternotomy is performed, the main goal is achieving control of the aorta and, both cava veins and the outflow graft, so, cardiopulmonary bypass (CPB) can be started. Most groups suggest completing the device dissection while on CPB support. It is important to stop the LT-MCS device and occlude its outflow graft when starting the CPB machine to avoid backward flow. In cases of different outflow graft implant sites, for example, in the descending aorta, control of it should also be achieved before starting the CPB machine. Once CPB is supported, the pump removal can be performed. The cardiectomy is completed in the usual way, making sure the outflow anastomotic site is removed.

After completion of the implant, it is mandatory to achieve proper hemostasis to minimize the need for blood products and reduce the risk of postoperative tamponade.

Following protamine administration, the driveline should be removed. In cases of driveline infection, as previously mentioned, the driveline exit site would be kept in a different surgical field to minimize the contamination of the mediastinum; thus, the internal part of the driveline would be removed from the inside and the infected part would be pulled once the chest is closed. As all foreign material should be removed, two incisions may be necessary to remove the totality of the driveline; we suggest doing extensive debridement of the exit site in cases of infection and ensure proper closing of the wounds to reduce the risk of collection development, even with the use of vacuum-assisted therapy.

3.5 Results

With the development of LT-MCS, several transplant programs report their concern regarding the impact of this bridging strategy on the transplant outcomes [36, 37]. However, long-term devices have proved themselves as successful bridge-to-transplant devices. Despite being a challenging surgery, survival results are comparable to direct transplant strategies in recent publications [23, 38, 39]and recent publications only showed a higher post-transplant transfusion need in the bridged group [23, 36].

Recent ISHLT data from its transplant registry show 90% 1-year survival in either direct transplant or bridge with left ventricular assist device; these same data showed decreased initial survival if patients were bridged with either biventricular support or total artificial heart, probably due to a worse preoperative status [40].

In addition to survival, the other main concern with this bridging strategy is post-transplant vasoplegia. Contradictory results have been published in this regard [41, 42].

3.6 Bridge-to-bridge

As previously developed, recent changes in the allocations systems give the highest priority to the sickest patients. However, this might lead to transplant patients who have had not enough time to recover organ function or who could have not been fully evaluated worsening transplant results. A way of avoiding this phenomenon would be the bridge-to-bridge strategy, which means that a patient under ST-MCS would be transitioned to a long-term device and transplanted once fully recovered and rehabilitated.

Before the surgery, a careful assessment of right ventricular function and associated valvular lesions, such as significant aortic regurgitation or tricuspid regurgitation, must be performed. The presence of intracavitary thrombi should also be evaluated. The presence of any of these lesions in addition to the initial device would impact the surgical technique and the approach. For example, if the patient is under ECMO support, the long-term device implant could be performed under the same support. In these cases, if concomitant lesions have been discarded, it is even possible to perform a minimally invasive device insertion. However, teams must keep in mind that right ventricular function is difficult to evaluate while on ECMO support. Thus, in addition to potential pulmonary congestion leads to a significantly higher incidence of postoperative right ventricular failure [43].

When the initial device is an Impella®, due to its peripheral implant, it is possible to perform the insertion both through a minimally invasive approach or through a median sternotomy. If the surgical team prefers to follow the minimally invasive approach without CPB support, we would suggest to have the femoral vessels prepared for cannulation in case the patient collapses at the time of stopping the Impella® device.

Once the implant of the new device has been finished, it is important not to forget to repair the cannulation site, ensuring the proper distal flow of the extremity to minimize vascular complications, which may have a high impact on survival.

If the patient is bridged from a Levitronix Centrimag®, the most probable approach would be through a median sternotomy; in these cases, we would suggest to transition the temporary support to cardiopulmonary bypass and then perform the implant. This strategy will allow to lift the heart without instability and to inspect the left ventricular chambers to remove any potential debris.

Despite ST-MCS allowing for rapid recovery, these patients can still be considered the sickest ones. As mentioned, the incidence of post-device right ventricular failure may reach up to 20%, higher than in the non-bridged population [43]. In addition, 1-year survival after the implant is also worse compared to the general LVAD population (1-year survival 70% vs. 91%) [39]. Despite these initial poorer results, when these patients recover and are transplanted, results are as successful as transplant after primary LVAD insertion, with 1-year survival around 90% [39].

4. Discussion

Heart transplant remains the gold-standard treatment for end-stage heart failure since the first case was performed in 1967. Once the initial issues with rejection were solved after the introduction of cyclosporine, results significantly improved and several transplant programs developed.

Simultaneously, several therapeutic advances led to significant improvement of pathologies previously lethal. This new chronicity of several cardiomyopathies in addition to an aging population made heart failure one of the most prevalent diseases, thus increasing the number of heart transplant candidates. On the other hand, the number of potential donors for a heart transplant was actually maintained or even diminished; this situation caused a clear disbalance and the shortage of donors became a reality.

Mechanical circulatory support was initially developed for patients who could not be weaned from CPB, such as the first implant performed by Dr. DeBakey and it became a field in continuous development. However, it was not until the early 2000s when the REMATCH trial [44] showed better survival with LT-MCS than with conventional treatment for end-stage heart failure patients. These results led to a tremendous expansion of the therapy with different devices being developed. Since the first generation XVE to the current HeartMate 3, devices have become smaller and more hemocompatible, significantly improving the results, both of survival and adverse effects. With the huge advances in the field, in addition to the shortage of donors, the heart failure community realized that LT-MCS, despite requiring additional surgery and the inherent technical complexities at the time of the transplant, was the best option to allow patients to reach the transplant in the best clinical situation possible; until the last allocation system modification, nearly 50% of the recipients in the USA had a previous long-term device.

In addition to the chronic heart failure population, as physicians, we face a significant proportion of patients with acute heart failure. In these circumstances, short-term MCS would be the preferred option. Short-term devices allow for rapid patient stabilization and organ recovery. In some cases, patients' myocardial function would recover and the device would be explanted, while in other cases, patients would need further therapies, such as heart transplants. This situation might be tricky as the transplant evaluation has to be performed under support, which might limit its depth, and the treating physicians should find the appropriate moment to list the patient finding a weak balance between patient recovery and avoidance of complications. As ST-MCS patients can be considered the sickest ones, the different allocations systems give these patients the highest priority on the transplant list, so they can have more opportunities of being transplanted. However, this strategy also increases the risk of transplanting patients not fully recovered or fully evaluated, which has proved to worsen transplant results [45], especially if ECMO is the bridging device.

The initial impairment of survival using the ST-MCS bridging strategy let to consider alternative strategies; the most used one, whenever possible, would be the bridge-to-bridge, which means transitioning a patient from short-term to a long-term device to allow for complete recovery. In these cases, patients undergo an additional surgical procedure, such as the LT-MCS implant, but they can be fully evaluated and be listed when they are completely recovered. Groups that follow this strategy have already published results comparable to the patients bridged directly with an LT-MCS device.

Aside from the device used, their common goal is to ensure the patient reaches the transplant in the best possible clinical condition. To ensure it, it is fundamental that patients' physical status is improved with adequate nutrition and adapted physical therapy, which should be started as soon as possible, to avoid muscle mass loss. In addition to recovery, the avoidance of adverse effects is of extreme importance; accurate blood pressure control would help to reduce the incidence of neurologic events and also the development of aortic regurgitation. It would also reduce afterload, which would improve the left ventricular unloading and signs of congestion. Prevention of infections is another striking aspect; it starts in the same operating theater with the implant of the driveline and it continues during the whole time on support, with accurate dressing changes and accurate follow-up [25, 26]. In the cases of ST-MCS, the same rules apply; in these cases, removal of unnecessary lines and careful assessment of the cannulas exit site might help in the reduction of infections.

Once at the time of the transplant, the surgical team should be aware of the different particularities of each device and plan the procedure accordingly. Dissection of long-term devices might need additional time compared to other cardiac reinterventions or ST-MCS devices may need an earlier aortic clamp than other cases. As important as surgical timing is planning additional procedures that might be required, such as vascular repair, wound debridement, or removal of an infected driveline. In this last case, special care should be taken to avoid mediastinal contamination.

Post-transplant care has no differences compared to non-bridged patients; immunosuppression regimens and rejection surveillance are kept the same; the only specific situation would be the extension of antibiotic treatment in cases of device infection and it should be individually discussed with the ID team.

Despite the initial concerns regarding transplant outcomes after the use of a mechanical device, results have proved to be excellent, with survival rates similar to the non-bridged population in the case of LT-MCS. ST-MCS might not seem a good strategy due to worse initial results. However, physicians should take into consideration that we are facing the sickest patients and that these temporary devices may be the only option available for these acute patients [39].

5. Conclusions

Mechanical circulatory support as a bridge-to-transplant strategy allows for patient recovery, increased functional capacity, and a reduction in wait-list mortality.

Despite the surgical challenges the different support strategies associate, post-transplant survival results have proved them a good strategy to safely bridge patients to heart transplant.

Conflict of interest

None of the authors has any conflict of interest regarding this manuscript.

Author details

Elena Sandoval* and Daniel Pereda
Cardiovascular Surgery Department, Hospital Clínic, Barcelona, Spain

*Address all correspondence to: esandova@clinic.cat

References

[1] Barnard CN. Human heart transplantation. Canadian Medical Association Journal. 1969;**100**:91-104

[2] Baumgartner WA, Reitz BA, Bieber CP, Oyer PE, Shumway NE, Stinson EB. Current expectations in cardiac transplantation. The Thoracic and Cardiovascular Surgeon. 1978;**75**:525-530

[3] Oyer PE, Stinson EB, Jamieson SW, et al. Cyclosporine a in cardiac allografting: A preliminary experience. Transplantation Proceedings. 1983;**15**: 1247-1252

[4] Khush KK, Cherikh WS, Chambers DC, Goldfarb S, Hayes D, Kucheryavava AY, et al. The international thoracic organ transplant registry of the International Society for Heart and Lung Transplantation: Thirty-fifth adult heart transplantation report- 2018; focus theme: Multiorgan transplantation. The Journal of Heart and Lung Transplantation. 2018;**37**(10):1155-1206

[5] Samsky MD, Patel CB, Owen A, Schulte PJ, Jentzer J, Rosember PB, et al. Ten-year experience with extended criteria cardiac transplantation. Circulation. Heart Failure. 2013;**6**(6): 1230-1238. DOI: 10.1161/ CIRCHEARTFAILURE.113.000296

[6] Schüler S, Parnt R, Warnecke H, Matheis G, Hetzer R. Extended donor criteria for heart transplantation. The Journal of Heart Transplantation. 1988;7(5):326-330

[7] Gil-Jaurena JM, Perez-Caballero R, Murgoitio U, Pardo C, Pita A, Camino M, et al. A neonatal ABO non-compatible heart transplant from a circulatory-determined death donor using NRP/ cold storage. Pediatric Transplantation. 2021;**Oct 18**:e14169. DOI: 10.1111/ petr.14169

[8] Woolley AE, Singh SK, Goldberg HJ, Mallidi HR, Givertz MM, Mehra MR, et al. Heart and lung transplants from HCV-infected donors to uninfected recipients. The New England Journal of Medicine. 2019;**380**(17):1606-1617

[9] Dhital KK, Chew HC, Macdonald PS. Donation after circulatory death heart transplantation. Current Opinion in Organ Transplantation. 2017;**22**:189-197

[10] Messer S, Page A, Colah S, et al. Human heart transplantation from donation after circulatory-determined death donors using normothermic regional perfusion and cold storage. The Journal of Heart and Lung Transplantation. 2018;**37**:865-869

[11] Dhital K, Ludhani P, Scheuer S, Connellan M, Macdonald P. DCD donations and outcomes of heart transplantation; the Australian experience. Indian. The Journal of Thoracic and Cardiovascular Surgery. 2020;**36** (Suppl. 2):224-232. DOI: 10.1007/ s12055-020-00998

[12] UNOS/OPTN. Adult Heart Allocation Changes. https://optn.transplant.hrsa.gov/learn/professional-education/adult-heart-allocation/

[13] McDonagh TA, Metra M, Adamo M, Gardner RS, Baumbach A, Böhm M, et al. 2021 ESC guidelines for the diagnosis and treatment of acute and chronic heart failure. European Heart Journal. 2021;**42**:3599-3726. DOI: 10.1093/ eurheartj/ehab368

[14] ELSO anticoagulation guidelines. 2015. www.elso.org

[15] Beavers CJ, DiDomenico RJ, Dunn SP, Cox J, To L, Weeks P, et al. Optimizing anticoagulation for patients receiving Impella support. Pharmacotherapy. 2021;**41**(11):932-942. DOI: 10.1002/pharm.2629

[16] ELSO ID Taskforce recommendation summary. www.elso.org

[17] Biffi S, DiBella S, Scaravilli V, Peri AM, Graselli G, Alagna L, et al. Infections during extracorporeal membrane oxygenation: Epidemiology, risk factors, pathogenesis and prevention. International Journal of Antimicrobial Agents. 2017;**50**:9-16. DOI: Doi.org/10.1016/j.antimicag.2017.02.025

[18] Solla-Buceta M, González-Vílchez F, Almenar-Bonet L, Lambert-Rodríguez JL, Segovia-Cubero J, González-Costello J, et al. Infectious complications associated with short-term mechanical circulatory suport in urgent heart transplantation candidates. Revista Española de Cardiología (English Edition). 2021;**26**:S1885-S5857. DOI: 10.1016/jrec.2020.11019

[19] Sandoval E, Fernández-Cisneros A, Pereda D. Asian Cardiovascular & Thoracic Annals. 2020;**28**(9):604-606. DOI: 10.1177/0218492320951014

[20] Barge-Caballero E, Almenar-Bonet L, González-VílchezF,Lambert-RodríguezJL, González-Costello J, Segovia-Cubero J, et al. Clinical outcomes of temporary mechanical circulatory support as a direct bridge to heart transplantation: A nationwide Spanish registry. European Journal of Heart Failure. 2018;**20**:178-186

[21] Yin MY, Wever-Pinzon O, Mhera MR, Selzman CH, Toll AE, Cherikh WS, et al. Post-transplant outcome in patients bridged to transplant with temporary mechanical circulatory support devices. The Journal of Heart and Lung Transplantation. 2019;**38**(8):858-869. DOI: 10.1016/j.healun.2019.04.003

[22] Moonsamy P, Axtell AL, Ibrahim NE, Funamoto M, Tolis G, Lewis GD, et al. Survival after heart transplantation in patients bridged with mechanical circulatory support. JACC. 2020;**75**(23):2892-2905. DOI: 10.1016/j.jacc.2020.04.037

[23] Finnan MJ, Bakir NH, Itoh A, Kotkar KD, Pasque MK, Damiano RJ, et al. 30 years of heart transplant: Outcomes after mechanical circulatory support from a single center. The Annals of Thoracic Surgery. 2021;**113**(1):41-48. DOI: 10.1016/j.athoracsur.2021.01.064

[24] Pagani F, Schueler S, Uriel N, Maltais S. ISHLT Monograph Series: Mechanical Circulatory Support Series. Vol. 14. Birmingham, Alabama: UAB; 2020

[25] Potapov E, Antonides C, Crespo-Leiro MG, Combes A, Färber G, Hannan MM, et al. 2019 EACTS expert consensus on long-term mechanical circulatory support. European Journal of Cardio-Thoracic Surgery. 2019;**56**(2):230-270. DOI: 10.1093/ejcts/ezz098

[26] Kirklin JK, Pagani FD, Goldstein DJ, John R, Rogers JG, Atturi P, et al. American Association for Thoracic Surgery/International Society for Heart and Lung Transplantation guidelines on selected topics in mechanical circulatory support. The Journal of Heart and Lung Transplantation. 2020;**39**(3):187-219. DOI: 10.1016/j.healun.2020.01.1329

[27] Hannan MM, Husain S, Mattner F, Danziger-Isakov L, Drew RJ, Corey GR, et al. Working formulation for the standardization of definitions of infections in patients using ventricular

assist devices. The Journal of Heart and Lung Transplantation. 2011;**30**(4):375-384. DOI: 10.1016/j.healu.2011.01.717

[28] Hannan MM, Xie R, Cowger J, Schueler S, de By T, Dipchand AI, et al. Epidemiology of infection in. Mechanical circulatory support: A global analysis from the ISHLT mechanically assisted circulatory support registry. The Journal of Heart and Lung Transplantation. 2019;**38**:364-373. DOI: doi.org/10.1016/j.healun.2019.01.007

[29] Jiritano F, Serraino GF, Rossi M. Ventricular assist device driveline infection: Treatment with platelet-rich plasma. The Annals of Thoracic Surgery. 2013;**96**:e37-e38. DOI: 10.1016/j.athoracsur.2013.01.093

[30] Tchoukina I, Smallfield MC, Shah KB. Device management and flow optimization on left ventricular assist device support. Critical Care Clinics. 2018;**34**(3):453-463. DOI: 10.1016/j.ccc.2018.03.002

[31] Saeed O, Jermyn R, Kargoli F, Madan S, Mannem S, Gunda S, et al. Blood pressure and adverse events during continuous flow left ventricular assist device support. Circulation. Heart Failure. 2015;**8**(3):551-556. DOI: 10.1116/CIRCHEARTFAILURE.114.002000

[32] Kocher A, Coti I, Laufer G, et al. Minimally invasive aortic valve replacement through an upper hemisternotomy: The Vienna technique. European Journal of Cardio-Thoracic Surgery. 2018;**53**(suppl. 2):ii29-ii31

[33] Leprince P, Rahmati M, Bonnet N, et al. Expanded polytetrafluoroethylene membranes to wrap surfaces of circulatory support devices in patients undergoing bridge to heart transplantation. European Journal of Cardio-Thoracic Surgery. 2001;**19**:302-306

[34] Vitali E, Russo C, Tiziano C, Lanfranconi M, Bruschi G. Modified pericardial closure technique in patients with ventricular assist device. The Annals of Thoracic Surgery. 2000;**69**:1278-1279

[35] Schmitto JD, Krabtasch T, Damme L, Netuka I. Less invasive HeartMate 3 left ventricular assist device implantation. Journal of Thoracic Disease. 2018;**10** (Suppl. 15):S1692-S1695. DOI: 10.21037/jtd.2018.01.26

[36] Russo MJ, Hong KN, Davies RR, et al. Posttransplant survival is not diminished in heart transplant recipients bridged with implantable left ventricular assist devices. The Journal of Thoracic and Cardiovascular Surgery. 2009;**138**:1425-1432

[37] Fukuhara S, Takeda K, Polanco AR, Takayama H, Naka Y. Prolonged continuous-flow left ventricular assist device suport and posttransplantation outcomes: A new challenge. The Journal of Thoracic and Cardiovascular Surgery. 2016;**151, 3**:872-880.e5. DOI: 10.1016/j.jtcvs.2015.10.024. Epub 2015 Oct 22

[38] Maltais S, Jaik NP, Feurer ID, Wigger MA, DiSalvo TG, Schlendorf KH, et al. Mechanical circulatory support and heart transplantation: Donor and recipient factors influencing graft survival. The Annals of Thoracic Surgery. 2013;**96**:1252-1258

[39] Yoshioka D, Li B, Takayama H, Garabn RA, Yopkata VK, Han J, et al. Outcomes of heart transplantation after bridge to-transplant strategy using various mechanical circulatory support devices. Interactive Cardiovascular and Thoracic Surgery. 2017;**25**:918-924. DOI: 10.1093/icvts/ivx201

[40] Khush KK, Hsich E, Potena L, Cherikh WS, Chambers DC, Harhay MO, et al. International Society for Heart and Lung Transplantation: Thirty-eight adult heart transplantation report-2021; focus on recipient characteristics. The Journal of Heart and Lung Transplantation. 2021;**40**(10):1023-1072. DOI: 10.1016/j.healun.2021.07.022

[41] Chan JL, Kobashigawa JA, Aintablian TL, Dimbil SJ, Perry PA, Patel JK, et al. Characterizing predictors and severity of vasoplegia syndrome after heart transplantation. The Annals of Thoracic Surgery. 2018;**105**(3):770-777. DOI: 10.1016/j.athoracsur.2017.09.039. Epub 2017 Dec 28

[42] Clerkin KJ, Mancini DM, Stehlik J, Cherikh WS, Hund LH. Continuous-flow mechanical circulatory support is not associated with early graft failure: An analysis of the International Society for Heart&lung transplantation registry. Clinical Transplantation. 2019;**33**(12):e13752. DOI: 10.1111/ctr.13752

[43] Shah P, Pagani FD, Desai SS, Rongione AJ, Maltais S, Haglund NA, et al. Outcomes of patients receiving temporary circulatory support before durable ventricular assist device. The Annals of Thoracic Surgery. 2017;**103**(1):106-112. DOI: 10.1016/j.athoracsurg.2016.06.002

[44] Rose EA, Gelijns AC, Moskowitz AJ, Heitjan DF, Stevenson LW, Dembitsky W, et al. Randomized evaluation of mechanical assistance for the treatment of congestive heart failure (REMATCH) study group. The New England Journal of Medicine. 2001;**345**(20):1435-1443. DOI: 10.1056/NEJMoa.012175

[45] Cogswell R, John R, Estep JD, Duval S, Tedford RJ, Pagani FD, et al. An early investigation of outcomes with the new 2018 donor heart allocation system in the United States. The Journal of Heart and Lung Transplantation. 2020;**39**(1):1-4. DOI: doi.10.1016/j.healun.2019.11.002

Chapter 6

The Role of Large Impella Devices in Temporary Mechanical Circulatory Support for Patients Undergoing Heart Transplantation

Yukiharu Sugimura, Sebastian Bauer, Moritz Benjamin Immohr, Arash Mehdiani, Hug Aubin, Ralf Westenfeld, Udo Boeken, Artur Lichtenberg and Payam Akhyari

Abstract

Large microaxial pump systems (Impella 5.0, or Impella 5.5; i.e., Impella 5+) (Abiomed Inc., Danvers, MA, USA) have gained increasing levels of attendance as valuable tools of mechanical circulatory support (MCS). Patients undergoing heart transplantation (HTX) often need temporary MCS in the perioperative course, either as a preoperative bridge or occasionally in the early post-transplant period. Here we present our experience using Impella 5+ support for patients designated to undergo HTX, describe technical aspects of implantation and removal, and further analyze factors influencing the overall patient outcome. Significant factors are discussed in front of the background of contemporary international literature, and current scientific questions are highlighted.

Keywords: cardiogenic shock, heart failure, Impella, heart transplantation, bridge to transplant, temporary mechanical circulatory support

1. Introduction

Impella (Abiomed Inc., Danvers, MA, USA) is a microaxial pump catheter inserted retrogradely into the left ventricle (LV) via the aortic valve to support antegrade blood flow from LV to the ascending aorta by the lifting force of rotation. Due to less invasive closed-chest application and convenient profile, Impella 5+ has attracted an increasing level of attention and widespread use to stabilize CS patients and to provide temporary mechanical circulatory support (MCS) combined with LV unloading.

Patients undergoing heart transplantation (HTX) often need large Impella 5+ as part of temporary mechanical circulatory support (tMCS) in the perioperative course, either as a preoperative bridge or occasionally in the early post-transplant period. However, despite some observational studies the evidence supporting this is yet limited, particularly in the specific cohort of patients awaiting HTX [1].

Therefore, we summarize the reported articles that focused on large Impella for a bridge to transplantation (BTT). Further, we present our experience using Impella 5+ support for patients undergoing HTX and further analyze factors influencing the overall patient outcome.

2. ECMELLA strategy for a bridge to candidacy

Impella 5+ plays a significant role as part of tMCS in patients considered eligible for a bridge to candidacy. In crash and burn patients suffering from acute cardiogenic shock or refractory decompensated heart failure, physicians are faced with four clinical therapy choices: (1) conservative therapy with adequate inotrope support, (2) tMCS using va-ECMO implantation, (3) tMCS by Impella implantation, and (4) the combination of the latter two represented by so-called ECMELLA concept.

Traditionally, va-ECMO is preferred as the first choice of tMCS for acute or sustained CS, e.g., in the setting of cardiopulmonary resuscitation (CPR), because of its convenience, rapid initiation effect, and stable mode of action. Moreover, patients can be not only supported hemodynamically but also regarding the respiratory situation. However, va-ECMO does not unload the left ventricle (LV), and by increasing the afterload, it may lead to LV congestion, pulmonary edema, and secondary right ventricular (RV) failure. To compensate for these limitations of va-ECMO, a large microaxial pump catheter, i.e., Impella 5+, maybe additionally administrated to obtain the concept of "ECMELLA" support. Herein, Impella enables to provide antegrade flow and unload LV to reduce myocardial oxygen consumption and increase coronary perfusion, which leads to improving pulmonary congestion [2]. Simultaneous use of Impella with va-ECMO contributes to a shift of LV pressure-volume loops to the left, which is particularly effective when a larger microaxial pump is used. This is supported by a simulation study, in which a 23% decrease in end-diastolic LV volume and a 41% decrease in pulmonary capillary wedge pressure has been demonstrated [3].

Regarding the superiority of clinical outcomes of ECMELLA over va-ECMO, a recent meta-analysis sheds new light on patient outcomes [4]. A total of 425 patients (only va-ECMO (n = 312 (73.4%)) and ECMELLA (n = 113 (26.6%)) arising from five retrospective observational comparative studies were selected for this analysis [5–9]. Although most of ECMELLA cohorts received "small" Impella, i.e., (Impella CP or Impella 2.5; n = 95 (84.1%), Impella 5.0; n = 18 (15.9%)), study results prompted the authors to suggest that ECMELLA strategy might contribute to lower mortality with a reasonable potential to improve the hemodynamic status and promote bridge to recovery or to the next therapy, i.e., pMCS or HTX. Further observational/meta-analysis studies support this hypothesis [10–12]. Further, the multicenter cohort study "STOP-SHOCK" shows a 21% reduction in 30-day mortality in propensity-score matched patients with LV unloading by Impella (thereof n = 14 with Impella 5.0; (5.5%)) despite a higher rate of bleeding or ischemic complications *versus* controls with ECMO alone (n = 255 per each group) [13]. At present, although no randomized, controlled trial exists, we can conclude that a growing body of evidence may favor the effectiveness of ECMELLA strategy on clinical outcomes. As far as timing of Impella implantation under va-ECMO is concerned, "STOP-SHOCK" has indicated that early LV unloading, i.e., before or within 2 hours after va-ECMO initiation, was associated with lower 30-day mortality (hazard ratio 0.76, P = 0.03). In contrast, delayed LV unloading, i.e., >2 hours post va-ECMO, revealed no significant effect of LV venting on 30-day mortality according to subanalysis. In another prospective observational study termed

"HACURE" from Hannover in Germany, the efficacy and safety of early MCS escalation therapy, i.e., ECMELLA has been evaluated. Although the authors did not specify the exact time window between the first MCS device and the implementation of the second MCS device, the study showed a reasonable survival rate (survival on MCS 61%, at 30 days 49%, 6 months 40%) and acceptable safety (hemolysis in 55%, major TIMI bleeding in 1%, limb ischemia in 9%) [14]. In summary, ECMELLA strategy involving an early initiation of LV unloading with large Impella under va-ECMO is a promising approach for better clinical outcomes, and this strategy may contribute to improved progression to the next therapy step beyond "bridge to candidacy", i.e., "bridge to pMCS" or "bridge to transplant."

3. Role for a bridge to pMCS/HTX strategy

In fact, how many Impella 5+ patients could be successfully bridged to pMCS/HTX? A comprehensive search of the database "Pubmed" up to September 20, 2021 in English has been conducted. Studies that focused on clinical outcomes inclusive transition to pMCS/HTX in consecutive series of adult patients (>18 years) with CS utilizing a large Impella system, i.e., Impella 5+, were included. Case reports were excluded. In the interest of comparable results, studies that did not mention the size of applied Impella were also excluded. Some studies contained patients with various sizes of Impella or with other LV unloading systems. These were also excluded because of a small cohort of large Impella systems and mixed effects. Finally, a total of 6 observational studies were signed up (**Table 1**) [15–20].

Because the patient cohort of each study was heterogeneous, e.g., proportion of ECMELLA patients varying between 10 and 74%, the mortality rate of each study also differed (23.5–50%). However, patients who were successfully weaned from Impella 5+ were 13.1–38.2% of total patients. On the other hand, 16–61% of patients were successfully bridged to pMCS/HTX. Of note, patients who were successfully bridged to pMCS/HTX obtained favorable clinical outcomes. Strikingly, almost all patients who underwent HTX survived until discharge. Seese *et al.* reported that 24% (n = 57) of all patients on the waiting list for HTX being on Impella 5.0 support (n = 236) finally experienced HTX, in whom post-transplant survival rate was excellent as 96.5% at 30-day, 93.8% at 90-day, and 90.3% at 1-year follow-up [19]. Despite no information of simultaneous use of va-ECMO (ECMELLA), Lima *et al.* also reported that 75% of patients in the bridge to pMCS/HTX group treated with Impella 5.0 were successfully transferred to subsequent therapy (left ventricular assist device (LVAD) or HTX), and survival rate at discharge was 93% (HTX) and 87% (LVAD) in these groups, respectively [21].

As a study for the superior function of preconditioning of Impella 5+ for direct bridging to HTX, Nordan *et al.* performed a retrospective analysis comparing MCS by Impella with IABP support. In this study, all patients were supported with either "solo" LV unloading (most of all; Impella 5.0) or IABP. They observed that the post-transplant survival rate is comparable between Impella-bridged patients and IABP-bridged patients despite higher operative risk in Impella-bridged patients.

In summary, although there are no randomized comparative studies about clinical outcomes between groups with and without Impella 5+ in CS patients and we cannot make definitive statements in this field yet, we suppose that large Impella systems most likely offer a valuable contribution to preconditioning of CS patients and to

Publication			**Patients**								
Author	**Year**	**Impella**	**Total**	**ECMELLA**	**Deceased at discharge**	**Successfully weaned**	**Transition to pMCS**				
							Total	**LVAD**		**HTX**	
								Total	Living	Total	Living
Chung *et al.*	2020	5.0	100	10 (10.0)	38 (38.0)	14 (14.0)	51 (51.0)	14 (14.0)	11 (78.6)	37 (37.0)	37 (100)
Tarabichi *et al.*	2020	5.0	40	9 (22.5)	21 (52.5)	11 (27.5)	8 (20.0)	6 (15.0)	N/A	2 (5.0)	N/A
Seese *et al.*	2020	5.0	236	14 (5.8)	N/A	31 (13.1)	144 (61.0)	87 (37.0)	N/A	57 (24.1)	55 (96.5)
Nelson *et al.*	2021	5.0	34	4 (11.8)	8 (23.5)*	13 (38.2)*	10 (29.4)	8 (23.5)	8 (100)	2 (5.9)	2 (100)
Bernhardt *et al.*	2021	5.5	46	14 (30.4)	13 (28.3)	16 (34.8)	20 (43.5)	19 (41.3)	17 (89.5)**	1 (2.2)	1 (100)
Sugimura *et al.*	2021	5+	50	38 (74.0)	25 (50.0)	17 (34.0)	8 (16.0)	6 (12.0)	6 (100)	2 (4.0)	2 (100)

*Data documented as n (%). ECMELLA, venous–arterial extracorporeal membrane oxygenation+Impella; HTX, heart transplantation; LVAD, left ventricular assist device; N/A, no available data; pMCS, permanent mechanical circulatory support; *, at 30 days; **, at 90 days; 5+, Impella 5.0 or 5.5.*

Table 1.
Overview and outcomes of large Impella with a focus on the transition to pMCS/HTX.

bridging strategies to pMCS/HTX, and furthermore, these strategies are associated with excellent postoperative clinical outcome.

4. Expected role for a bridge to recovery in post-transplant phase

After HTX, comprehensive therapy is required for recovery. We sometimes encounter life-threatening complications. Primary graft dysfunction (PGD) is one of the critical complications and might occur in 2-28% of patients in the acute phase after HTX [22]. In PGD, mortality is reported to be as high as up to 85% [22]. The primary clinical manifestation of PGD is LV failure, which is affected by various factors, e.g., age and ischemic time of donor, acute rejection [23, 24]. Thus, most patients require MCS, e.g., va-ECMO support or temporary ventricular assist device (VAD) in PGD. A recent study has indicated that va-ECMO initiation due to "early graft failure," defined as the need of va-ECMO within the first 24-hours post-HTX, might be associated with a worse survival rate at 1 year (36%) and 5 years (28%) when compared to outcome in patients without early graft failure [25]. On the other hand, as far as temporary extracorporeal centrifugal VAD, i.e., CentriMag (Levitronix, LLC, Waltham, MA, USA) is concerned, a retrospective study of CentriMag utilization in the setting of PGD in 34 post-HTX patients reported that CentriMag support contributed to the salvage of 32% patients with severe PGD (survival rate at 30 days; 50%, at 1 year; 32%) [26].

The efficacy of Impella is theoretically comparable to that of CentriMag when used as a temporary VAD. Because of its convenient use, Impella will be the preferred system for the management of PGD. However, no studies have been yet reported, to the best of our knowledge. We suppose that Impella certainly must have been used as a bridge to recovery tool in the early post-HTX phase in clinical practice. Due to limited cases of PGD, no robust data have been published so far. More studies are warranted to evaluate the role of standard and primary utilization of Impella for PGD.

5. Our experience

5.1 Background

At our institute, Impella 5+ has been utilized since November 2018. We reported our initial experience with the first 50 consecutive cases treated with Impella 5+, in which patients were enrolled in the observation period between November 2018 and August 2020 [15]. However, meanwhile more patients have been treated with Impella 5+ at our institution. In front of this background, we would like to discuss the clinical role and the clinical outcomes of Impella 5+ in the setting of a bridge to HTX. As described, reports on the role of Impella 5+ in the context of the bridge to HTX are still scarce. Thus, we designed a single-center observational retrospective study to identify the clinical outcome of large Impella-bridged HTX and to elucidate the usefulness of the large Impella system as a temporary MCS in a larger patient cohort.

5.2 Study population

At our institute from November 2018 up to September 2021, a total of 102 Impella 5+ were utilized for MCS in 89 patients. Finally, pMCS implantation or HTX were

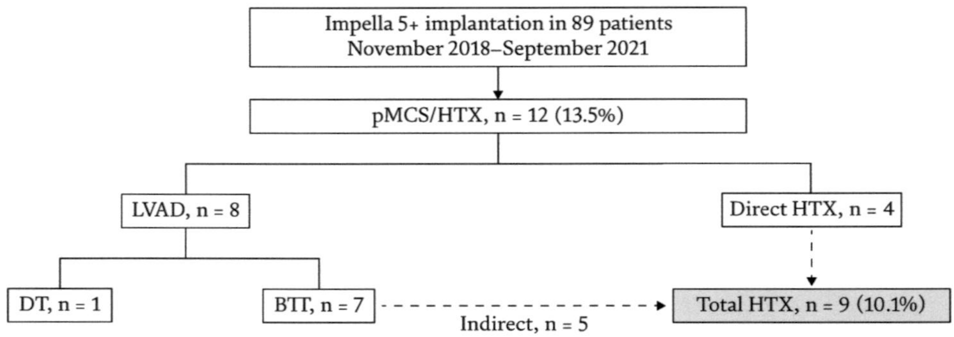

Figure 1.
Flow chart of the study population for analysis. BTT, bridge to transplant; DT, destination therapy; HTX, heart transplantation; LVAD, left ventricular assist device.

	Patients (n = 11)
Age (y)	52.4 ± 9.8
Male, n (%)	10 (90.9)
Arterial hypertension, n (%)	5 (45.5)
Hyperlipidemia, n (%)	5 (45.5)
Diabetes, n (%)	4 (36.4)
Peripheral vascular disease, n (%)	1 (9.1)
Arrhythmia, n (%)	3 (27.3)
COPD, n (%)	0 (0.0)
Nicotine abuses, n (%)	5 (45.5)
Drug abuses, n (%)	0 (0.0)
Dialysis, n (%)	0 (0.0)
History of PCI, n (%)	3 (27.3)
post CPR, n (%)	3 (27.3)
Biventricular failure, n (%)	7 (63.6)
ICM, n (%)	7 (63.6)
DCM, n (%)	2 (18.2)
Myocarditis, n (%)	1 (9.1)
Heart transplant rejection, n (%)	1 (9.1)
va-ECMO implantation, n (%)	7 (63.6)
Upgrade from Impella CP, n (%)	4 (36.4)

Data documented as n (%) or mean ± standard deviation. COPD, chronic obstructive pulmonary disease; CPR, cardiopulmonary resuscitation; DCM, dilatative cardiomyopathy; ICM, ischemic cardiomyopathy; PCI, percutaneous coronary intervention; va-ECMO, venous–arterial extracorporeal membrane oxygenation.

Table 2.
Baseline clinical characteristics.

performed in 12 of them (13.5%), in whom 11 patients were directly bridged to pMCS/HTX under Impella 5+ support, whereas 1 patient underwent HTX after successfully weaning of Impella 5 at the current admission.

LVAD implantation as primary pMCS was performed in 8 patients whose therapy concept was "BTT" for 7 patients and "destination therapy (DT)" for 1 patient because of his advanced age (76 years old).

Direct HTX were performed in 4 patients (primary HTX; n = 3, secondly HTX; n = 1). Further, HTX following LVAD after Impella 5+ support was also performed in 5 patients, who build up 62.5% of patients who underwent LVAD implantation as primary tMCS after Impella 5+ support. Thus, a total of 9 patients (10.1%) underwent HTX after Impella 5+ support (**Figure 1**).

5.3 Patients characteristics

Table 2 shows baseline clinical characteristics of 11 patients (BTT n = 7, direct HTX n = 4), without 1 DT patient. The most common underlying disease for Impella implantation was ischemic cardiomyopathy (ICM) (n = 7, 63.6%), followed by dilated cardiomyopathy (DCM; n = 2, 18.2%). Three patients were post-CPR, and a combination of va-ECMO plus Impella, referred to as 'ECMELLA' was administrated in 7 patients (63.6%). In all eleven cases, implantation of Impella 5 was performed via the right subclavian artery.

5.4 Clinical outcomes

Table 3 shows the clinical course of MCS in 11 patients successfully bridged to pMCS/HTX. Impella 5+ support time was 17.4 ± 15.6 days (median 12 days) for bridge to pMCS/HTX in 11 patients. It means that patients underwent either LVAD implantation or HTX on average after 17.4 days following Impella 5+ initiation.

Patient	Pre pMCS/HTX				pMCS/HTX	
	ECMELLA	va-ECMO ex?	Impella ex?	tRVAD?		
1	Yes	No	No	—	LVAD/tRVAD	(HTX)
2	Yes	Yes	No	No	LVAD/tRVAD	(HTX)
3	No	—	No	—	LVAD	(HTX)
4	Yes	Yes	Yes	No	—	HTX
5	Yes	Yes	No	Yes	—	HTX
6	Yes	Yes	No	No	LVAD/tRVAD	(HTX)
7	Yes	No	No	—	LVAD/tRVAD	(HTX)
8	No	—	No	—	LVAD	—
9	No	—	No	—	—	HTX
10	No	—	No	—	LVAD	—
11	Yes	Yes	No	No	—	HTX

ECMELLA, venous–arterial extracorporeal membrane oxygenation+Impella; ex, explantation; HTX, heart transplantation; LVAD, left ventricular assist device; pMCS, permanent mechanical circulatory support; tRVAD, temporary right ventricular assist device; va-ECMO, venous–arterial extracorporeal membrane oxygenation; –, not applicable; (HTX), indirect HTX.

Table 3.
Clinical course in 11 patients successfully bridged to pMCS/HTX.

In 5 of 7 ECMELLA patients, va-ECMO explanation was performed before pMCS/HTX, of whom 1 patient required a temporary right ventricular assist device (tRVAD). As described, 1 patient underwent HTX after successful weaning of Impella 5 at the same admission (patient 4).

Among LVAD patients (n = 7), simultaneous tRVAD was required in 4 patients for postoperative management.

All 11 patients survived the first 30 days after pMCS/HTX operations. However, 2 patients (patients 9, 11) died of septic shock (after 129 days, 122 days, respectively) after HTX. The latter patient was after secondly HTX due to heart transplant rejection.

As far as complications of Impella 5+, a re-implantation of Impella 5+ was necessary total in 3 patients due to (1) Impella thrombosis (n = 2), and (2) Impella dislocation (n = 1). Additionally, Impella dislocation occurred in one more patient. The patient (Patient 10. in **Table 3**) was directly implanted LVAD.

6. Conclusion

Our experience shows (1) successful transition to pMCS/HTX of 13.5% (n = 12/89), (2) 30 days survival after bridging to pMCS/HTX of 100%, (3) HTX of 10.1% (n = 9/89), and (4) 30 days survival rate of 100% and in-hospital mortality of 22.2% (n = 2/9) after HTX.

According to already published articles, a large Impella system seems to contribute to preconditioning of CS patients not only for a bridge to pMCS/HTX but also for the excellent postoperative clinical outcome. This hypothesis is supported by 100% post-transplant 30 days survival rate in patients who underwent HTX on Impella 5+ in our study. Using Impella 5+ the majority of patients with ECMELLA due to CS could be successfully weaned from va-ECMO before pMCS/HTX installation. This fact also indicates favorable clinical outcomes of Impella 5+ in CS patients awaiting HTX. However, patient selection and choice of size and timing of Impella support remain the subject of future studies for bridging strategies to pMCS/HTX. As a caution, Impella dysfunction due to thrombosis or dislocation of the pump could occur with the long-term utilization of Impella 5+ for bridge to pMCS/HTX.

Acknowledgements

We gratefully acknowledge the work of the members of the heart failure team at the University Hospital Duesseldorf.

Conflict of interest

The authors declare no conflict of interest.

Author details

Yukiharu Sugimura[1], Sebastian Bauer[1], Moritz Benjamin Immohr[1], Arash Mehdiani[1], Hug Aubin[1], Ralf Westenfeld[2], Udo Boeken[1], Artur Lichtenberg[1] and Payam Akhyari[1]*

1 Department of Cardiac Surgery and Research Group for Experimental Surgery, Medical Faculty and University Hospital Düsseldorf, Heinrich Heine University Hospital, Düsseldorf, Germany

2 Division of Cardiology, Pulmonology and Vascular Medicine, Medical Faculty, Heinrich-Heine University, Düsseldorf, Germany,

*Address all correspondence to: Payam.Akhyari@med.uni-duesseldorf.de

References

[1] Wernly B, Bhatt DL, Thiele H, Jung C. Impella in cardiogenic shock: Is it time to hit the break? Shock. 2021;**55**(5):693-694

[2] Donker DW, Brodie D, Henriques JPS, Broome M. Left ventricular unloading during veno-arterial ECMO: A review of percutaneous and surgical unloading interventions. Perfusion. 2019;**34**(2):98-105

[3] Donker DW, Brodie D, Henriques JPS, Broome M. Left ventricular unloading during veno-arterial ECMO: A simulation study. ASAIO Journal. 2019;**65**(1):11-20

[4] Vallabhajosyula S, O'Horo JC, Antharam P, Ananthaneni S, Vallabhajosyula S, Stulak JM, et al. Venoarterial extracorporeal membrane oxygenation with concomitant impella versus venoarterial extracorporeal membrane oxygenation for cardiogenic shock. ASAIO Journal. 2020;**66**(5):497-503

[5] Patel SM, Lipinski J, Al-Kindi SG, Patel T, Saric P, Li J, et al. Simultaneous venoarterial extracorporeal membrane oxygenation and percutaneous left ventricular decompression therapy with impella is associated with improved outcomes in refractory cardiogenic shock. ASAIO Journal. 2019;**65**(1):21-28

[6] Akanni OJ, Takeda K, Truby LK, Kurlansky PA, Chiuzan C, Han J, et al. EC-VAD: Combined use of extracorporeal membrane oxygenation and percutaneous microaxial pump left ventricular assist device. ASAIO Journal. 2019;**65**(3):219-226

[7] Mourad M, Gaudard P, De La Arena P, Eliet J, Zeroual N, Rouviere P, et al. Circulatory support with extracorporeal membrane oxygenation and/or impella for cardiogenic shock during myocardial infarction. ASAIO Journal. 2018;**64**(6):708-714

[8] Tepper S, Masood MF, Baltazar Garcia M, Pisani M, Ewald GA, Lasala JM, et al. Left ventricular unloading by impella device versus surgical vent during extracorporeal life support. The Annals of Thoracic Surgery. 2017;**104**(3):861-867

[9] Pappalardo F, Schulte C, Pieri M, Schrage B, Contri R, Soeffker G, et al. Concomitant implantation of Impella((R)) on top of veno-arterial extracorporeal membrane oxygenation may improve survival of patients with cardiogenic shock. European Journal of Heart Failure. 2017;**19**(3):404-412

[10] Grajeda Silvestri ER, Pino JE, Donath E, Torres P, Chait R, Ghumman W. Impella to unload the left ventricle in patients undergoing venoarterial extracorporeal membrane oxygenation for cardiogenic shock: A systematic review and meta-analysis. Journal of Cardiac Surgery. 2020;**35**(6):1237-1242

[11] Russo JJ, Aleksova N, Pitcher I, Couture E, Parlow S, Faraz M, et al. Left ventricular unloading during extracorporeal membrane oxygenation in patients with cardiogenic shock. Journal of the American College of Cardiology. 2019;**73**(6):654-662

[12] Schrage B, Burkhoff D, Rubsamen N, Becher PM, Schwarzl M, Bernhardt A, et al. Unloading of the left ventricle during venoarterial extracorporeal membrane oxygenation therapy in cardiogenic shock. JACC Heart Failure. 2018;**6**(12):1035-1043

[13] Schrage B, Becher PM, Bernhardt A, Bezerra H, Blankenberg S, Brunner S, et al. Left ventricular unloading is associated with lower mortality in patients with cardiogenic shock treated with venoarterial extracorporeal membrane oxygenation: Results from an international, Multicenter Cohort Study. Circulation. 2020;**142**(22):2095-2106

[14] Tongers J, Sieweke JT, Kuhn C, Napp LC, Flierl U, Rontgen P, et al. Early escalation of mechanical circulatory support stabilizes and potentially rescues patients in refractory cardiogenic shock. Circulation. Heart Failure. 2020;**13**(3):e005853

[15] Sugimura Y, Katahira S, Immohr MB, Sipahi NF, Mehdiani A, Assmann A, et al. Initial experience covering 50 consecutive cases of large Impella implantation at a single heart centre. ESC Heart Fail. 2021. DOI:10.1002/ehf2.13594

[16] Nelson DW, Sundararajan S, Klein E, Joyce LD, Durham LA, Joyce DL, et al. Sustained use of the impella 5.0 heart pump enables bridge to clinical decisions in 34 patients. Texas Heart Institute Journal. 2021;**48**(3):e207260

[17] Bernhardt AM, Potapov E, Schibilsky D, Ruhparwar A, Tschope C, Spillmann F, et al. First in man evaluation of a novel circulatory support device: Early experience with the Impella 5.5 after CE mark approval in Germany. The Journal of Heart and Lung Transplantation. 2021;**40**(8):850-855

[18] Tarabichi S, Ikegami H, Russo MJ, Lee LY, Lemaire A. The role of the axillary Impella 5.0 device on patients with acute cardiogenic shock. Journal of Cardiothoracic Surgery. 2020;**15**(1):218

[19] Seese L, Hickey G, Keebler ME, Mathier MA, Sultan I, Gleason TG, et al. Direct bridging to cardiac transplantation with the surgically implanted Impella 5.0 device. Clinical Transplantation. 2020;**34**(3):e13818

[20] Chung JS, Emerson D, Ramzy D, Akhmerov A, Megna D, Esmailian F, et al. A new paradigm in mechanical circulatory support: 100-patient experience. The Annals of Thoracic Surgery. 2020;**109**(5):1370-1377

[21] Lima B, Kale P, Gonzalez-Stawinski GV, Kuiper JJ, Carey S, Hall SA. Effectiveness and safety of the impella 5.0 as a bridge to cardiac transplantation or durable left ventricular assist device. The American Journal of Cardiology. 2016;**117**(10):1622-1628

[22] Kobashigawa J, Zuckermann A, Macdonald P, Leprince P, Esmailian F, Luu M, et al. Report from a consensus conference on primary graft dysfunction after cardiac transplantation. The Journal of Heart and Lung Transplantation. 2014;**33**(4):327-340

[23] Russo MJ, Chen JM, Sorabella RA, Martens TP, Garrido M, Davies RR, et al. The effect of ischemic time on survival after heart transplantation varies by donor age: an analysis of the United Network for organ sharing database. The Journal of Thoracic and Cardiovascular Surgery. 2007;**133**(2):554-559

[24] Del Rizzo DF, Menkis AH, Pflugfelder PW, Novick RJ, McKenzie FN, Boyd WD, et al. The role of donor age and ischemic time on survival following orthotopic heart transplantation. The Journal of Heart and Lung Transplantation. 1999;**18**(4):310-319

[25] Loforte A, Fiorentino M, Murana G, Gliozzi G, Cavalli GG, Mariani C, et al. Mechanically supported early graft failure after heart transplantation.

Transplantation Proceedings. 2021;**53**(1): 311-317

[26] Thomas HL, Dronavalli VB, Parameshwar J, Bonser RS, Banner NR. Steering group of the UKCTA. Incidence and outcome of Levitronix CentriMag support as rescue therapy for early cardiac allograft failure: A United Kingdom national study. European Journal of Cardio-Thoracic Surgery. 2011;**40**(6):1348-1354

Section 3

Heart Transplantation in Pediatrics

Chapter 7

Pediatric Heart Transplantation

Estela Azeka

Abstract

Despite advances in medical management, patients submitted for heart transplantation procedures still are at risk to development of complications. This chapter will discuss some specific topics of pediatric heart transplantation, focusing on perioperative care: (i) recipient management, (ii) donor evaluation, (iii) immunosuppression, (iv) early postoperative management, (v) complications, and (vi) conclusions.

Keywords: heart transplantation, child, complications, immunosuppression, management, perioperative period, heart failure, mechanical circulatory support, pediatric

1. Introduction

Heart transplantation (HT) has been the therapeutic option for patients with complex congenital heart disease and cardiomyopathies with heart failure (HF) refractory to conventional treatment [1–4].

Despite advances in molecular biology, immunosuppressive drug therapy, the knowledge of the potential complications that may occur after the procedure are essential to improve the quality of life of patients and their survival.

In this chapter we will discuss:

1. Recipient management

2. Donor evaluation

3. Immunosuppression

4. Early postoperative management

5. Complications

6. Conclusions

2. Recipient management

The main types of pediatric heart diseases considered for heart transplantation are [1]:

- cardiomyopathies with refractory heart failure (**Figures 1** and **2**);
- congenital heart diseases with or without ventricular dysfunction and/or in natural history evolution that do not present the possibility of a new therapeutic intervention;
- patients undergoing heart transplantation due to graft vascular disease, rejection and/or graft failure.

The clinical manifestations of heart failure in children vary according to age of the patient and severity of disease. In infants, the most common signs and symptoms are poor weight gain, tachypnea and diaphoresis during feeding and fatigability. Young children may present abdominal pain, vomiting, nausea, poor appetite, fatigability,

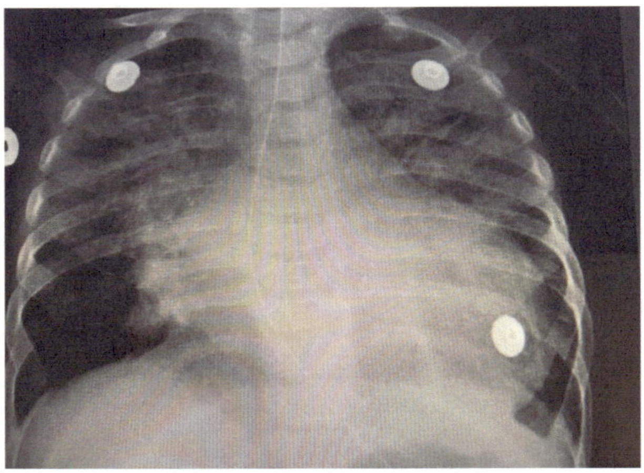

Figure 1.
Chest X-ray showing enlargement cardiac área in a child with dilated cardiomyopathy.

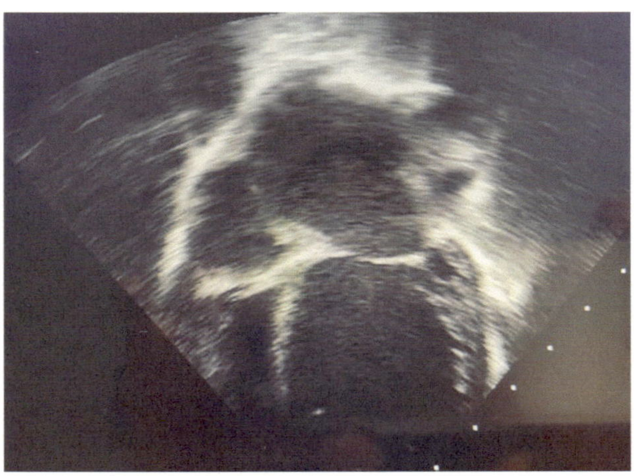

Figure 2.
Echocardiogram showing enlargement of left ventricle chamber in a child with dilated cardiomyopathy.

Clinical status
Pulmonary hypertension
Frailty
Pre-transplant vaccination/immunization
Mechanical assist device
Multidisciplinary approach

Table 1.
Specific topics for evaluation.

recurrent cough and failure to thrive. In adolescents, abdominal pain, anorexia, exercise intolerance, dyspnea, oedema or syncope may be found. Nowadays, heart failure in children can be classified and categorize of the stage and severity by the modified NYHA, stages of heart failure infants and children and recommended therapy (stage A, B, C and D), modified Ross classification and by INTERMACS, which can help in decision making. The INTERMACS classification was initially developed to consider the patient for mechanical circulatory support [5–8]. Pediatric patients with stage D heart failure are listed for heart transplantation [1, 6].

There are some important topics [1] to be addressed at the moment to evaluate a pediatric recipient for heart transplantation (**Table 1**):

1. The clinical status of patient: if the patient is in the intensive care unit receiving drugs with continuous infusions such as phosphodiesterase 3 (PDE3) inhibitors (milrinone) or epinephrine and anti-congestive medications; if the patient is with ventricular assist device or if the patient is at outpatient clinics.

   The clinical status will determine if the patient is in priority or not for heart transplantation when listed;

2. The type of anti-congestive medications for heart failure: diuretics, drugs that reduce afterload (angiotensin-converting enzyme inhibitors), ivabradine, sacubitril/valsartan and beta-blockers (metoprolol succinate and carvedilol) for improvement of symptoms and reduction of cardiac work;

3. Pulmonary vascular resistance index (PVRI): children who are candidates for heart transplantation and who present a high pulmonary vascular resistance index should be considered for the use of pulmonary vasodilators inhaled and intravenous (nitric oxide, prostacyclins, nitroprusside and milrinone). Prolonged use of inotropic agents may reduce pulmonary resistance to pulmonary vascular resistance índex < 6 Woods units/m^2 or transpulmonary gradient < 15 mmHg. Patients with pulmonary hypertension are refractory to medical therapy can be a candidate for mechanical assist devices to try to reduce the PVRI;

4. Nutritional assessment and support must be performed so that the patient can be adequately prepared for the surgical procedure and its recovery. Moderate to severe wasting and elevated weight/height are considered a risk for mortality during the waitlist. The restriction of fluids and sodium is part of the recommendations in the treatment of HF.

5. Physical rehabilitation: a physical rehabilitation regimen should also be part of the treatment;

6. Anticoagulation: children with severe ventricular dysfunction are at risk of thrombus formation therefore anticoagulation or anti-platelet aggregation should be considered if the patient has previous history of thrombus.

7. Immunizations: immunizations must be carried out according to the vaccination schedule.

8. Frailty is one of the major concerns due to chronic heart failure and is considered a prognostic factor of morbidity and mortality;

   - Pre-transplant specific assessments are in **Table 1**. They are performed according to the patient's history and clinical conditions.

   - Laboratory tests for initial evaluation for heart transplantation are in **Table 2**. HLA antibody level greater than 70% is considered high and may compromise short- and medium-term survival outcomes after transplantation.

   - The assessment of the multidisciplinary team is fundamental for the success of long-term follow-up. The multidisciplinary team including nurse, psychologist, social worker, physiotherapist, dentist and nutritionist provides information about the patient as well as the family's suitability for the transplant procedure. Psychosocial support is vital when the child becomes a candidate for heart transplantation, as there is a need to restructure the family routine as a result of outpatient follow-up.

Mechanical circulatory support has been an option for children with refractory heart failure.

ECMO in children should be considered to provide adequate systemic perfusion and oxygenation for myocardial recovery after cardiopulmonary bypass or in patients as a bridge for heart transplantation and considered for long-term mechanical circulatory support (MCS). The use of ventricular assist device (VAD) has been increased for bridge to heart transplantation, decision or destination. The type of VAD depends on the weight, body superface área and pulmonary hypertension. In general, infants

Chest radiology
Electrocardiogram
Echocardiogram
VO_2 measurement
Magnetic cardiac resonance
Endomyocardial biopsy
Cardiac catheterization
Angiotomography

Table 2.
Pre-transplant specific cardiac assessment.

Complete blood count
Biochemistry
Liver and kidney profile
Lipid profile
Albumin and total proteins
BNP and pro-BNP
PCR
Urine I
Parasitological examination of faeces
Serology for infections such as hepatitis, HIV, toxoplasmosis, Epstein-Barr virus, Chagas disease, PCR for CMV and EBV
Blood typing
Panel reactive antibody percentage: magnitude of sensitization of the pre-transplant patient (immune panel) with HLA typing

Table 3.
Laboratory tests for initial evaluation of heart transplantation.

are candidates for paracorporeal MCS and adolescents for implanted ones. The prevalence of children waiting for heart transplantation with MCS has been increased in the last years (**Table 3**).

3. Donor assessment

The potential donor must be evaluated in relation to the recipient. The topics for donor evaluation in children are in **Table 4**. Pre-existing cardiac anomalies such as coronary artery disease, valve anomalies, left ventricular hypertrophy, donor cardiac function, donor-recipient size matching should be addressed before accepting the potential donor.

Blood type
Weight and height
Determination of cause of death
Ischemic time
Age
Past medical history
Electrocardiogram
Chest X-ray
Echocardiogram
Serology for infections such as hepatitis, HIV, toxoplasmosis, Epstein-Barr virus, Chagas disease, PCR for CMV and EBV

Table 4.
Donor evaluation.

Recently, ISHLT Pediatric Consensus (DOAM) describes the principal recommendations for acceptance of the pediatric donor [9].

Donation after Circulatory Death (DCD) should be performed in centres with experience in marginal donor hearts, perioperative mechanical support, the use of ex-situ organ perfusion devices for preservation and transportation.

ABO-incompatible heart transplant procedure has been performed in children in some centres with results similar to ABO compatible due to the scarcity of donors.

4. Immunosuppression

Immunosuppression regimens are generally defined according to the period of transplantation and the presence of rejection [10, 11]:

- Induction
- Maintenance
- Rejection treatment

Induction therapy can be defined as prophylactic immunosuppressive therapy in the perioperative period, usually with cytolytic agents, to reduce the incidence of early rejection (**Table 5**). Nowadays, the use of induction therapy has increased and is not associated with an increase in infection and malignancy [12].

Different classes of drugs are used for initial and maintenance immunosuppression in children.

The most used initial regimens are composed of the association of corticosteroids, calcineurin inhibitors and antiproliferative agents (**Table 5**).

The use of tacrolimus as a calcineurin inhibitor and the replacement of Azathioprine as an antiproliferative agent with mycophenolate is the current trend in most centres worldwide.

Induction therapy
Thymoglobulin rabbit
Maintenance regimen
1. Calcineurin inhibitors a) Tacrolimus b) Cyclosporin
2. Antiproliferative regimen: a) Mychophenolate b) Azathioprine
3. Corticosteroids
4. Proliferation signal inhibitors a) Sirolimus b) Everolimus

Table 5.
Most common immunosuppression drugs.

EKG
Systemic blood pressure
Central venous pressure
Pulmonary artery wedge pressure
Arterial oxygen saturation
Mixed venous saturation
Urinary output
Lactate
Vital signs (temperature, heart rate, respiratory rate)

Table 6.
Monitoring in Early post-operative care.

Proliferation signal inhibitors (everolimus and sirolimus) are used in renal failure, graft vascular disease and lymphoproliferative disease in combination with a calcineurin inhibitor or in monotherapy (**Table 5**).

In children, it is important to address the avoidance of steroids as maintenance drug therapy due to failure to adequate height development.

5. Perioperative management

Perioperative management consists of some topics that are listed in **Table 6** [11–16].

6. Complications

In perioperative period, the main complications of transplantation can be inherent to transplantation, such as early graft dysfunction, right ventricular dysfunction,

Tricuspid valve regurgitation
Pericardial effusion
Vasoactive drugs
Vasoplegia
Right ventricular dysfunction
Pulmonary hypertension
Mechanical circulatory support
Early allograft dysfunction
Arrhythmias
Renal function
Hyperglicemia
Antibiotics prophylaxis
Fontan-patients management

Table 7.
Topics of perioperative care.

Clinical findings
Chest X-ray
EKG
Echocardiogram
Endomyocardial biopsy
Biomarkers

Table 8.
Methods for rejection diagnosis.

hyperacute rejection as well as due to the immunosuppressive medication itself: infection, systemic arterial hypertension and renal failure (**Tables** 7 and **8**). In the late postoperative period, coronary allograft vasculopathy, tumour, primary graft dysfunction are some causes of long-term complications.

Rejection has been reported as the main cause of death after transplantation. The diagnosis of rejection is made by a combination of clinical signs and symptoms, non-invasive tests and/or endomyocardial biopsy, using the International Society of Cardiac and Lung Transplantation (ISHLT) criteria [14]. Several noninvasive methods have been reported such as echocardiography, cardiac magnetic resonance, electrocardiogram, Gallium-67 as well as biomarkers of injury or immunoreactivity such as BNP, troponin and donor-specific antibodies (DSA) for rejection surveillance in pediatric heart transplantation. These non-invasive methods have been described as high degree of specificity and low sensitivity and are useful for identifying those without rejection episodes. Therefore, endomyocardial biopsy is still the gold standard for rejection although there are risks related to the procedure such as venous occlusion, radiation and perforation.

6.1 Rejection treatment

Treatment of rejection should be directed towards the underlying aetiology, as well as the severity of the condition based on clinical, laboratory and pathological findings.

6.2 Acute cellular rejection

- Mild and asymptomatic (1R)—does not require treatment due to the high rate of spontaneous resolution and the absence of association with reduced long-term survival and graft vascular disease.

- Moderate and severe cell rejection (ISHLT $\geq$ 2R) (**Figure 3**)—should be treated with enhanced immunosuppression. If a patient with signs of ventricular dysfunction and needs vasoactive drugs, methylprednisolone therapy and anti-thymocyte globulin association is recommended. MCS should be considered if there is hemodynamic instability.

6.3 Humoral rejection

It includes the same schemes used to treat cell rejection, with high doses of corticosteroids and lymphocytolytic agents. Additionally, intravenous immunoglobulin

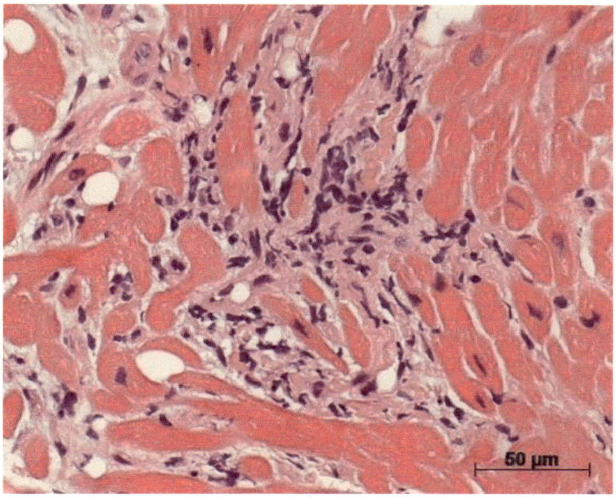

Figure 3.
Cellular rejection: a focus of inflammatory infiltrate with cellular aggression and architectural distortion in acute cellular rejection grade 2R.

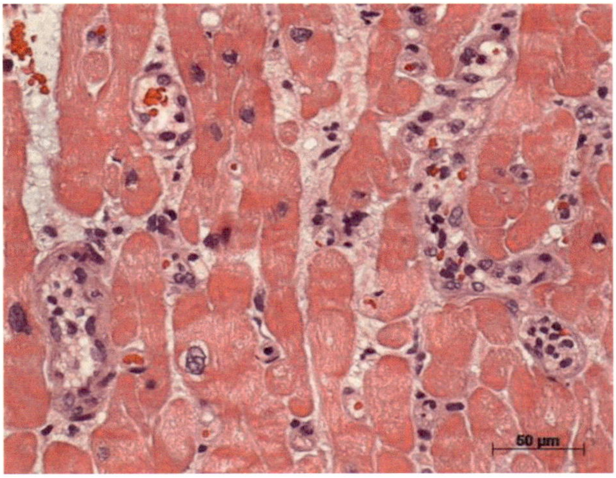

Figure 4.
Humoral rejection: interstitial edema and endothelial swelling of capillaries in antibody-mediated rejection. Note also the presence of mononuclear cells inside capillaries.

and plasmapheresis to remove circulating antibodies and specific therapies to target B cells (cyclophosphamide, mycophenolate and rituximab) can be used (**Figure 4**).

7. Conclusions

Heart transplantation is an option for refractory heart failure in children with cardiomyopathies and complex heart diseases. It is a highly complex clinical-surgical therapy that involves a specialized multidisciplinary team so that child care can be performed successfully. Nowadays, the Pediatric Heart Transplantation Society

(PHTS) has developed a database where clinical trials and robust research have been performed for the best care of this fragile pediatric population.

Acknowledgements

Dr. Luiz Benvenuti from the Pathology Department for the pictures of rejection.

Author details

Estela Azeka
Pediatric Cardiology and Adults with Congenital Heart Disease Unit, Instituto do Coração (InCor) HCFMUSP, Faculdade de Medicina da Universidade de São Paulo, São Paulo, Brazil

*Address all correspondence to: estela_azeka9@hotmail.com; estela.azeka@hc.fm.usp.br

References

[1] Kirk R, Dipchand AI, Rosenthal DN, et al. The International Society for Heart and Lung Transplantation Guidelines for the management of pediatric heart failure: Executive summary. The Journal of Heart and Lung Transplantation. 2014;**33**(9):888-909

[2] Lipshultz SE, Law YM, Asante-Korang A, et al. Cardiomyopathy in children: Classification and diagnosis: A scientific statement from the American Heart Association. Circulation. 2019;**140**. CIR000682

[3] Law YM, Lal AK, Chen S, et al. Diagnosis and management of myocarditis in children: A Scientific Statement from the American Heart Association. Circulation. 2021;**144**(6):e123-e135

[4] Roeleveld PP, Axelrod DM, Klugman D, et al. Hypoplastic left heart syndrome: From fetus to fontan. Cardiology in the Young. 2018;**28**(11):1275-1288

[5] Ross RD. The Rossclassification for heart failure in children after 25 years: A review and an age-stratified revision. Pediatric Cardiology. 2012;**33**(8):1295-1300. DOI: 10.1007/s00246-012-0306-8

[6] Rosenthal D, Chrisant MR, Edens E, et al. International Society for Heart and Lung Transplantation: Practice guidelines for management of heart failure in children. The Journal of Heart and Lung Transplantation. 2004;**23**:1313-1333

[7] Morales DLS, Rossano JW, VanderPluym C, et al. Third Annual Pediatric Interagency Registry for Mechanical Circulatory Support (Pedimacs) Report: Preimplant Characteristics and Outcomes. The Annals of Thoracic Surgery. 2019; **107**(4):993-1004

[8] Baumgartner H, DeBacker J, Babu-Narayan SV, et al. 2020 ESC guidelines for the management ofadult congenital heart disease. European Heart Journal. 2020;**00**:1-83

[9] Kirk R, Dipchand AI, Davies RR, et al. ISHLT consensus statement on donor organ acceptability and management in pediatric heart transplantation. The Journal of Heart and Lung Transplantation. 2020;**39**(4):331-341

[10] Daly KP. Contemporary transplantation immunosuppression: Balancing on the immunosuppression seesaw. Pediatric Transplantation;**13**:52

[11] Azeka E, Auler JO Jr, Marcial MB, et al. Heart transplantation in children: Clinical outcome during the early postoperative period. Pediatric Transplantation. 2005;**9**(4):491-497

[12] Gajarski R, Blume ED, Urschel S, et al. Infection and malignancy after pediatric heart transplantation: The role of induction therapy. The Journal of Heart and Lung Transplantation. 2011;**30**(3):299-308

[13] Mowers KL, Simpson KE, Gazit AZ, et al. Moderate-severe primary graft dysfunction after pediatric heart transplantation. Pediatric Transplantation. 2019;**23**(2):e13340

[14] Stewart S, Winters GL, Fishbein MC, et al. Revision of the 1990 working formulation for the standardization of nomenclature in the diagnosis of heart rejection. The Journal of Heart and Lung Transplantation. 2005;**24**(11): 1710-1720

[15] Dipchand AI, Edwards LB, Kucheryavaya AY, et al. The registry of the International Society for Heart and Lung Transplantation: Seventeenth official pediatric heart transplantation report--2014; focus theme: Retransplantation. The Journal of Heart and Lung Transplantation. 2014;**33**(10):985-995

[16] L'Huillier AG, Dipchand AI, Ng VL, et al. Posttransplant lymphoproliferative disorder in pediatric patients: Survival rates according to primary sites of occurrence and a proposed clinical categorization. American Journal of Transplantation. 2019

Section 4

Surgical Techniques

Chapter 8

Evolution of Heart Transplantation Surgical Techniques

Samuel Jacob, Anthony N. Pham and Si M. Pham

Abstract

Organ transplantation has kindled the human imagination since the beginning of time. Prehistorically, transplantation appeared as mythological stories: from creatures with body parts from different species, the heart transplant between two Chinese soldiers by Pien Ch'iao, to the leg transplant by physician Saints Cosmas and Damian. By 19th century, the transplantation concept become possible by extensive contributions from scientists and clinicians whose works had taken generations. Although Alexis Carrel is known as the founding father of experimental organ transplantation, many legendary names had contributed to the experimental works of heart transplantation, including Guthrie, Mann, and Demikhov. The major contribution to experimental heart transplantation before the clinical era were made by a team lead by Richard Lower and Norman Shumway at Stanford University in the early 1960s. They played the vital role in developing experimental and clinical heart transplantation as it is known today. Using Shumway biatrial technique Christiaan Barnard started a new era of clinical heart transplantation, by performing the first in man human-to-human heart transplantation in 1967. The techniques of heart transplant have evolved since the first heart transplant. This chapter will summarize the techniques that have been used in clinical heart transplantation.

Keywords: heterotopic heart transplantation, orthotopic heart transplant, bicaval technique, biatrial technique, cardiectomy, donor heart preparation

1. Introduction

Heart transplantation has captivated the human mind since the beginning of time. Prehistorically, transplantation appeared as mythological stories with creatures whose bodies consist of parts from different species. It is possible that chimeric beings, such as the Chimera of Greek mythology with a human head, snake tail, and lion heart and body, were created surgically through supernatural forces. Many transplant mythological tales suggested a surgical basis for these myths, with the most striking story reported by a Chinese doctor Pien Ch'iao in the 4th decade B.C. when he examined two sick soldiers and made the diagnosis that each had an imbalance of Yin and Yang; one had a strong will but weak spirit, while the other had the opposite. To correct the imbalance, he anesthetized them with powerful medication and cut open their chests and exchanged their hearts. Patients were unconscious for 3 days. After waking up they felt markedly improved [1].

IntechOpen

By the late 19th and early 20th century, the transplantation concept become possible by the development of surgical asepsis vascular anastomotic technique and understanding of the role of immunology in organ rejection. Alexis Carrel is known as the founding father of experimental organ transplantation. He was a French surgeon who developed the technique of vascular anastomosis in Lyon, France, and later he applied it to transplant a kidney into the necks of dogs [2].

Carrel left Lyons for the University of Chicago and began his collaboration with Charles Claude Guthrie. Together they established the foundation of organ transplantation using their vascular surgery technique. Their team described the first heterotopic heart transplant in mammals, were they connected a heart from a small dog into the neck of a larger one [3].

Frank C. Mann and his coworkers at the Mayo Clinic, modified the technique described by Guthrie and Carrel to create a heterotopic heart transplant in the dog neck to expand on the study of heart transplantation and make the seminal contribution to the field by describing that immunologic rejection was the main cause of graft failure. They also recognized the importance of ventricular distention and air embolism and the need for heparin to prevent thrombosis [4–6].

Vladimir Demikhov, a Russian physiologist, who's work was hidden from the west achieved a milestone in transplantation in the 1940s and 1950s. He performed a series of experimental operations on canines that's includes orthotopic heart transplantation, heterotopic heart transplantation, and heart-lung transplantation in bloc [7]. In the meantime, Wilford Neptune and his group at Hahnemann Medical College in Philadelphia, performed heart-lung transplantation in dogs without cardiopulmonary bypass using hypothermia in the recipient dog [8]. The major contribution to in experimental heart transplantation before the clinical era were made at Stanford in the early 1960s. Richard Lower and Norman Shumway and their team were responsible for developing heart transplantation as it is known today [9–12].

The first human heart transplant was performed with a chimpanzee donor. This was performed by Dr. James D. Hardy at the University of Mississippi Medical Center in January 1964, using Shumway technique [13]. Unfortunately, the small heart could not handle the large venous return of the recipient, and the patient died 1 hour after implantation of the heart [13].

On December 3, 1967, the first human-to-human heart transplantation took place at Groote Schuur Hospital, Cape Town, South Africa, by Christiaan Barnard and his team. They retrieved a heart from a donor after circulatory death (DCD), which is considered the first DCD heart, and implanted it into a 57-year-old patient with ischemic cardiomyopathy [14].

In today's clinical practice, orthotopic heart transplant (OHT) is the gold standard treatment for patients with refractory congestive heart failure from end stage heart diseases [15]. Many heart transplant techniques have been described. The bi-atrial technique, which was refined and popularized by Lower and Shumway in 1960 [9], was used to perform the first heart transplantation and was widely used for its relative simplicity. 'Wythenshawe' bi-caval technique of heart transplant, described by Sarsam et al. [16] had replaced the original biatrial technique in most transplant centers because it is more anatomical, associated with less sinus node dysfunction, and less tricuspid regurgitation, Yacoub and his colleagues introduced the total heart transplant technique in 1989 [17], however it did not gain much popularity because of its complexity without much physiological advantages. The heterotopic heart transplant techniques, described by Barnard in 1975 [18], was developed to treat patients with irreversible pulmonary hypertension, and as a way to keep the patient alive in case the donor heart fails due to primary graft dysfunction or severe rejection, the main cause of death after heart transplantation before cyclosporine era. Heterotopic heart transplant is rarely used today because of the advents in left ventricular assist device and immunosuppressants. However, it is still a useful technique as a biological left ventricular assistance (a new two-stage method) for heart failure treatment some specific circumstances [19].

In this chapter we will describe evolution of heart transplant techniques that have been used for patients with normal cardiac anatomy. Various modifications of these techniques have been adapted for patients with end-stage congenital heart diseases but will not be discussed in detail.

2. Clinical heterotopic heart transplantation

After a series of experimental techniques and studies on animals [20–23], clinical heterotopic heart transplantation was introduced by Barnard and colleagues at the Groote Schuur Hospital, Cape Town, South Africa in 1974 [18] in response to a clinical need that was not met by orthotopic heart transplantation, namely, heart failure with pulmonary hypertension. Currently, heterotopic heart transplants are performed rarely but may be indicated in patients with irreversible pulmonary hypertension or significant donor-recipient size mismatch, when left ventricular assist devices are not available or contraindicated [24].

In addition, this technique could be used as a temporary bridge to recovery in patients with cardiogenic shock. The other benefit is that the circulation of a patient could be maintained in case of rejection by the native heart. Furthermore, the graft could be removed by side-clamping the three anastomotic areas without the use of cardiopulmonary bypass in the setting of rejection or recovery.

2.1 Preparation of the donor heart

The heart is prepared on the back table in a sterile field and a basin of cold normal saline or cardioplegic solution. The stump of the IVC and the orifices of both right pulmonary veins are closed with continuous 5-0 polypropylene sutures, with care not to occlude the orifice of the coronary sinus. The bridge of tissue between the left superior and inferior pulmonary veins is excised to create a single opening into the left atrium. This opening may need to be extended to achieve a diameter of approximately 3.5–4 cm, or the equivalent of a normal mitral valve orifice. The midpoint of the posterior wall of this opening is marked with a suture as a reference during subsequent implantation into the recipient. The main pulmonary artery is divided at its bifurcation to allow extra length for implantation. A longitudinal 5 cm incision, just to the right of the interatrial septum, is made in the posterior aspect of the SVC and right atrium; at least half the length of this incision must involve the right atrial wall [25].

2.2 Preparation of the recipient

With the recipient in supine position, a median sternotomy is performed, and pericardium is opened longitudinally. Then a large right rectangular pericardial window is created in the right pleural cavity to accommodate the donor heart. Care is taken to avoid damaging the right phrenic nerve.

Hemostasis of the edges of this flap must be carried out carefully because the exposure will be difficult after the heart is in place. Next patient is fully heparinized, and the recipient is cannulated with an aortic cannula inserted at the level of the origin of the innominate artery, and venous cannulas in the SVC and the IVC (through the low atrial wall). Umbilical tapes snares are placed around the SVC and IVC to achieve total cardiopulmonary bypass (CPB) at some stage of the operation. Cardiopulmonary bypass is initiated, and a left upper pulmonary vein vent introduced. The patient is cooled to 28°C and cardioplegia is given through the aortic root.

2.3 Heterotopic implantation

The donor heart is placed in the right thoracic cavity in the window created anterior to the right lung and lying as a mirror image of the recipient's heart. An incision is made into the recipient's left atrium posterior to the interatrial groove, as in the mitral valve surgery incision. The midpoint of the posterior lip of the incision in the recipient left atrium is sutured using double-ended 4-0 polypropylene to the midpoint of the posterior lip of the donor left atrium at the site of the previously inserted marker stitch. The posterior aspect is completed first then the anterior aspect. The completed anastomosis will be totally inaccessible at the end of the operation therefore, it is essential that it be hemostatic. A 5 cm longitudinal incision is made into the lateral aspect of the recipient SVC and right atrium just anterior to the interatrial groove, beginning 2–3 cm above the junction of the vena cava and extending 3 cm into the right atrium. The midpoint of the posterior lip of the incision in the recipient atrium is sutured to the most caudal point of the incision in the donor atrium, using a double-ended 5-0 polypropylene suture (**Figure 1A**). The two right atria are then anastomosed by a continuous suture proceeding in each direction like a diamond shape, first posteriorly and then anteriorly. This allows the widest possible opening and prevents kinking of the right atrial anastomosis. At the completion of this anastomosis the ligated donor azygos vein remnant will lie at the midpoint of the anterior suture line.

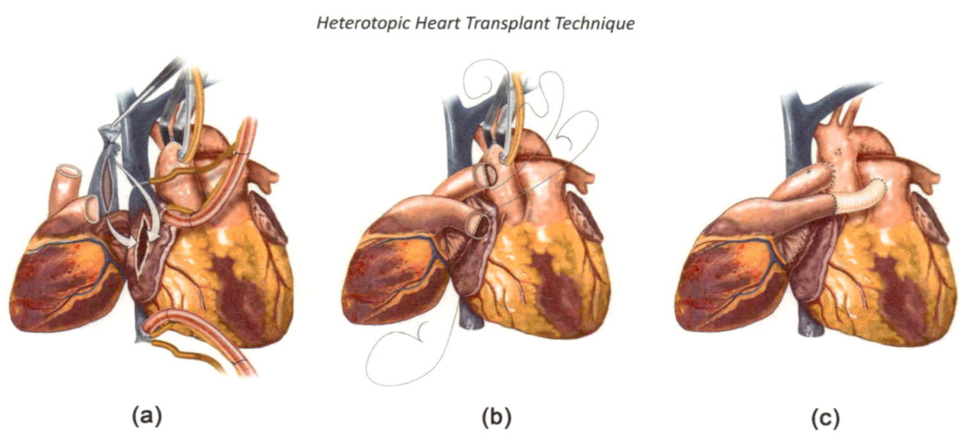

Figure 1.
(a) After finishing the left atrium anastomosis, a longitudinal incision is made on the recipient right atrium anterior to the interatrial groove, and the incision is extended superiorly into the SVC. After the donor right atrium is similarly incised, the donor recipient anastomosis is performed in a diamond shape. (b) The donor aorta is anastomosed to the recipient's by end-to-side anastomosis, and the PA is connected to the right atrium appendage for left heart support. (c) For bi-ventricular support configuration, the PA is connected, via a Dacron graft the recipient's PA.

Although the atrial anastomoses can be done with the beating recipient's heart, it is easier to perform these anastomoses with the native heart in an arrested state.

The donor's aorta is trimmed to the appropriate length and anastomosed in an end-to-side fashion to the recipients. It is important to trim the donor's aorta to the minimum length required, otherwise the donor heart will drop back into the right pleural cavity and cause compression atelectasis of the right lung. The cardioplegic catheter in the donor aorta is converted for use as an air vent, and the caval snares are released. For left ventricular support alone, the donor pulmonary artery is connected to the right atrial appendage (**Figure 1B**). For biventricular support the donor's pulmonary artery is connected to the recipient's main pulmonary trunk. To do that the donor pulmonary artery has to be extended with a conduit (usually Dacron graft) to prevent undue tension or distortion of the other anastomoses. The size of graft chosen will depend largely on the diameter of the donor pulmonary artery; this is usually on the order of 22 mm. The Dacron graft is anastomosed end-to side to the recipient pulmonary artery using continuous 5-0 polypropylene suture (**Figure 1C**). After assuring that all anastomoses are hemostatic, the SVC cannula is withdrawn into the right atrium and the IVC cannula is removed. Inotropic medications are started as needed, and if the hemodynamic status is stable, cardiopulmonary bypass is discontinued and all cannulas are removed from the patient.

2.4 Modifications of the heterotopic heart transplant techniques

In 2017, Copeland et al. [26] published an alternate heterotopic heart transplant technique as a biologic left ventricular assist device. The donor heart left pulmonary veins and inferior vena cava are oversewn, like original technique. The donor and recipient left atria are anastomosed first. Then, the donor aorta is anastomosed to the recipient aorta in an end-to-side fashion. The aortic cross clamp is removed, and the patient is placed in Trendelenburg position. The donor pulmonary artery is anastomosed to the recipient right atrium. The donor superior vena cava (SVC) is anastomosed to the recipient superior vena cava in an end-to-side fashion. The anastomosis of the SVC is marked with clips to facilitate identification of the anastomosis during future endomyocardial biopsy through the right internal jugular vein.

Recently, Gaiotto et al., proposed a two-stage approach that allows conversion of a heterotopic heart transplant into an orthotopic one in patients with secondary pulmonary hypertension due to left ventricular failure [19].

The intention of this new approach is to decompress the native left ventricle to allow reversal of pulmonary hypertension, (LV) while preserving the donor's right ventricular function by diverting the entire blood volume from the SVC flowing through the donor RV. They proposed a slight modification of the Copeland technique by an end-to-end connection of the donor's and recipient's SVC; the rest of the anastomoses are the same as in Copeland's description. This first stage allows the recipient to have a biological left ventricular assist device while preserve the donor right ventricle function by filling it with blood from the upper part of the body. Because the RV is a flow-dependent chamber, its function would be preserved as it will receive all blood from the superior vena cava (SVC). This will prevent the donor RV from undergoing atrophy that is associated with the reduced blood flow from the side anastomosis of the original Copeland's technique. This modification provides decompression of the recipient LV and gradual reduction of the pulmonary vascular resistance through the parallel connection of the donor and recipient's left ventricles via the left atrial anastomosis.

When the recipient pulmonary hypertension resolves, the patient will undergo a second stage operation, in which the native heart will be removed and the donor heart will be "twisted" into the orthotopic position, connecting end-to-end the donor's PA (via a Dacron graft extension) to the recipient PA, and anastomosing the stump of the donor's IVC to the recipient's IVC. The technique will obviate the associated complications from having the native heart in circulation, such as thrombus formation in the native left ventricle, needs for long-term systemic anticoagulation, and ventricular fibrillation [27, 28]. Of note is the fact that this is just a concept proposed by Gaiotto et al.; they have not reported any actual case yet. However, the concept is supported by a case report in which the native heart was removed from a heterotopic heart transplant patient with success. Pham et al. [29] first reported case of congestive heart failure due to regurgitation of the native aortic and mitral valves, causing a left-to-left shunting in a patient with a heterotopic heart transplant. The arterial blood recirculates from the ascending aorta through the incompetent native aortic and mitral valves to the native and transplanted donor left atria, then donor left ventricle causing volume overloading of the heterotopic donor heart and congestive heart failure. The patient underwent resection of the native heart and survived more than 2 years later. This case demonstrated that the heterotopic donor heart alone can sustain the recipient after pulmonary hypertension resolved.

3. Bi-atrial technique of heart transplantation

Bi-atrial heart transplant technique is the first technique used in clinical heart transplantation. Shumway and Lower at Stanford University refined this surgical technique, which later called "Shumway" or bi-atrial technique (BA) [9]; it became the standard heart transplant surgical technique until the 1990s. The Stanford group also introduced the use of cold (4°C) isotonic saline solution to preserve the donor heart and the use of cardiopulmonary bypass to support the transplanted heart temporarily after the completion of the operation to until the donor slowly took over the circulation [30].

3.1 Cardiectomy

Communication between recovery team and transplanting team is very important to reduce the ischemic time, cardiopulmonary bypass time, and unnecessary delay. Communication and timing between both teams is very critical. If the ischemic time is short, cardiectomy of recipient heart could be done when the donor heart in the operating room, or just before the donor heart arrive to the hospital.

The chest is opened in a normal fashion through median sternotomy, the pericardium is opened vertically and horizontally as reversed T shape, then a full dose of heparin is given. When the ATC level is reached above 400, then cannulation of the aorta, SVC, and IVC is performed.

Cannulation of the aorta should be high and optimal usually just proximal to the origin of brachiocephalic artery, and the CPB is initiated. Then the aorta is cross clamped the venous cannulation is snared with umbilical tapes to achieve complete CPB.

The cardiectomy starts by opening the right atrium along the atrio-ventricular groove toward and coronary sinus inferiorly and toward the roof of the left atrium (**Figure 2A**). The interatrial septum is open with a blade at the foremen ovale and extended inferiorly to the coronary sinus orifice and superiorly

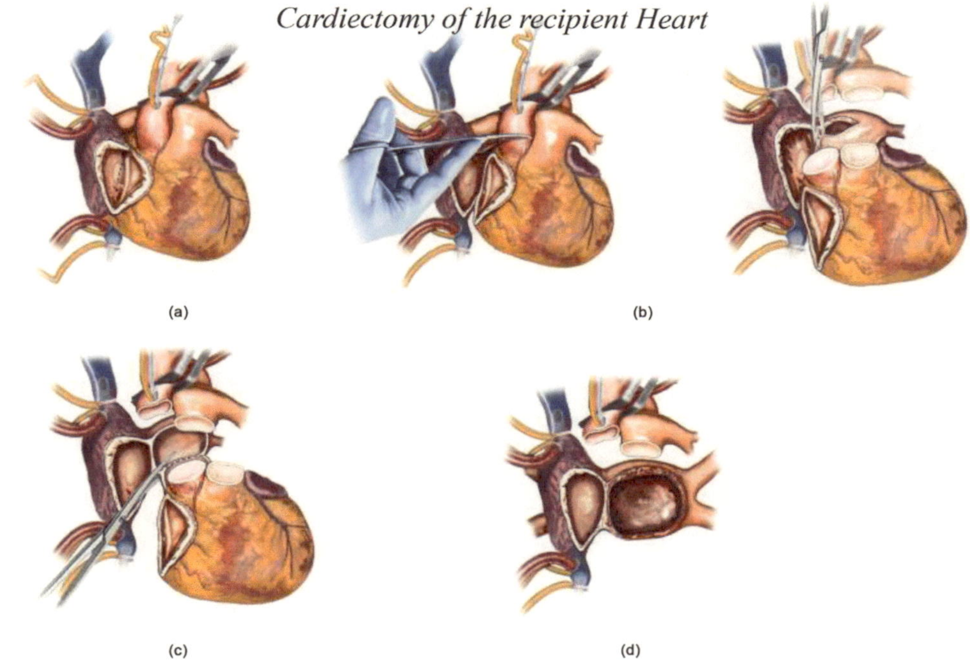

Figure 2.
Recipient's cardiectomy. (a) The recipient's cardiectomy is initiated by opening the right atrium along the atrio-ventricular groove. (b) The great vessels are transected above the semilunar commissures. (c, d), The atria are incised along the atrioventricular grooves, leaving cuffs for allograft implantation.

to the roof of the left atrium between the SCV and the root of the aorta. The great vessels are transected above the semilunar valves (**Figure 2B**). The recipient's cardiectomy is completed by continue to divide the left atrium along the atrioventricular grooves (**Figure 2C** and **D**). The left and right atrial cuffs are then trimmed, including removal of both atrial appendages (**Figure 2D**). Electrocautery is used to separate the proximal ends of the aorta and pulmonary artery to have a clear swing margin and to reduce the bleeding. Right pulmonary artery should be visualized to reduce damaging it during dissection. To achieve a dry field of blood a vent drain is placed at the left atrium remnant directly or through the right superior pulmonary vein.

The stumps of the recipient aorta and pulmonary artery are suspended with stay sutures to retract these structures away from the field to facilitate exposure of the left atrial cuff for anastomosis.

3.2 Donor heart preparation

The donor heart is removed from the transport cooler and placed in a basin of cold saline or cardioplegic solution at the back table. Sharp dissection is used to isolate the aorta from the PA.

The left atrium is tailored to the size of the recipient LA remnant, by connecting the left pulmonary veins orifices with the right pulmonary veins orifices and trimming the access tissues. The interatrial septum is inspected and a patent foramen ovale, if present, is closed. The SVC of the donor heart is ligated, and an incision is made in the

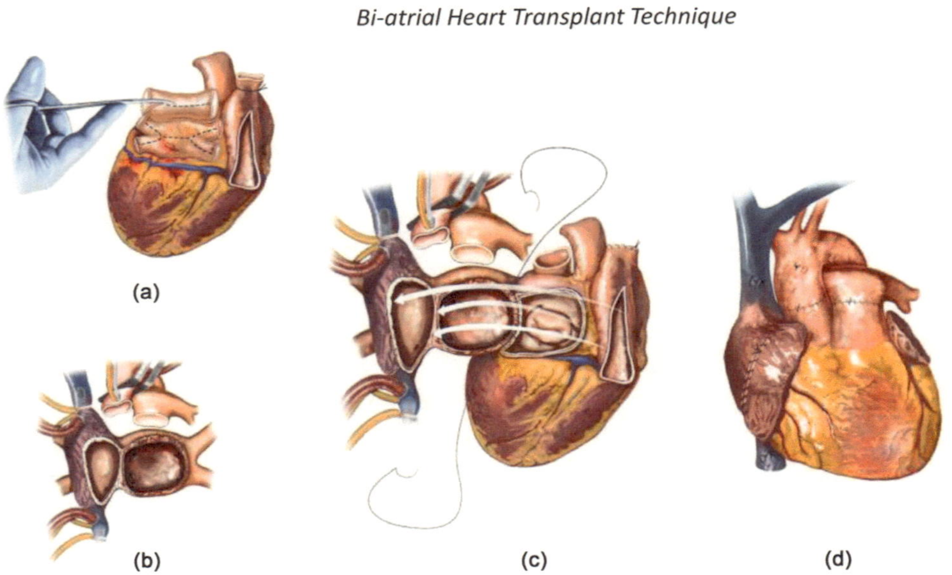

Figure 3.
Bi-atrial heart transplant technique. (a) Preparation of the donor heart at the back table. (b) Recipients atrial cuffs after cardiectomy. (c) Lines of anastomoses for left and right atriums. (d) Final sutures line as seen anteriorly after completion of aortic and PA anastomoses.

posterior wall of the stump of the inferior vena cava and continued toward the SVC and directed away from the sinus node either posteriorly (**Figure 3A**) or toward the right atrial appendage to prevent sinus dysfunction. All valves and cardiac chambers are inspected for vegetation, clots, or foreign bodies. Some surgeons perform donor left appendage ligation at the back table to reduce the risk of the embolization. After finishing this step, the heart is brought to the surgical field for implantation.

3.3 Implantation

Donor heart is held outside the recipient chest cavity on the left side, the back of the heart is faced up. Then implantation starts with running double-armed 3-0 polypropylene suture.

First suture is very important for orientation and runs from the remnant left atrial cuff at the confluence of the left superior and inferior pulmonary veins and through the donor left atrial cuff near the base of donor left appendage. After passing the suture multiple times, the allograft is parachuted into the chest cavity and suturing is continued in a running fashion posteriorly and medially to the inferior aspect of the interatrial septum. Then the second arm is run along the roof of the left atrium till meet with the other end. Assessment of size discrepancy is very important in each suture between the donor and recipient, plication of access tissues might be necessary to achieve good hemostasis and anatomical geometry. Most centers use constant insufflation of carbon dioxide into the mediastinum to reduce the amount of intracardiac air. The right atrial anastomosis is performed in a running fashion similar to the left, with the initial anchor suture placed either at the most superior or inferior aspect of the interatrial septum so that the ends of the suture meet in the middle of the anterolateral wall (**Figure 3C**).

The end-to-end pulmonary artery anastomosis is performed using a 5-0 polypropylene suture beginning with the posterior wall from inside of the vessel and then completing the anterior wall from the outside. It is crucial that the pulmonary artery ends be trimmed to the appropriate length to eliminate any redundancy in the vessel that may cause kinking.

Finally, the aortic anastomosis is performed using 4-0 polypropylene sutures with a technique similar to that for the pulmonary artery, except that some redundancy is desirable in the aorta to facilitate visualization of the posterior suture line. It is important to get good hemostasis for this suture line as bleeding in the posterior wall of the aortic anastomosis is difficult to repair after the heart is reperfused. Toward this end, some surgeons performed a two-layer aortic anastomosis with or without bolstering with a strip of recipient's pericardium (**Figure 3D**).

Re-warming usually is begun at the start of the pulmonary arterial anastomosis. Routine deairing techniques are then employed and temporary pacing wires are placed in the right ventricle and atrium. Lidocaine (100–200 mg intravenously) and methylprednisone (10 mg/kg) is administered, and the aortic cross-clamp is removed. Cardioversion and temporary pacing are usually needed in most patients. A needle vent is inserted in the ascending aorta for final deairing, and infusion of inotropes is initiated, and suture lines are inspected carefully for hemostasis. The patient is weaned from cardiopulmonary bypass, heparin is reversed, and after hemodynamic stability, the cannulas are removed. Following insertion of mediastinal and pleural tubes, the sternotomy incision is closed in the standard fashion.

The advantage of the biatrial technique is its simplicity that allow the operation to be performed quickly and less time on cardiopulmonary bypass. However, when compared with the bicaval technique it has several drawbacks, including a large common (combined donor's and recipient's) right and left atrium, with distorted geometry that can lead to lead to higher incidence of mitral and tricuspid valve incompetence, rhythm disturbances, and tendency of thrombus formation and septal aneurysm [31, 32]. Because of these drawbacks the biatrial technique has been mostly replaced by the bicaval technique.

4. Bi-caval technique of heart transplantation

Sievers and co-workers [33] in 1991, and the Wythenshawe group [16] in 1993, introduced into clinical practice the bi-caval transplantation technique (BC), characterized by two arterial, one left atrial, and two caval anastomoses. The recipient cardiectomy is performed similar as in the biatrial technique, except most of the wall of the right atrium is removed to create SVC and IVC stumps and a cuff of left atrium that contain orifices of all pulmonary veins.

The superiority of the BC technique has been shown in many publications; therefore it has been the preferred techniques in most transplant centers while the biatrial techniques are used only in selected cases [34–40].

4.1 Cardiectomy

Preparation for to place the recipient on cardiopulmonary bypass is as described in the biatrial technique. Native cardiectomy is started out as in the biatrial technique to remove the heart, leaving the left and right atrial cuffs (**Figure 3D**). The anterior and lateral walls of the right atrium are removed, and the SCV and IVC are completely

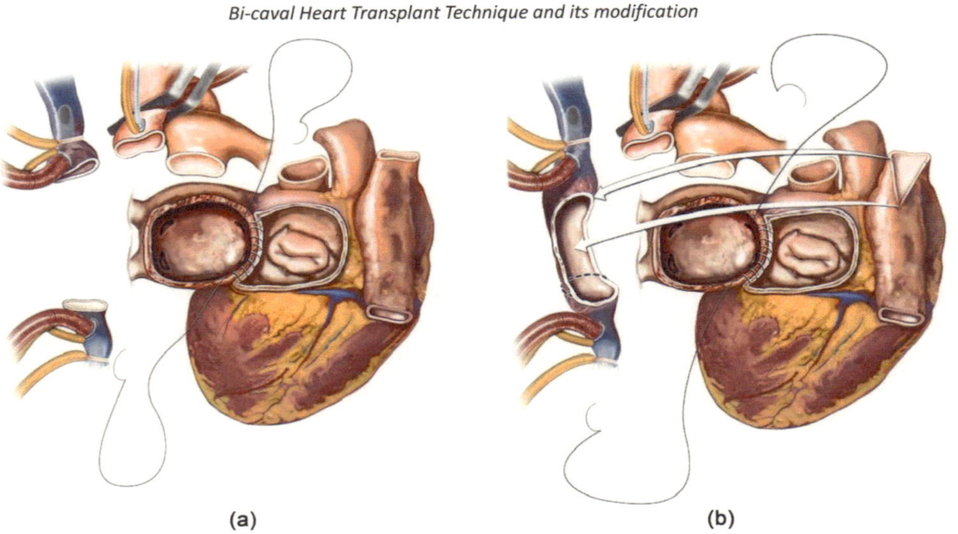

Figure 4.
Bicaval technique of heart transplant. (a) Standard bi-caval technique, which include complete excision of the right atrium and bicaval separation. (b) Modified bi-caval technique, include partial excision of the right atrium by keeping the posterior wall that connects the SVC and IVC.

disconnected from the right atrium in preparation for the end-to-end anastomosis to the corresponding donor cava (**Figure 4A**). Attention should be made to avoid damaging the recipient right pulmonary vein. In addition, the cutting edges of the right and left atria tend to bleed, therefore it is important to get good hemostasis with cautery, or suture ligatures because some areas will be inaccessible after implantation.

4.2 Donor heart preparation

The donor heart preparation for bicaval technique is similar to the to the one for biatrial technique with the exception that the donor right atrium is left intact; the SCV and IVC are not divided posteriorly, and their cut ends are left open (**Figure 4A**).

It is important to leave a generous the donor SCV remnant (usually at or above the azygous vein) to avoid tension on the SCV anastomosis. Therefore, during donor harvesting the SCV should be divided above the junction with the innominate vein.

4.3 Implantation

The most commonly used orthotopic heart transplant technique is today the bicaval technique (**Figure 4A**). As we described in the previous technique, donor heart is held outside the recipient chest cavity on the left side, the back of the heart is faced up. Then implantation starts with running double-armed 3-0 polypropylene suture. First suture is very important for orientation and runs from the remnant left atrial cuff at the confluence of the left superior and inferior pulmonary veins and through the donor left atrial cuff near the base of donor left appendage. After passing the suture multiple times, the allograft is parachuted into the chest cavity and suturing is continued in a running fashion posteriorly and medially to the inferior aspect of the interatrial septum. Then the second arm is run along the roof of the left atrium till meet with the other end. Assessment of size discrepancy is very important in each suture between the donor and recipient, plication of access tissues might be necessary to achieve good hemostasis and anatomical geometry. Individual end-to-end anastomoses of the IVC performed following the left atrial anastomosis. The aortic, pulmonary arterial and IVC and SCV anastomoses can be done in a single aortic cross-clamp. As an alternative, to shorten donor ischemic time, the aortic anastomosis is performed immediately after the left atrial anastomosis and the aortic clamp is removed, allowing the donor heart to be reperfused while the remaining anastomoses are done with the heart beating.

In our practice, after we finish the left atrial anastomosis, we suture the posterior wall of the IVC anastomosis (the anterior wall after removal of the aortic cross clamp). Next, we perform the aortic end-to-end anastomosis with 4-0 polypropylene sutures. We use a strip of recipient's pericardium and incorporated it with the suture line, especially the back wall, to bolster it. Some surgeons use a double layer suturing technique to achieve hemostasis. After completion of the aortic anastomosis, we place temporary pacing wires into the right ventricle, remove the aortic cross clamp after de-airing, and start re-perfusing the heart to reduce the ischemic time.

Most often, the heart needs cardioversion and temporary pacing to keep in an organized rhythm.

Next, the pulmonary arterial anastomosis is performed, using 5-0 polypropylene sutures. We do not tie the sutures it at this stage but use it to remove air from the right ventricle after the caval tapes are removed. To keep the operating field dry, we place a flexible sump suction in the right atrium via the SVC and another in the recipient's pulmonary artery stump. The SVC and the anterior portion of the IVC anastomosis are then completed.

If the donor IVC opening is small, an inverted V cut could be made in the donor IVC opening to accommodate the remaining recipient tissues. At the completion of all anastomoses, the caval tapes are removed, de-airing of the RV is done, and the patient is weaned off cardiopulmonary bypass. After hemostasis is achieved, the sternum is closed in a normal fashion.

5. Modified bi-caval heart transplantation

Modified bi-caval technique was first introduced by Kitamura and Kakuta in Japan, by leaving the posterior atrial bridge of tissue between SCV and IVC intact. The advantages of this technique are: (a) to prevent retraction of the caval stumps that make the anastomosis difficult, (b) to keep the orientation of the caval stumps to prevent twisting of the anastomosis, and (c) to allow for adjusting the sites where the caval anastomoses are done in case of extreme donor-recipient size mismatch with the donor heart much smaller than the recipient's. With the presence of caval snares, the anatomical orientation can be lost, thus the anastomoses may be twisted or kinked. Furthermore, the caval end-to-end anastomosis in the original bicaval technique may become stenotic due to inadequate donor intercaval length in size-mismatched donor, causing excessive tension on the suture line. By leaving a thin strip of the posterior wall of the right atrium as a bridge connecting the superior and inferior venae cavae, it is easy to adjust the amount of atrial excision to the donor heart size. The modified bicaval anastomosis technique allows for an adjustable caval anastomosis to compensate for the size mismatch. The modified bicaval technique may result is lower incidence of late caval anastomotic stricture because the anastomosis can be performed with no tension or kinking. Its advantages have been elucidated in several studies [41–43].

5.1 Cardiectomy

Cardiectomy in modified bi-caval is very similar to the original bi-caval techniques. The only difference is not to completely transect the right atrium. Most of the lateral and anterior walls of the right atrium are resected, leaving the posterior wall intact to connect to the SVC and IVC (**Figure 4B**). The end-to-end caval anastomoses are performed by incorporated the posterior wall of the right atrium into the suture line. In some cases, it is easier to perform the IVC anastomosis if the recipient IVC is disconnected from the native right atrium (**Figure 4B**, dotted line).

This technique will facilitate the orientation of the bicaval anastomoses. In addition, the anastomoses will be easier to perform because there is no retraction of the SVC and IVC cuffs into the caval cannulae. Furthermore, with a V-shape cut in the donor SVC stump (**Figure 4A**), the SVC anastomosis is widened, with less chance of becoming stenotic.

5.2 Donor heart preparation

The donor heart preparation is similar to the bi-caval technique. The only difference is to make a longitudinal (about 3 cm) V shape incision in the posterior aspect of the donor SVC, using the azygos vein as a marker. This incision will help create a wide SVC anastomosis and help orienting the donor SVC (with the apex V corresponding to the posterior midline of the recipient SVC) to prevent twisting.

5.3 Implantation

Implantation of modified bi-caval is very much similar to the original bi-caval technique. However, care should be taken to ligate all opening of thebesian veins in the remnant of the right atrial wall to prevent bleeding.

In our experience, the posterior wall of the IVC anastomosis is better sutured from the assistant's side starting lateral to medial posteriorly and using the other arm the same way anteriorly. The SVC anastomosis starts from the most caudal part of the V shaped cut in the donor side to the middle part of the back wall of the RA with 4-0 polypropylene suture. It is better to tie down the first stitch, then run one arm anterior-lateral, and the other arm anterior-medial, then tie both in the front. As previous techniques, the SVC, IVC, and pulmonary anastomoses can be done after the cross-clamp is removed, which is our preferred technique. Hemostasis is achieved and CPB is weaned, chest is closed in a normal fashion as mentioned before.

6. Total heart transplantation

Yacoub, Banner, and Dreyfus [17, 44, 45] proposed a more anatomical surgical technique of bi-caval implantation, with complete excision of the recipient's right and left atria and direct anastomoses to the left pulmonary veins, right pulmonary veins, IVC and SVC. The rationale for this technique is to avoid non physiological geometry, which can lead to higher incidence of mitral and tricuspid valve incompetence, rhythm disturbances and tendency of thrombus formation and septal aneurysm [31].

6.1 Cardiectomy

Following median sternotomy, vertical pericardiotomy, and CPB establishment as explained previously. Cardiectomy is started in similar way as bicaval technique. The great vessels are transected above the semilunar valves, whereas the atria are incised along the atrioventricular grooves, leaving the right and left atrial cuffs behind. The lateral and anterior wall of the right atrium are removed, and the SVC and IVC are disconnected from the posterior remnant of the right atrium. The special feature of this technical is to separate the left pulmonary veins from the right veins, be excising the back wall of the left atrium to create two separate left atrial cuffs: one on the right that contains the right superior and inferior pulmonary veins, and one on the left with the left superior and inferior pulmonary veins.

6.2 Donor heart preparation

The donor heart preparation is similar as in bi-caval technique. However, harvesting of the donor heart is slightly modified to include the four pulmonary veins intrapericardially. The tissue bridge between the superior and inferior pulmonary veins on each side is divided to create a single left and right orifices. At the end of preparation, the donor left atrium should have two oval openings on each side (**Figure 5**).

6.3 Implantation

This procedure is more technically difficult than the standard bi-caval orthotopic transplantation.

The total anastomosis in this technique is six, including two in left atria. The procedure starts by implanting the left recipient pulmonary vein button to the corresponding orifice on the donor left atrium. Next the right pulmonary vein button is

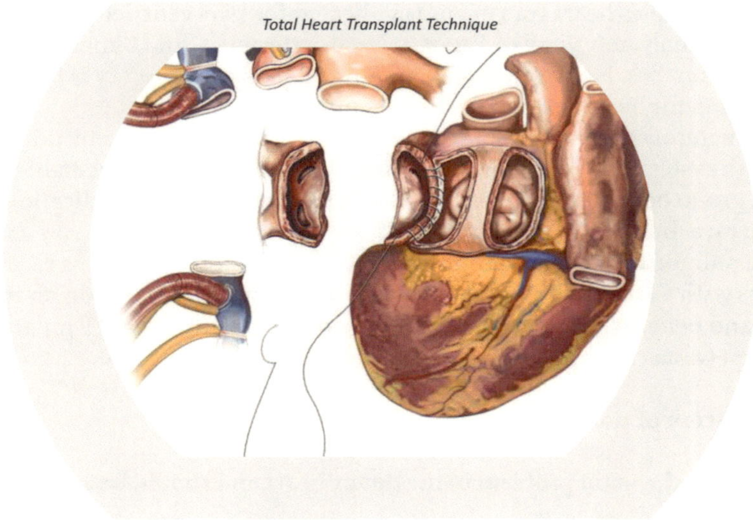

Figure 5.
Total heart transplant include; complete excision of the recipient's left and right atria, leaving separated SVC, IVC, and separate left atrial cuffs around left and right pulmonary veins.

anastomosed to the corresponding orifice on the donor left atrium. The suture line is started on the posterior aspect of both orifices. After finishing this step, the inferior vena cava anastomosis is completed and the rest of the procedure as described before for the bi-caval technique (**Figure 5**).

The disadvantage of this technique includes the marginally prolonged ischemic transplantation time, which is likely of no clinical relevance, as well as the potential for stenosis at the level of the venous anastomoses. Both problems, however, can be avoided with experience. Bleeding in the back wall of the left atrium is more difficult to control. The technique of total heart transplantation is more challenging but without convincing evidence of physiological of clinical advantages over the bicaval technique. Furthermore, with the advance of lung transplantation, a donor often donates a heart and both lungs, making preservation of an intact left atrium during organ retrieval difficult. Therefore, the technique of total heart transplantation has never been widely adopted.

7. Special considerations for heart transplantation in patients with end-stage congenital heart diseases

Techniques of heart transplant in patients with end-stage congenital heart diseases (CHD) is complicated and depends on the anatomical abnormalities. These techniques are beyond the scope of this chapter. However, will go through some special considerations.

CHD are diagnosed during infancy with 59% of the cases during the first year of life, 37% of children age 1–10 years, 23% of adolescent patients age 11–17 years, and 3% of adults [46, 47]. Heart transplant for CHD has some unique challenges, particularly those who have had previous repair or palliation. Over the years, indications for heart transplant in children and infants has changed as most of the CHD advanced recently. Fewer complex single ventricle anomalies required HT as a primary treatment. Many examples heart transplant is indicated for two-ventricle anomalies such as Ebstein's anomaly, tetralogy of Fallot, truncus arteriosus, and Shone's complex, and d-, 1-TGAs anomalies. However, failure of surgical palliative surgery is becoming the main indication for heart transplant in congenital heart diseases.

Visceral heterotaxia may add to surgical complexity but do not contraindicate HT. Patients with systemic complications of Fontan physiology represent a unique and expanding group being referred for HT. Absolute anatomic contraindications to HT in CHD are rare, but may include severe diffuse hypoplasia or pulmonary arteries or irreparable pulmonary venous malformations. The decision on when to recommend HT patients with CHD can be difficult, requiring serious consideration on the long-term risks and benefits. In general, the classic timing of listing for HT for any indication has been when the expected survival at 2 years is 50% [48, 49].

7.1 Consideration of donor heart

Oversizing is the main problem in the donor heart and should be avoided when is selected.

Specially in patient with fixed and scarred mediastinum. The ratio between donor-recipient should not be more than 2:1, with exception in recipients with elevated PAP.

Cardiac and vascular tissues recovered during procurement are very much dependent on recipient anatomy, anomalies, and prior intervention. In general, it is advised to obtain en bloc tissues with the heart such as innominate vein with the SVC, full length of the pulmonary artery including right and left pulmonary arteries branches. Most of the time it is preferred not to have a lung team during recovery and to share tissues.

As we mentioned before, communication between recovery team and transplanting team is very important to reduce the ischemic time, cardiopulmonary bypass time, and unnecessary delay. Communication and timing between both teams is very critical.

7.2 Consideration of operative techniques

As we mentioned HT in CHD usually performed after multiple palliative surgeries, and that could be very challenging due to adhesions and identifying anomalies and corrections previously performed. In addition, vascular access for lines placements can be challenging as will, and sometimes needs direct cutdowns. Topical cooling measures are initiated early, same with defibrillator pads. Extra cushion is taken when performing sternotomy to avoid massive bleeding and air embolization. Most of the time central cannulation is possible in pediatric heart transplantation. However, alternative access should be considered and prepared, such as groins and subclavian or axillaries. It is possible to simplify the CPB by placing a single venous cannula. In difficult cases, deep systematic cooling and circulatory arrest might be needed to finish the transplant. If the pericardial space is small, the left side of the pericardium is excised, and pleural cavity is opened to expand the cavity. Minimizing dissection in that aria is desirable to avoid damaging the phrenic nerve. Multiple techniques have been described for complex cardiac malformation [50, 51]. In the case of abnormal situs and bilateral SVCs, atrial flaps and donor brachycephalic vein, cavo-caval connection could be performed. If the recipient had reconstruction of the brachiocephalic vein, the ascending aorta is kept long to perform retro-aortic vein placement or short to perform ante-aortic vein placement. Usually, the extra donor pulmonary artery tissues are used to correct the native pulmonary anomalies.

In some cases, anastomosis of the pulmonary artery laterally may be required with dextrocardia.

In patients with visceral heterodoxy or situs inversus, where the pulmonary atrium is midline or shifted to the right, the donor heart left pulmonary veins are oversewn, the left atrium is opened between the right pulmonary veins, and then anastomosed to the recipient's right-sided left atrium.

Multiple factors contribute to increased risk of bleeding after HT for CHD. These factors include chronic anticoagulation, liver dysfunction, dense adhesions, multiple thoracotomies, collateral vessels, splanchnic venous congestion, prolonged operative and CPB times, cyanosis, and thrombocytopenia.

8. Summary

The technique of heart transplantation has evolved over more than a century, from an experimental procedure to test the vascular anastomosis to the biatrial, bicaval and total heart transplantation techniques (**Figure 6**). The field has been built on the creativity and tenacity of many people of different disciplines to provide a therapeutic

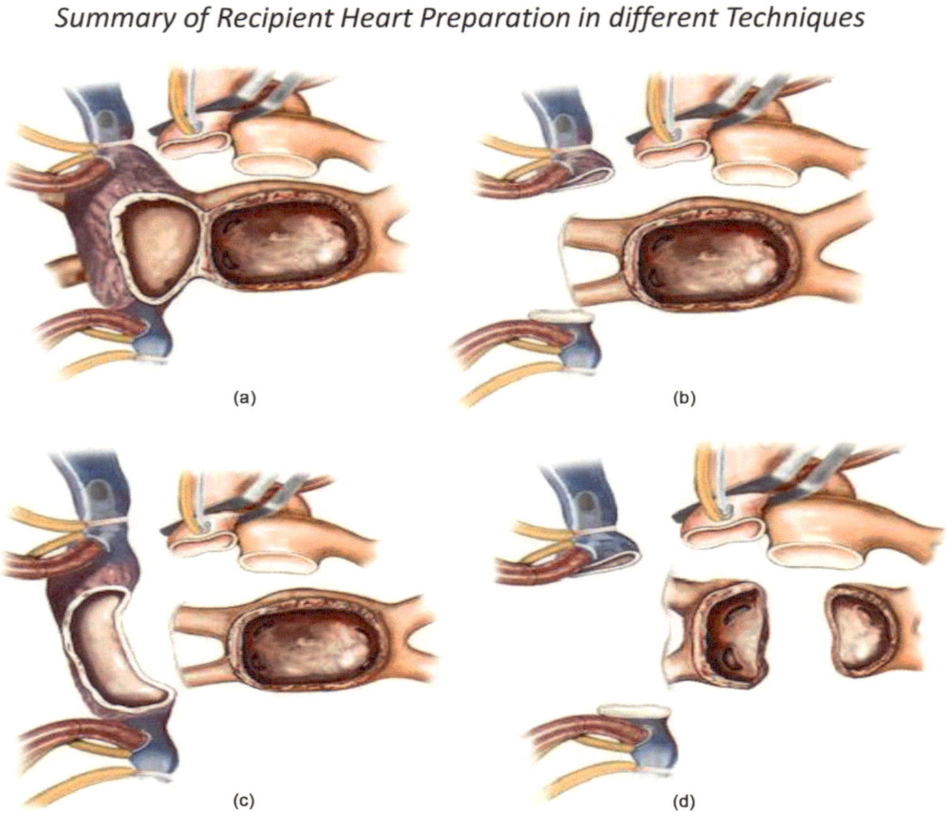

Figure 6.
Summary of recipient's preparation for different heart transplant techniques. Preparations for bi-atrial (a), bi-caval (b), modified bi-caval (c), and total heart transplant (d) techniques.

option that has improved and prolong the lives of many. The field needs similarly talented people and resources to overcome the next frontiers to make the organ last longer with transplantation tolerance, and to expand the donor pool, including donation after circulatory death, and xenografts.

Author details

Samuel Jacob[1,2]*, Anthony N. Pham[3] and Si M. Pham[1,2]

1 Heart and Lung Transplant Program, Mayo Clinic, Jacksonville, FL, United States

2 Mayo Clinic School of Medicine and Science, Rochester, MN, United States

3 Lake Erie College of Osteopathic Medicine, Erie, PA, United States

*Address all correspondence to: jacob.samuel@mayo.edu

References

[1] Kahan BD, Ch'iao P. The legendary exchange of hearts, traditional Chinese medicine, and the modern era of cyclosporine. Transplantation Proceedings. 1988;**20**:2-12

[2] Comroe JH. Who was Alexis who? Bulletin of the Texas Heart Institute. 1979;**6**:251-270

[3] Carrel A, Guthrie CC. The transplantation of veins and organs. American Journal of Medicine. 1905;**10**:1101-1102

[4] Sterioff S, Rucker-Johnson N, Frank C. Mann and transplantation at the Mayo Clinic. Mayo Clinic Proceedings. 1987;**62**:1051-1055

[5] Wu PPT, Mann FC. Histologic studies of autogenous and homogenous transplants of the kidney. Archives of Surgery. 1934;**28**:889-908

[6] Mann FC, Priestley JT, Markowitz J, Yater WM. Transplantation of the intact mammalian heart. Archives of Surgery. 1933;**26**:219-224

[7] Matskeplishvili S. Vladimir Petrovich Demikhov (1916-1998): A pioneer of transplantation ahead of his time, who lived out the end of his life as an unknown and in poor circumstances. European Heart Journal. 2017;**38**(46):3406-3410

[8] Neptune WB, Cookson BA, Bailey CP, Appler R, Rajkowski F. Complete homologous heart transplantation. Archives of Surgery. 1953;**66**:174-178

[9] Lower RR, Shumway N. Studies on the orthotopic homotransplantation of the canine heart. Surgical Forum. 1960;**11**:18-19

[10] Hurley EJ, Dong E, Stofer RC, Shumway NE. Isotopic replacement of the totally excised canine heart. The Journal of Surgical Research. 1962;**2**:90-94

[11] Dong E, Hurley EJ, Lower RR, Shumway NE. Performance of the heart two years after autotransplantation. Surgery. 1964;**56**:270-273

[12] Lower RR, Dong E, Shumway NE. Suppression of rejection crises in the cardiac homograft. The Annals of Thoracic Surgery. 1965;**1**:645-649

[13] Hardy J, Chavez CM, Kurrus FD, Neeley WA, Eraslan S, Turner MD. Heart transplantation in man. JAMA. 1964;**188**:1132-1140

[14] Barnard CN. A human cardiac transplant. An interim report of a successful operation performed at Groote Schuur Hospital, Cape Town. South African Medical Journal. 1967;**41**:1271-1274

[15] Metra M, Ponikowski P, Dickstein K, et al. Advanced chronic heart failure: A position statement from the Study Group on Advanced Heart Failure of the Heart Failure Association of the European Society of Cardiology. European Journal of Heart Failure. 2007;**9**:684-694

[16] Sarsam MA, Campbell CS, Yonan NA, Deiraniya AK, Rahman AN. An alternative surgical technique in orthotopic cardiac transplantation. Journal of Cardiac Surgery. 1993;**8**(3):344-349

[17] Yacoub M, Mankad P, Ledingham S. Donor procurement and surgical techniques for cardiac transplantation. Seminars in Thoracic and Cardiovascular Surgery. 1990;**2**:153-161

[18] Barnard CN, Losman JG. Left ventricular bypass. South African Medical Journal. 1975;**49**(9):303-312

[19] Gaiotto FA, Barbosa Filho ACA, Tenório DF, Steffen SP, Jatene FB. Heterotopic heart transplantation as a left ventricular biological assistance: A new two-stage method proposal. Brazilian Journal of Cardiovascular Surgery. 2020;**35**(6):986-989. DOI: 10.21470/1678-9741-2020-0506

[20] Ono K, Lindsey ES. Improved technique of heart transplantation in rats. The Journal of Thoracic and Cardiovascular Surgery. 1969;**57**:225-229

[21] Adams DH, Chen RH, Kadner A, Nancy S. Technique for heterotopic pig heart xenotransplantation in primates. The Annals of Thoracic Surgery. 1999;**68**:265-268

[22] Reitz B. The history of heart and heart-lung transplantation. In: Baumgartner WR, Achuf SC, editors. Heart and Heart-Lung Transplantation. Philadelphia, PA: WB Saunders; 1990. pp. 1-14

[23] Konstantinov IE. A mystery of Vladimir P. Demikhov: The 50th anniversary of the ®rst intrathoracic transplantation. The Annals of Thoracic Surgery. 1998;**65**:1171-1177

[24] Losman JG, Levine H, Campbell CD, et al. Changes in indications for heart transplantation: An additional argument for the preservation of the recipient's own heart. The Journal of Thoracic and Cardiovascular Surgery. 1982;**84**:716

[25] Novitzky D, Cooper D, Barnard C. The surgical technique of heterotopic heart transplantation. The Annals of Thoracic Surgery. 1983;**36**:476-482

[26] Copeland J, Copeland H. Heterotopic heart transplantation: Technical considerations. Operative Techniques in Thoracic and Cardiovascular Surgery. 2017;**21**:269-280

[27] Tagusari O, Kormos RL, Kawai A, Yamazaki K, Pham SM, Hattler BG, et al. Native heart complications after heterotopic heart transplantation: Insight into the potential risk of left ventricular assist device. The Journal of Heart and Lung Transplantation. 1999;**18**(11):1111-1119

[28] Kotliar C, Smart FW, Sekela ME, Pacifico A, Pratt CM, Noon GP, et al. Heterotopic heart transplantation and native heart ventricular arrhythmias. The Annals of Thoracic Surgery. 1991;**51**(6):987-991

[29] Pham SM, Kormos RL, Griffith BP. Native cardiectomy in a heterotopic heart transplant recipient. The Journal of Thoracic and Cardiovascular Surgery. 1996;**112**(4):1109-1111

[30] DiBardino DJ. The history and development of cardiac transplantation. Texas Heart Institute. 1999;**26**:198-205

[31] Jacob S, Sellke F. Is bicaval orthotopic heart transplantation superior to the biatrial technique? Interactive Cardiovascular and Thoracic Surgery. 2009;**9**:333-342

[32] Fernandez-Gonzales AL, Llorens R, Herreros JM, et al. Intracardiac thrombi after orthotopic heart transplantation: Clinical significance and etiologic factors. The Journal of Heart and Lung Transplantation. 1994;**13**:236-240

[33] Sievers HH, Weyand M, Kraatz EG, Bernhard A. An alternative technique for orthotopic cardiac transplantation, with preservation of the normal anatomy of the right atrium. The Thoracic and Cardiovascular Surgeon. 1991;**39**:70-72

[34] Schnoor M, Schafer T, Luhmann D, Sievers HH. Bicaval versus standard technique in orthotopic heart transplantation: A systematic review and meta-analysis. Journal of Thoracic and Cardiovascular Surgery. 2007;**134**(5):1322-1331

[35] Sun JP, Niu J, Banbury MK, et al. Influence of different implantation techniques on longterm survival after orthotopic heart transplantation: An echocardiographic study. The Journal of Heart and Lung Transplantation. 2007;**26**:1243-1248

[36] Davies RR, Russo MJ, Morgan JA, et al. Standard versus bicaval techniques for orthotopic heart transplantation: An analysis of the united network for organ sharing database. The Journal of Thoracic and Cardiovascular Surgery. 2010;**140**:700

[37] Weiss ES, Nwakanma LU, Russell SB, Conte JV, Shah AS. Outcomes in bicaval versus biatrial techniques in heart transplantation: An analysis of the UNOS database. The Journal of Heart and Lung Transplantation. 2008;**27**:178-183

[38] Czer LS, Cohen MH, Gallagher SP, Czer LA, Soukiasian HJ, Rafiei M, et al. Exercise performance comparison of bicaval and biatrial orthotopic heart transplant recipients. Transplantation Proceedings. 2011;**43**(10):3857-3862

[39] Aleksic I, Freimark D, Blanche C, et al. Does total orthotopic heart transplantation offer improved hemodynamics during cellular rejection events? Transplantation Proceedings. 2003;**35**(1532):2000

[40] Locali RF, Matsuoka PK, Cherbo T, Gabriel EA, Buffolo E. Should biatrial heart transplantation still be performed? A meta-analysis. Arquivos Brasileiros de Cardiologia. 2010;**94**(6):829-840

[41] Kitamura S, Nakatani T, Bando K, Sasako Y, Kobayashi J, Yagihara T. Modification of bicaval anastomosis technique for orthotopic heart transplantation. The Annals of Thoracic Surgery. 2001;**72**(4):1405-1406

[42] Kakuta T, Fukushima S, Shimahara Y, Yajima S, Kawamoto N, Tadokoro N, et al. Benefits of the modified bicaval anastomosis technique for orthotopic heart transplantation from a size-mismatched marginal donor. Circulation Journal. 2019;**84**(1):61-68

[43] Kitamura S, Nakatani T, Kato T, Yanase M, Kobayashi J, Nakajima H, et al. Hemodynamic and echocardiographic evaluation of orthotopic heart transplantation with the modified bicaval anastomosis technique. Circulation Journal. 2009;**73**(7):1235-1239

[44] Banner NR, Khaghani A, Fitzgerald M, Mitchell AG, Radley-Smith R, Yacoub MH. The expanding role of cardiac transplantation. In: Unger F, editor. Assisted Circulation. Berlin: Springer-Verlag; 1989

[45] Dreyfus G, Jebara V, Mihaileanu S, Carpentier AF. Total orthotopic heart transplantation: An alternative to the standard technique. The Annals of Thoracic Surgery. 1991;**52**:1181-1184

[46] Kirk R, Dipchand AI, Edwards LB, et al. The registry of the international society for heart and lung transplantation: Fifteenth pediatric heart transplantation report—2012. The Journal of Heart and Lung Transplantation. 2012;**31**:1065-1086

[47] Stehlik J, Edwards LB, Kucheryavaya AY, et al. The registry of the society for international heart and lung transplantation: 29th official adult heart transplant report—2012. The Journal of Heart and Lung Transplantation. 2012;**31**:1052-1064

[48] Pincott ES, Burch M. Indications for heart transplantation in congenital heart disease. Current Cardiology Reviews. 2011;7:51-58

[49] Almond CSD, Thiagarajan RR, Piercey GE, et al. Waiting list mortality among children listed for heart transplantation in the United States. Circulation. 2009;**119**:717-727

[50] Vricella LA, Razzouk AJ, Gundry SR, et al. Heart transplantation in infants and children with situs inversus. The Journal of Thoracic and Cardiovascular Surgery. 1998;**116**:82-86

[51] del Nido PJ, Bailey LL, Kirklin JK. Surgical techniques in pediatric heart transplantation. ISHLT Monograph Series. 2007;**2**:83-102

Section 5

Immunosupprresive Therapy

Chapter 9

Induction Therapy in the Current Immunosuppressive Therapy

Takuya Watanabe, Yasumasa Tsukamoto, Hiroki Mochizuki, Masaya Shimojima, Tasuku Hada, Satsuki Fukushima, Tomoyuki Fujita and Osamu Seguchi

Abstract

The current immunosuppressive therapy including calcineurin inhibitors, mycophenolate mofetil, and steroids, has substantially suppress rejections and improved clinical outcomes in heart transplant (HTx) recipients. Nevertheless, the management of drug-related nephrotoxicity, fatal acute cellular rejection (ACR), antibody-mediated rejection and infections remains challenging. Although previous some studies suggested that perioperative induction immunosuppressive therapy may be effective for the suppressing ACR and deterioration of renal function, increased incidence of infection and malignancy was concerned in recipients with induction immunosuppressive therapy. The international society of heart and lung transplantation (ISHLT) guidelines for the care of heart transplant recipients do not recommend routine use of induction immunosuppressive therapy, except for the patients with high risk of acute rejection or renal dysfunction, however, appropriate therapeutic regimen and indication of induction immunosuppressive therapy remains unclear in HTx recipients. We review current evidence of induction immunosuppressive therapy in HTx recipients, and discuss the appropriate therapeutic regimen and indication of induction therapy.

Keywords: induction therapy, interleukin-2 receptor antagonists, polyclonal anti-thymocyte antibodies, acute cellular rejection, renal dysfunction

1. Introduction

Triple immunosuppressive therapy including calcineurin inhibitors (CNI), anti-metabolites, and steroids, has substantially improved clinical outcomes for heart transplant (HTx) recipients. Nevertheless, the management of CNI-related nephrotoxicity, fatal acute cellular rejection (ACR), antibody-mediated rejection (AMR), and infections remains challenging [1]. Immunosuppressive regimens for organ transplantation can be generally characterized as induction, maintenance, or rescue therapies [2]. Recently, desensitization therapy has also been considered for recipients who are highly sensitized to Human leukocyte antigen (HLA) or have donor specific HLA antibodies [3]. Induction immunosuppressive therapy is a powerful and prophylactic therapy that is used perioperatively to prevent episodes of acute rejection, which is expected to improve the clinical prognosis or make their managements easier in high-risk HTx recipients. Currently, approximate 50% of HTx recipients employ a strategy of induction therapy, however, international clinical guidelines do not recommend the routine use of induction immunosuppressive therapy since the impact of induction therapy on survival in HTx recipients remains unclear [1]. In the more recent clinical situation, tacrolimus, which is recent alternative choice of cyclosporine, significantly reduces the incidence of ACR. And desensitization therapy is also becoming an established medical treatment for sensitized HTx recipients. Appropriate indications and therapeutic regimens for administering induction immunosuppressive therapy to HTx recipients requires further consideration in the recent clinical situations.

This manuscript will provide an overview of the induction immunosuppressive therapy up to now, and future perspective of the induction immunosuppressive therapy in the new era of the current more established immunosuppression.

2. Induction immunosuppressive therapy in HTx

2.1 Immune response system in transplant recipients

Immune response system that influences the rejection in transplant recipients is divided into two categories depending on the immune cells that primarily work, although each response influences the other; T-cell-mediated and antibody-mediated immune response.

2.1.1 T-cell mediated immune response

T-cell mediated immune response system in transplanted recipients is generally explained from three pathway; direct and semi-direct pathway which donor antigen presentation cell (APC) affect, and indirect pathway which recipient APC (**Figure 1**) [2]. Thymic selection in the native thymus occurs without regard for donor-specific allo-antigens. The naïve T cell has a relatively high allo-specific precursor frequency (**Precursor frequency**). This process can be nonspecifically reduced by depletion induction immunosuppressive agents including anti-thymocyte antibodies (ATG), muromonab-CD3 (OKT3), and alemtuzumab (**Figure 1a**). Allo-antigen is presented via donor (direct or semi-direct) or recipient-itself (indirect) APCs in the secondary lymphoid tissues inducing naïve T cell activation (**Antigen presentation**). In transplantation, graft derived APCs likely dominate this process early through reperfusion induced mobilization to the secondary lymphoid tissue and direct pathway. This pathway gives way to recipient derived migratory APCs later through indirect mechanisms and may also be influenced by semi-direct presentation of intact donor HLA by recipient cells. T-cell depleting agents, Interleukin 2 receptor (IL2R) blockage, and methylprednisolone limit this process (**Figure 1b**). T-cell activation occurs as an aggregate effect of many spectral processes (**Activation threshold**). Given that T cells have long been known to be important in rejection, some maintenance immunosuppressive agents including CNI, anti-metabolites and mammalian target of rapamycin (mTOR) inhibitors also alter the threshold of activation of T-cell also affect this process (**Figure 1b** and **c**). T-cells activation in the secondary lymphoid and injured endothelium and ischemic injury (**Figure 1A**) attenuates platelet and

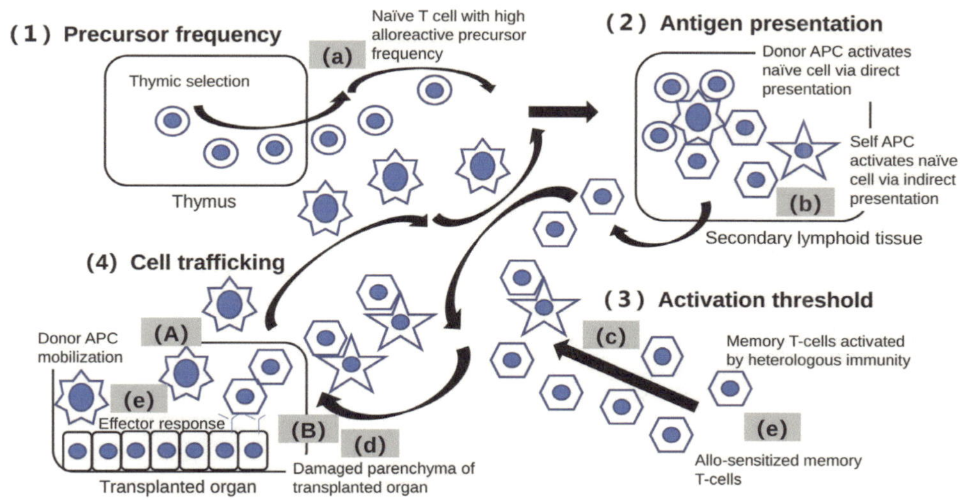

Figure 1.
T-cell mediated immune response.

complement binding and activation thus activating endothelial cells and donor APCs, initiating chemotactic signals, and providing signals to lower the activation threshold of local effector cells (**Figure 1B**). The local cytokine milieu reinforces local cell activation and can be inhibited by IL2R-specific agents, methylprednisolone, CNIs and mTOR inhibitors (**Figure 1d**). Allo-sensitized memory cells and cells activated through heterologous immunity or homeostatic proliferation bypass the need for nodal presentation. Depletion agents can both attenuate and augment this effect (**Figure 1e**). Activated T cells and recipient APCs are attracted to the graft site by chemokines and adhesion molecule expression (**Cell Trafficking**). Reperfusion injury initiates donor derived APCs to mobilize toward the nodes for direct pathway. Depletion agents, polyclonal antibody and methylprednisolone limit chemotaxis and/or adhesion. Cytotoxic T lymphocyte (CTL) encounter the graft in sufficient numbers to cause clinical damage, and are reenforced by a milieu rich in T cell derived cytokines (e.g. IL-2) (**Effector response**). Damage to the organ occurs through contact dependent CTL activity and through the direct effect of cytolytic cytokines (e.g. TNF-α). Depletion agents and selective IL-2 receptor antibodies limits the productiveness of this response and prevents the attainment of milieu that is supportive of CTL activity (**Figure 1e**).

2.1.2 Antibody-mediated immune response

Anti-body mediated rejection (AMR) is a major limitation to long-term HTx survival and is mainly driven by antibodies directed against the mismatched HLA Class I and Class II antigens (HLA antibodies) expressed on the allograft. Pre-sensitized patients who possess HLA antibodies are disadvantaged by having to wait longer to receive an organ from suitably matched donor. The number of pre-sensitized patients has been increasing, a trend that is likely due to the increased use of mechanical circulatory assist devices [4]. The humoral immune system is responsible for antibody production, which leads to AMR (**Figure 2**) [5]. Naïve B-cells are produced in the bone marrow and become activated in secondary lymphoid tissues when antigen

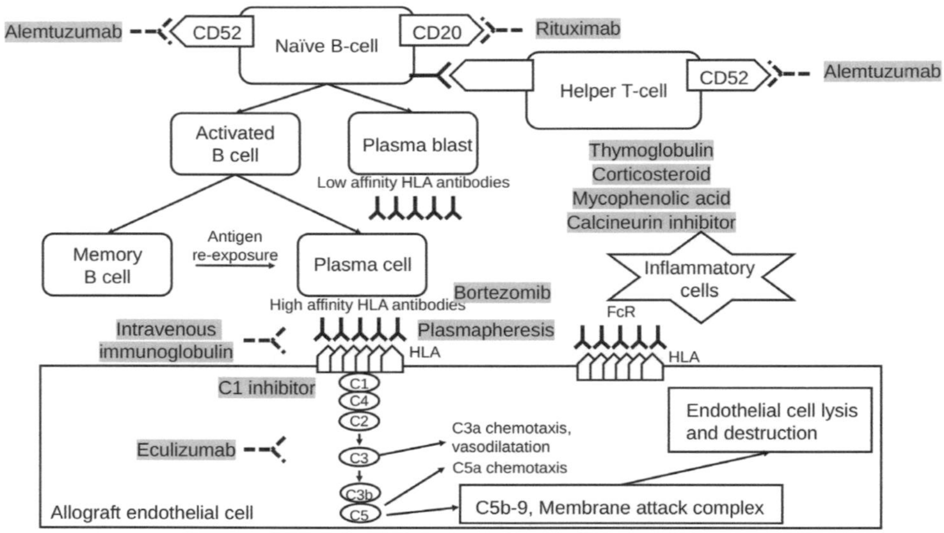

Figure 2.
Antibody-mediated immune response.

is encountered in the presence of APC and T-helper cells. Activated B-cells develop either into plasma blast secreting low-affinity antibody or interact with follicular dendritic and T-helper cells to form germinal centers [6]. Within germinal centers, B-cells undergo proliferation, hypermutation and affinity maturation to become high-affinity antibody-secreting plasma cells or memory B-cells. Plasma cells migrate back to the bone marrow, whereas memory B-cells circulate through secondary lymphoid organs and in the peripheral circulation. Upon re-exposure to antigen, memory B-cells rapidly proliferate and differentiate into plasma cells, producing high-affinity class-switched antibodies. Sensitized patients, who have already donor-specific antibodies pre-transplantation or memory B-cells against donor HLA by previous exposure, have high risk of hyperacute humoral rejection after HTx. In addition, antibody-mediated allograft injury occurs through complement pathway activation. HLA antibody-antigen complexes on allograft endothelial cells activate C1 triggering complement cascade activation and formation of the C5b-9 membrane attack complex to cause endothelial-cell lysis and destruction. Complement products also cause injury through recruitment of inflammatory cells (C3a, C4a, C5a), mast-cell histamine release (C5a), upregulation of endothelial adhesion molecules (C5a), tissue factor synthesis and thrombotic injury (C5a, C5b-9) and Weibel-Palade bodies (WPB) exocytosis [7]. DSA also exert harmful effects independent of complement activation through Fc-receptor recruitment of inflammatory cells and release of inflammatory mediators. The resulting cellular inflammation, thrombosis, hemorrhage and lysis cause allograft injury and dysfunction.

Desensitization therapy is a specific and important option for increasing donor pool and access to transplantation for the sensitized patient, which reduces or eliminates HLA antibody and/or facilitates transplantation in the presence of DSA. Since T-B-cell interaction is also associated with the plsma-cell antibody production, T-cell directed therapy including mycophenolate acid is also considered as a desensitization therapy. ATG, an option for induction therapy, binds to cell surface antigens on T cells to injure and reduce T cells. Since humoral immune responses are suppressed when helper T cell function is reduced, ATG has the effect of decreasing sensitization by suppressing T-B cell interactions. Other agents specific to desensitization do not necessarily suppress the T dell mediated immune response. Previous consensus report suggests that post-transplant induction therapy as well as standard maintenance immunosuppression is recommended to prevent rejection in patients who have undergone desensitization [8].

2.2 Induction therapy in the current clinical situation

Historically, all organ transplantation employed induction regimens using some immunosuppressive agents [2]. Their strategies include preoperative high dose therapy with maintenance drugs, including glucocorticosteroids, antimetabolites and intravenous CNI, or specialized induction agents such as antibodies or infusion proteins. The concept that more immunosuppression is required early after transplantation is well established regarding induction therapies to prevent rejections. Specialized induction immunosuppressive agents which do not affect worsening renal function are used in the early perioperative management of patients with known or worsening renal insufficiency, as it may enable delayed initiation with calcineurin inhibitors to prevent the development of acute renal failure. Major concerns of induction therapy may be increased risk of infection and malignancy. Specialized induction immunosuppressive agents can largely be divided into two categories: depleting antibodies and non-depleting antibodies [2]. Depleting antibodies include both monoclonal (OKT3 and alemtuzumab) and polyclonal (ATG) antibodies. Depleting antibodies reduce alloreactive T cells at the time of transplantation, in turn suppressing host response to the allograft. As depleting antibodies acts primitive T-cell and also indirectly suppresses the anti-body mediated response via B-cell, resulting in a stronger suppression of immune responses more than non-depleting antibodies. While, as nondepleting antibodies inhibit T-cell activities which acts against a downstream of immune-response cascade (such as IL-2-driven cell proliferation), it may suppress rejections more specifically.

2.2.1 Current trend of Induction therapy regimens

Cai and Terasaki reviewed renal transplant recipients in the United Network for Organ Sharing (UNOS) database, [9] there had been three distinct time periods of induction regimens: (1) 1987–1993, the old, low-induction antibody era, when fewer than 30% of all kidney recipients received induction therapy, consisting mostly (80%) of anti-lymphocyte globulin or OKT3; (2) 1994–2002, the transitional, high-induction antibody era, when approximately 80% of kidney transplant recipients received induction therapy, and anti-lymphocyte globulin and OKT3 starting to be replaced by daclizumab (1998), basiliximab (1998), and rATG (1999); and (3) 2003–2010, the modern high-induction antibody era, with induction therapy remaining high, more than 80% of all transplant patients receiving induction therapy, mostly rATG, basiliximab, daclizumab, or alemtuzumab (2003). Regarding to HTx recipients, Whitson et al. evaluated the usefulness of induction therapy using UNOS database from 2001 to 2012 in HTx recipients [10]. Of the 17,857 HTx recipients, 8216 (46%) recipients had induction therapy; 55% were IL-2R antibodies (IL-2RA), 40% some depletion agents including ATG, and 4% alemtuzumab. Nozohoor et al., reviewed 27,369 adult HTx recipients in the International Society for Heart and Lung Transplantation (ISHLT) registry database, showed that 11,681 (43%) recipients had induction therapy; 59% were ATG and 41% basiliximab [11]. Tzani et al. showed the trend in induction therapy utilization in patients who underwent HTx from 1990 to 2020, using UNOS Registry Standard Analysis and Research database [12]. The utilization of induction therapy gradually increased, reaching almost 50% in 2006, and then maintained similarly until 2016, with a recent gradual decrease to almost 40 % of all HTx in 2020. The use of alemtuzumab and OKT3 decreased significantly while the use of IL-2RA and ATG increased, and since 2003, IL-2RA has been used primarily as induction therapy. The international registry data base has also showed that almost 50% of HTx programs employ a strategy of induction therapy. Although multitude induction agents are available as mentioned above, IL-2RA and polyclonal ATG were commonly used [1].

2.2.2 Current clinical implication of induction therapy

The purpose of induction therapy is primarily to achieve high intensity immunosuppression early in the postoperative period to reduce the incidence of rejection and to delay the initiation of nephrotoxic immunosuppression with CNI in recipients with compromised renal function [9]. In addition, reduced risk of incidence of rejection may result in suppressing the development of cardiac allograft vasculopathy [13]. The potential disadvantage of induction therapy is the increased risk of infection in early phase and malignancy in the long-term post-HTx [13]. A previous meta-analysis showed that acute rejection might be reduced by induction therapy compared with no induction, and did not show other clear survival benefits or harms associated with the use of any kind of T-cell antibody induction agents compared with no induction [14]. Another systematic review showed that patients receiving induction therapy had similar risk of moderate-to-severe rejection, all-cause death, infection, and cancer with patients who did not receive induction therapy [15]. A more recent retrospective analysis using large cohort date of UNOS registry showed that induction therapy was associated with lower mortality and treated rejection episodes than no induction therapy [12].

In the current clinical situation, the improvement and establishment of new maintenance immunosuppression agents such as tacrolimus replaced cyclosporine and mycophenolate mofetil replaced azathioprine have significantly reduced risk of acute T-cell mediated rejection in acute phase post-HTx, which may lead that previously observed benefits of induction therapy tend to decrease overtime. Thus, although the clinical need of induction therapy to suppress T-cell mediated rejection may be decreasing, younger patients, multiparous women, African Americans, patients with longer term ventricular assist device, [16] and patients with long ischemic time [17] may be still good indication for the induction therapy in HTx. On the other hand, long awaiting time for HTx due to the severe donor shortage and increasing in the implantation of left ventricular assist device pre-HTx have increased risk of sensitization and pre-existing renal dysfunction before HTx. Highly sensitized patients, and those with positive cross-match may also have been considered as the candidate for the induction therapy in the past, however, since evidence for desensitization therapy is being established, truly high risk patients for hyperacute antibody-mediated rejection with high intensity of donor-specific should be considered more specific desensitization rather than introduction immunosuppressive therapy. And induction therapy may be generally used in combination with desensitization therapy, not induction therapy alone [3, 5]. Patients with pre-existing renal dysfunction may still be the best indication of induction therapy in the current clinical situation [17–20].

2.3 Specific agents for induction therapy

There are many specialized induction agents that are now being used to target the components of immunity heightened during transplantation. Although there is positive evidence in randomized trials and prospective studies comparing with standard maintenance regimens, no-induction or methylprednisolone induction, most trials use the surrogate endpoint of acute rejection, rather than more definitive outcome measures such as patient or graft survival. Several induction regimens have shown to measurably increase the risk of posttransplant lymphoproliferative disease (PTLD) and death from malignancy when combined with conventional maintenance immunosuppression [21]. This manuscript focuses on two specific induction immunosuppressive agents which were commonly used in current clinical situations; ATG and IL-2RA.

2.3.1 Polyclonal antibody

ATG is a polyclonal antibody derived from immunization of mainly rabbits with human thymocytes. The final product includes antibodies against multiple cell surface proteins, and HLA class 1 heavy chains, and is effective in preventing cellular immune responses against a variety of antigenic stimuli, through substantial lymphocyte depletion. Namely, ATGs bind to several antigens on T- and B-cells, causing T- and B-lymphocyte depletion. Given their broad spectrum of specificity, they have frequently been suggested to mediate their anti-rejection properties through means other than depletion, including costimulation blockade, adhesion molecule modulation, and B cell depletion. ATG is the most commonly used induction agent. Around 20% of HTx recipients receive ATG as induction therapy. There are no studies comparing ATG induction therapy with no induction therapy [15], and the efficacy of ATG induction therapy has been investigated in comparison with induction therapy with IL-2RAs which already showed the significant reduction of rejections. A large multicenter study has observed lower rates of rejection and an increased risk of infection with ATG [22].

The xenogeneic (horse or rabbit) origin of ATG may induce a host antibody response leading to acute hypersensitivity response or rarely, serum sickness on subsequent exposure, which is characterized by fevers, chills, tachycardia, hypertension or hypotension, myalgias, and rash, and may occur after the first dose. Rarely, cytokine release syndrome can occur. Furthermore, these ATGs cannot be used repeatedly for rejection to avoid a second or subsequent allergic reaction. ATG mat be left aside for future refractory rejections, not using for introduction.

2.3.2 Interleukin 2 receptor antibody

The high affinity alpha chain IL2 receptor (CD25) was the first molecule to be successfully targeted with a humanized monoclonal antibody in solid organ transplantation. IL-2RA act through the binding of the IL-2 receptor located on activated T-cells, thereby inhibiting the proliferation and differentiation of T-lymphocytes. Basiliximab is a monoclonal antibody that selectively binds to the IL-2 receptor of T-lymphocytes, blocks binding of IL-2 to the receptor complex, and inhibits IL-2 mediated T-lymphocyte proliferation [23]. Daclizumab is a humanized anti-IL-2R (CD25) monoclonal antibody that has the murine antigen-binding sequences molecularly engrafted onto a human antibody [24]; however, daclizumab has since been discontinued by the manufacturer due to diminishing use. Basiliximab is notable for a significantly lower incidence in drug-related adverse events [25], compared with other specialized agents for induction therapy. Cytokine release syndrome has not been reported after administration of this type of drug.

Three randomized trials have compared with IL-2RA vs. no induction [23, 24, 26]. A systematic review including these randomized trials showed that IL-2RAs significantly reduced the risk of acute rejection. However, because these randomized trials had a high risk of bias despite randomization, this significant superiority of the IL-2 receptor was not clear according to the random effects model. Its survival benefits were also not found [27]. Furthermore, most of the studies to date have been in HTx recipients who received cyclosporine rather than tacrolimus for primary immunosuppression, with limited evidence in the new immunosuppression era. Watanabe et al. in HTx recipients receiving tacrolimus showed that basiliximab-based induction immunosuppressive therapy might suppress mild acute cellular rejection, and improve renal function in recipients with deteriorated renal function, and resulting in the its non-inferior outcome as compared to no-induction group even in recipients with any comorbidity [17].

2.3.3 Current evidence of comparison ATG vs. IL-2 RA

Although two randomized controlled trials demonstrated that the IL-2RA, daculizmab, effectively reduced the rate of moderate and severe rejections within first year after HTx [12, 23, 24], such effect could not be observed in trials for ATG. Previous systematic review which evaluated four randomized trials comparing of ATG with IL-2RA [28–31] showed that the use of IL-2RA was associated with significantly higher risk of moderate-to-severe rejection than ATG, but similar risk of death, infections, and malignancy [15]. In the retrospective analyses using large registry or cohort data in HTx, Nozohoor et al. [11] suggested that the recipients receiving ATG showed the better survival as compared with those receiving IL-2RA, however, found more malignancy post-HTx with ATG compared with basiliximab. Tzani et al. [12] showed that ATG has lower risk of treated rejection and mortality as compared with IL-2RA. And Ansari et al. in the retrospective analysis showed similar one-year survival between ATG and IL-2RA, but IL-2RA exhibited decreased long-term survival compared with ATG at 5 years and 10 years post-HTx [32]. On the other hand, Mazimba et al. [33] showed a conflict results when patients were stratified using risk of infection and rejection; IL-2RA was lower incidence of rejection but increased costs for infection in the patients with low risk of rejection and high risk of infection, and had significant lower incidence of rejection in patients with high risk of rejection and low risk infection as compared with ATG. A potential disadvantage of induction therapy is a risk of malignancies induced by its excessive immunosuppression in the long-term post-HTx [34]. ATG depletes cytotoxic T lymphocytes against organisms and virus infected cells as well as transplant organs. Therefore, ATG-based induction therapy may cytotoxic T lymphocytes against Epstein Barr virus (EBV) and EBV infected B lymphocytes which may result in primary-like EBV infection and EBV related B cell type posttransplant lymphoproliferative disorder (PTLD). Most previous studies did not show the difference of the incidence of malignancy between ATG- and IL-2RA-based induction therapies. Nozohoor et al. showed that the use of ATG may be associated with increased malignancy-related mortality, compared with no-induction [11]. Especially in pediatric HTx, ATG-based induction therapy tends to be preferred to IL-2RA-based induction therapy in younger patients, in those with congenital heart diseases, in patients requiring pre-transplant inotropic or mechanical support, and in more sensitized patients or those with longer ischemic time [35]. Children are at greatly increased risk of PTLD versus adults, and PTLD is the most common form of post-transplant malignancy in children [36]. Although the relative rarity of PTLD makes an accurate assessment of the effect of specific immunosuppressive agents difficult, a recent review concluded no increased risk of PTLD in children given ATG after pediatric HTx [35]. They speculated that it is possible that this reduction in risk may have arisen from the general trend towards less intensive maintenance therapy in recent years. ATG-based induction may also have been used to facilitate CNI-sparing or steroid sparing therapy in pediatric HTx, potentially lowering risk the risk for PTLD.

Regarding maintenance immunosuppression, tacrolimus is more potent than cyclosprone and has proven to reduce rejection rates as well as an effective rescue agent for patients with recurrent or refractory acute allograft rejection. Tacrolimus has replaced cyclosporine in many transplant centers and currently. This raises the question about effectiveness of induction therapy in current tacrolimus-based immunosuppression era. Ali et al. performed meta-analysis to explore the effect of IL-2RA vs ATG on morbidity and mortality in renal transplant patients receiving tacrolimus-based maintenance immunosuppressive therapy, which revealed no significant difference in patient and graft survival when using IL-2RA vs ATG with the tacrolimus-based maintenance immunosuppression. The difference in efficacy between ATG and basiliximab in the era of newer immunosuppressive agents needs to be explored in HTx recipients.

ATG and IL-2RA may not be compared identically as induction therapy because the pharmacological mechanisms of action, response range, and safety of the two immunosuppressive agents are very different. Induction therapy with desensitization in highly sensitized patients or patients with donor specific antibodies may be not sufficient for basiliximab, and ATG should be selected as induction therapy. On the other hand, if induction therapy is administered because of concerns about worsening renal function immediately after transplantation in non-sensitized recipients, ATG may not be appropriate because it may lead to excessive immunosuppression, and the use of safer may be appropriate. Furthermore, since xenogeneic origin of ATG, ATGs cannot be used repeatedly for rejection to avoid a second or subsequent allergic reaction, ATG may require to be left aside for future refractory rejections.

3. Future perspective regarding the induction therapy

3.1 Appropriate indication for induction therapy

The appropriate indications for administering induction therapy have not been established. Previous studies suggested that recipients with an increased risk of rejection, which were younger patients, multiparous women, African Americans, patients with longer term ventricular assist device [16], and patients with long ischemic time [17], are good indication for the induction therapy in HTx, as well as recipients with deteriorated renal function. Watanabe et al. proposed the original indication criteria which included potential difficulty in patient management including donor or recipient older age, impairment of cardiac function or pre-existing coronary atherosclerosis of donor heart in early phase after HTx which may cause intolerance to immunosuppression.

3.2 Appropriate regimens for induction therapy

There is currently no consensus regarding the dose or duration of induction agents in different types of HTx recipients, or the timing and intensity of initial CNI therapy in recipients receiving induction therapy. The immunosuppression protocols for administering induction therapy varies according to the dosage of CNI administered and applies to those recipients who require CNI withdrawal with cytolytic therapy for renal dysfunction or as a modification of the standard triple immunosuppression regimen [23, 24, 27]. And these regimens influence perioperative over- or under immunosuppression particularly, and need to be careful in patients with administered induction therapy. Minimization and optimization of baseline immunosuppressive agents may be useful for improving clinical outcomes. Regarding the optimization of maintenance immunosuppression, some landmark trials in CNI minimization and withdrawal shows the clinical usefulness, however, perioperative optimization in immunosuppression in patients with induction therapy is still controversial [23, 24, 27]. When considering the optimal immunosuppressive regimen with induction therapy, it may be useful to monitor the degree of immunosuppression. Previous review paper suggested that CD3 monitoring, or absolute lymphocyte count is useful to guide ATG dosing [35]. Where this approach is applied, the previous ISHLT guideline advise targeting a CD3 count in the range of 25–50 cells/mm^3, or an absolute total lymphocyte count <100–200 cells/mm^3 [37]. A previous small sample retrospective study showed the patient group managed with CD3 monitoring received a significantly lower total ATG dose, although clinical outcome including survival, rejection and infection did not differ [38]. Regarding IL-2RA based induction therapy, CD25 which expressed on activated T lymphocytes may be useful for assessing the effects of IL-2RA. A previous study monitoring the CD25 count to evaluate the effect of IL2-RA showed that a 2-dose regimen of basiliximab-based induction therapy administered on Day 0 and Day 4 after transplantation still suppressed T-lymphocyte activation for an average 40–50 days after renal transplantation [39]. Watanabe et al. performed an original regimen that CNI dosage was slowly increased to prevent further deterioration of renal dysfunction due to CNI-induced kidney injury for the recipients with renal dysfunction, and to prevent over-immunosuppression for the pretransplant sensitized recipients; trough level of tacrolimus in the induction group was significantly lower than that in the no-induction group until 3 weeks post-HTx. However, recipients receiving induction therapy showed significantly higher incidence of infectious disease. Further investigation is needed for appropriate regimens for induction therapy.

4. Conclusions

This manuscript reviews previous and more current evidence of induction therapy in HTx recipients, and discussed the appropriate therapeutic regimen and indication of induction therapy in the current clinical situation. In previous evidence, conflicting results have been reported with regard to the effect of induction therapy on long-term survival, also the comparison between ATG and IL-2RA. Appropriate patient selection and agent selection may maximize the efficacy of induction therapy. The proper use of induction therapy is still being determined. Recent advances in immunosuppressive agents have changed the clinical course of HTx recipients. Induction therapy should be selected, specifically based on their mechanism of action to specific clinical need and aim.

Acknowledgements

This work was supported by a Japan Heart Foundation Research Grant and by the JSPS KAKENHI [grant number JP19K09256] to T.W., and was supported by the JSPS KAKENHI [grant number 21H0921] to Yasunori Shintani.

Conflict of interest

The authors declare no conflict of interest.

Author details

Takuya Watanabe[1*], Yasumasa Tsukamoto[1], Hiroki Mochizuki[1], Masaya Shimojima[1], Tasuku Hada[1], Satsuki Fukushima[2], Tomoyuki Fujita[2] and Osamu Seguchi[1]

1 Department of Transplant Medicine, National Cerebral and Cardiovascular Center, Osaka, Japan

2 Department of Cardiovascular Surgery, National Cerebral and Cardiovascular Center, Osaka, Japan

*Address all correspondence to: watanabe.takuya@ncvc.go.jp

References

[1] Khush KK, Potena L, Cherikh WS, Chambers DC, Harhay MO, et al. The International Thoracic Organ Transplant Registry of the International Society for Heart and Lung Transplantation: 37th adult heart transplantation report-2020; focus on deceased donor characteristics. The Journal of Heart and Lung Transplantation: The Official Publication of the International Society for Heart Transplantation. 2020;**39**:1003-1015

[2] Kirk AD. Induction immunosuppression. Transplantation. 2006;**82**:593-602

[3] Habal MV. Current desensitization strategies in heart transplantation. Frontiers in Immunology. 2021;**12**: 702186

[4] Kobashigawa J, Colvin M, Potena L, Dragun D, Crespo-Leiro MG, et al. The management of antibodies in heart transplantation: An ISHLT consensus document. The Journal of Heart and Lung Transplantation: The Official Publication of the International Society for Heart Transplantation. 2018;**37**:537-547

[5] Chih S, Patel J. Desensitization strategies in adult heart transplantation-Will persistence pay off? The Journal of Heart and Lung Transplantation: The Official Publication of the International Society for Heart Transplantation. 2016;**35**:962-972

[6] Stegall MD, Dean PG, Gloor J. Mechanisms of alloantibody production in sensitized renal allograft recipients. American Journal of Transplantation: Official Journal of the American Society of Transplantation and the American Society of Transplant Surgeons. 2009; **9**:998-1005

[7] Murata K, Baldwin WM 3rd. Mechanisms of complement activation, C4d deposition, and their contribution to the pathogenesis of antibody-mediated rejection. Transplantation Reviews (Orlando, FL.). 2009;**23**:139-150

[8] Kobashigawa J, Mehra M, West L, Kerman R, George J, et al. Report from a consensus conference on the sensitized patient awaiting heart transplantation. The Journal of Heart and Lung Transplantation: The Official Publication of the International Society for Heart Transplantation. 2009;**28**:213-225

[9] Cai J, Terasaki PI. Induction immunosuppression improves long-term graft and patient outcome in organ transplantation: An analysis of United Network for Organ Sharing registry data. Transplantation. 2010;**90**:1511-1515

[10] Whitson BA, Kilic A, Lehman A, Wehr A, Hasan A, et al. Impact of induction immunosuppression on survival in heart transplant recipients: A contemporary analysis of agents. Clinical Transplantation. 2015;**29**:9-17

[11] Nozohoor S, Stehlik J, Lund LH, Ansari D, Andersson B, Nilsson J. Induction immunosuppression strategies and long-term outcomes after heart transplantation. Clinical Transplantation. 2020;**34**:e13871

[12] Tzani A, Van den Eynde J, Doulamis IP, Kuno T, Kampaktsis PN, et al. Impact of induction therapy on outcomes after heart transplantation. Clinical Transplantation. 2021;**35**:e14440

[13] Ruan V, Czer LS, Awad M, Kittleson M, Patel J, et al. Use of anti-thymocyte globulin for induction therapy in cardiac transplantation: A

review. Transplantation Proceedings. 2017;**49**:253-259

[14] Penninga L, Moller CH, Gustafsson F, Gluud C, Steinbruchel DA. Immunosuppressive T-cell antibody induction for heart transplant recipients. The Cochrane Database of Systematic Reviews. 2013;**12**:Cd008842

[15] Briasoulis A, Inampudi C, Pala M, Asleh R, Alvarez P, Bhama J. Induction immunosuppressive therapy in cardiac transplantation: A systematic review and meta-analysis. Heart Failure Reviews. 2018;**23**:641-649

[16] Higgins R, Kirklin JK, Brown RN, Rayburn BK, Wagoner L, et al. To induce or not to induce: Do patients at greatest risk for fatal rejection benefit from cytolytic induction therapy? The Journal of Heart and Lung Transplantation: The Official Publication of the International Society for Heart Transplantation. 2005;**24**:392-400

[17] Watanabe T, Yanase M, Seguchi O, Fujita T, Hamasaki T, et al. Influence of induction therapy using Basiliximab with delayed tacrolimus administration in heart transplant recipients—comparison with standard tacrolimus-based triple immunosuppression. Circulation Journal: Official Journal of the Japanese Circulation Society. 2020;**84**:2212-2223

[18] Cantarovich M, Metrakos P, Giannetti N, Cecere R, Barkun J, Tchervenkov J. Anti-CD25 monoclonal antibody coverage allows for calcineurin inhibitor "holiday" in solid organ transplant patients with acute renal dysfunction. Transplantation. 2002; **73**:1169-1172

[19] Delgado DH, Miriuka SG, Cusimano RJ, Feindel C, Rao V, Ross HJ. Use of basiliximab and cyclosporine in heart transplant patients with pre-operative renal dysfunction. The Journal of Heart and Lung Transplantation: The Official Publication of the International Society for Heart Transplantation. 2005;**24**:166-169

[20] Rosenberg PB, Vriesendorp AE, Drazner MH, Dries DL, Kaiser PA, et al. Induction therapy with basiliximab allows delayed initiation of cyclosporine and preserves renal function after cardiac transplantation. The Journal of Heart and Lung Transplantation: The Official Publication of the International Society for Heart Transplantation. 2005;**24**:1327-1331

[21] Cherikh WS, Kauffman HM, McBride MA, Maghirang J, Swinnen LJ, Hanto DW. Association of the type of induction immunosuppression with posttransplant lymphoproliferative disorder, graft survival, and patient survival after primary kidney transplantation. Transplantation. 2003;**76**:1289-1293

[22] Emin A, Rogers CA, Thekkudan J, Bonser RS, Banner NR. Antithymocyte globulin induction therapy for adult heart transplantation: A UK national study. The Journal of Heart and Lung Transplantation: The Official Publication of the International Society for Heart Transplantation. 2011;**30**:770-777

[23] Beniaminovitz A, Itescu S, Lietz K, Donovan M, Burke EM, et al. Prevention of rejection in cardiac transplantation by blockade of the interleukin-2 receptor with a monoclonal antibody. The New England Journal of Medicine. 2000;**342**:613-619

[24] Hershberger RE, Starling RC, Eisen HJ, Bergh CH, Kormos RL, et al. Daclizumab to prevent rejection after cardiac transplantation. The New England Journal of Medicine. 2005;**352**:2705-2713

[25] Nashan B, Moore R, Amlot P, Schmidt AG, Abeywickrama K, Soulillou JP. Randomised trial of basiliximab versus placebo for control of acute cellular rejection in renal allograft recipients. CHIB 201 International Study Group. Lancet (London, England). 1997;**350**:1193-1198

[26] Mehra MR, Zucker MJ, Wagoner L, Michler R, Boehmer J, et al. A multicenter, prospective, randomized, double-blind trial of basiliximab in heart transplantation. The Journal of Heart and Lung Transplantation: The Official Publication of the International Society for Heart Transplantation. 2005;**24**:1297-1304

[27] Moller CH, Gustafsson F, Gluud C, Steinbruchel DA. Interleukin-2 receptor antagonists as induction therapy after heart transplantation: Systematic review with meta-analysis of randomized trials. The Journal of Heart and Lung Transplantation: The Official Publication of the International Society for Heart Transplantation. 2008;**27**:835-842

[28] Bonaros N, Dunkler D, Kocher A, Imhof M, Grimm M, et al. Ten-year follow-up of a prospective, randomized trial of BT563/bb10 versus anti-thymocyte globulin as induction therapy after heart transplantation. The Journal of Heart and Lung Transplantation: The Official Publication of the International Society for Heart Transplantation. 2006;**25**:1154-1163

[29] Carrier M, Leblanc MH, Perrault LP, White M, Doyle D, et al. Basiliximab and rabbit anti-thymocyte globulin for prophylaxis of acute rejection after heart transplantation: A non-inferiority trial. The Journal of Heart and Lung Transplantation: The Official Publication of the International Society for Heart Transplantation. 2007;**26**:258-263

[30] Mattei MF, Redonnet M, Gandjbakhch I, Bandini AM, Billes A, et al. Lower risk of infectious deaths in cardiac transplant patients receiving basiliximab versus anti-thymocyte globulin as induction therapy. The Journal of Heart and Lung Transplantation: The Official Publication of the International Society for Heart Transplantation. 2007;**26**:693-699

[31] Mullen JC, Kuurstra EJ, Oreopoulos A, Bentley MJ, Wang S. A randomized controlled trial of daclizumab versus anti-thymocyte globulin induction for heart transplantation. Transplantation Research. 2014;**3**:14

[32] Ansari D, Lund LH, Stehlik J, Andersson B, Hoglund P, et al. Induction with anti-thymocyte globulin in heart transplantation is associated with better long-term survival compared with basiliximab. The Journal of Heart and Lung Transplantation: The Official Publication of the International Society for Heart Transplantation. 2015;**34**:1283-1291

[33] Mazimba S, Tallaj JA, George JF, Kirklin JK, Brown RN, Pamboukian SV. Infection and rejection risk after cardiac transplantation with induction vs. no induction: A multi-institutional study. Clinical Transplantation. 2014;**28**:946-952

[34] Lindenfeld J, Miller GG, Shakar SF, Zolty R, Lowes BD, et al. Drug therapy in the heart transplant recipient: Part I: Cardiac rejection and immunosuppressive drugs. Circulation. 2004;**110**:3734-3740

[35] Schweiger M, Zuckermann A, Beiras-Fernandez A, Berchtolld-Herz M, Boeken U, et al. A review of induction with rabbit antithymocyte globulin in pediatric heart transplant

recipients. Annals of Transplantation. 2018;**23**:322-333

[36] Opelz G, Döhler B. Lymphomas after solid organ transplantation: A collaborative transplant study report. American Journal of Transplantation: Official Journal of the American Society of Transplantation and the American Society of Transplant Surgeons. 2004;**4**:222-230

[37] Costanzo MR, Dipchand A, Starling R, Anderson A, Chan M, et al. The International Society of Heart and Lung Transplantation Guidelines for the care of heart transplant recipients. The Journal of Heart and Lung Transplantation: The Official Publication of the International Society for Heart Transplantation. 2010;**29**:914-956

[38] Thrush PT, Gossett JG, Costello JM, Matthews KL, Nubani R, et al. Role for immune monitoring to tailor induction prophylaxis in pediatric heart recipients. Pediatric Transplantation. 2014;**18**:79-86

[39] Haba T, Uchida K, Katayama A, Tominaga Y, Sato T, et al. Pharmacokineticsandpharmacodynamics of a chimeric interleukin-2 receptor monoclonal antibody, basiliximab, in renal transplantation: A comparison between Japanese and non-Japanese patients. Transplantation Proceedings. 2001;**33**:3174-3175

Chapter 10

Role of the Transplant Pharmacist

Megumi Ikura, Kazuki Nakagita, Takaya Uno, Hiromi Takenaka, Sachi Matsuda, Miho Yoshii, Rikako Nagata, Ichiro Nakakura, Naoki Hayakawa, Tsutomu Nakamura, Kyoichi Wada and Osamu Seguchi

Abstract

At the National Cerebral and Cardiovascular Center, Japan, pharmacists have been involved in drug treatment management and patient care as members of multidisciplinary heart transplant teams that include surgeons, physicians, recipient transplant coordinators, and nurses during the waiting period for heart transplantation (HTx), HTx surgery, and post-HTx. During the waiting period, pharmacists play an important role in adjusting the use of antibiotics, anticoagulants, and antiarrhythmics by patients receiving a ventricular assist device (VAD). During HTx surgery and post-HTx, pharmacists advise physicians regarding the individualized medication protocol for immunosuppression and infection prevention to be used for each patient based on the patient's pre-HTx characteristics as well as gene polymorphisms. They thus contribute to reducing the burden on the physician through the sharing of tasks. Throughout all three phases of HTx, pharmacists repeatedly provide medication and adherence education to the patients and caregivers. It is hoped that an academic society-led training protocol as well as transplant pharmacists will be established in Japan and other developed countries, and that these specialized transplant pharmacists would then provide individualized pharmacotherapy for the use of various antibiotics, anticoagulants, and immunosuppressive agents that have a narrow range of treatment in VAD and HTx patients.

Keywords: transplant pharmacist, individualized therapy, patient education, immunosuppressive agents

1. Introduction

In 1997, the Act on Organ Transplantation was enacted in Japan, and the first heart transplantation (HTx) under the law was performed in 1999 [1]. However, the number of organ donors has been quite low in Japan, and therefore, many HTx candidates have no choice but to travel overseas to seek the opportunity for HTx [2]. Meanwhile, the Declaration of Istanbul was set out at the Transplantation Society in 2008, in which patients awaiting HTx need to wait for donor opportunities in their own countries, sidestepping efforts by many individuals related to organ transplantation to amend and revise the Act on Organ Transplantation in 2010. Over the last decade, although the number of brain-dead organ donors has increased gradually, the number of patients awaiting HTx has been increasing year by year [2]. Furthermore, the COVID-19 pandemic reduced the frequency of the organ transplantation procedures, and the number of organ donors has decreased. Consequently, the waiting period for HTx has become longer, at 5 years or more in most cases in Japan [3].

At the National Cerebral and Cardiovascular Center (NCVC), Japan, the multidisciplinary HTx team, including surgeons, physicians, pharmacists, recipient transplant coordinators (RTC), nurses, nutritional support teams (NSTs), physical therapists, and medical engineers, has supported the patients during the waiting period for HTx, HTx surgery, and post-HTx. In this situation, pharmacists play the role of a specialist providing pharmaceutical care to patients awaiting HTx as well as heart transplant recipients (HTRs). The pharmacist stationed in the ward participates in morning and evening conferences as a member of the medical team to monitor the patient's daily condition, provides pharmacological management, and actively provides prescription support and patient education, and it is expected that the transplant pharmacist also actively contributes to individualized pharmacotherapy for various patient groups, from those suffering from severe heart failure to those in the post-transplantation phase.

In this chapter, the role and responsibilities of pharmacists are described from the perspective of drug treatment management and patient education in preoperative and postoperative HTx patients, and individualized pharmacotherapy is also discussed.

2. Waiting for an HTx

Patients awaiting HTx have terminal circulatory failure, and ventricular assist devices (VADs), which can mechanically propel blood from the heart to the central circulation and temporarily augment the cardiac output, have been recognized as essential treatment options as "bridge to transplant" (BTT) [1–3]. VADs include intracorporeal or paracorporeal devices, and the former can not only improve the functional status and quality of life of the patients awaiting HTx, but also enable them to return to almost normal lives [4, 5].

On the other hand, VADs often cause pump thrombosis by forming blood clots in the device, and therefore patients receiving VADs require long-term anticoagulation treatment to prevent thromboembolic complications. In addition, although intracorporeal VADs are fully implantable pumps in the body, a driveline attached to the pump penetrates the skin and connects to an external controller and battery, thereby potentially increasing the risk of infectious diseases that may require hospitalization.

At NCVC, intracorporeal VADs have been used in more than 90% of the patients awaiting HTx. The pharmaceutical management and patient education by pharmacists are described below.

2.1 Pharmaceutical management

2.1.1 Warfarin (WF)

Warfarin (WF) is most frequently used as a prophylactic antithrombotic drug after VAD implantation [6]. In general, the dose of WF is routinely adjusted according to the prothrombin time international normalized ratio (PT-INR). At the start of an urgent anticoagulant therapy for VAD implantation, heparin or dalteparin is used in combination with WF while paying attention to heparin-induced thrombocytopenia until stable PT-INR can be maintained. Meanwhile, antimicrobial agents such as linezolid (LZD), daptomycin (DAP), and levofloxacin, and antiarrhythmic agents such as amiodarone (AMD), may result in drug–drug interactions with WF, which could lead to unexpected anticoagulation and bleeding risk [7–9]. Pharmacists check classical clinical factors (age, sex, weight, height, and concomitant medication) and request the physicians in charge to take blood samples for additional PT-INR monitoring and provide prescription support, if a potential drug interaction between WF and concomitant medication is a concern.

WF produces an anticoagulant effect by interfering with the interconversion of vitamin K (VK) to its reduced form, which is required for γ-carboxylation of several vitamin-K-dependent proteins that regulate blood coagulation [6]. VK is present in many kinds of foods and beverages, and it has been reported that meals affect PT-INR in patients taking WF [7–9]. Therefore, careful attention should be paid to foods and drinks for the control of PT-INR. On the other hand, VK plays an important role in bone formation through activation of osteocalcin as well as maintenance of normal blood coagulation [10, 11], and excessive restriction of VK intake may lead to decreased quality of life. At NCVC, an interdisciplinary NST, composed of physicians, dieticians, pharmacists, and nurses, participates in the routine assessment of the patient's energy, protein, fluid, mineral, and electrolyte requirements as well as vitamins, and pharmacists explain the importance of dietary management to obtain stable PT-INR to the patients receiving VAD and their families/relatives during hospitalization [12]. A certified dietician also controls every HTR's VK intake through the meals not only during hospitalization but also after release from the hospital.

Recently, genetic polymorphisms of genes encoding cytochrome (CYP) 2C9, a metabolic enzyme of *S*-WF, and those of the VK epoxide reductase complex (VKORC1), a target enzyme of WF in vitamin K recycling, have also been reported as key factors affecting the pharmacokinetics (PK) and pharmacodynamics (PD) of WF, respectively. These factors may be useful for the control of PT-INR through dose adjustments [10, 11]. At NCVC, we often observe that some patients with an implanted VAD have difficulties in controlling the dose of WF. In such a case, pharmacists suggest the physician additional tests to determine the genotypes of CYP2C9 and VKORC with the consent of the patient and carefully adjust the WF dosage [11]. Because dose adjustments based on gene polymorphisms are not covered by the universal health insurance system in Japan so far, further evidence-based data accumulation is needed.

Meanwhile, when the patient with VAD undergoes urgent surgery or experiences severe or life-threatening bleeding, the dose of WF should be reduced immediately, and anticoagulation reversal is required. The International Society for Heart and Lung Transplantation (ISHLT) guidelines recommend that anticoagulation therapy should be held in patients with mechanical circulatory support in the setting of clinically significant bleeding [13]. In such emergency cases, in addition to the cessation of WF treatment, intravenous administration of vitamin K2 as an antagonist of the anticoagulant activity of WF and that of human prothrombin complex supplemented with VK-dependent blood coagulation factors are performed to improve the excessively enhanced anticoagulant state.

2.1.2 Antimicrobial agents

During the waiting period for HTx, VAD-associated infections can often be a problem. Pharmacists help physicians select appropriate antimicrobial agents and maintain their dosing adjustments. In addition, pharmacists routinely monitor side effects and sometimes utilize therapeutic drug monitoring (TDM) [14]. LZD and DAP are effective for

Gram-positive bacteria such as *Enterococcus faecium*, *Staphylococcus aureus*, *Streptococcus agalactiae*, *Streptococcus pneumoniae*, *Streptococcus pyogenes*, and others, which are resistant to other antibiotics [15]. However, LZD may induce pancytopenia, which makes it difficult to continue the administration of the drug. DAP is also used to treat various bacterial infections caused by Gram-positive bacteria, including methicillin-resistant *S. aureus* (MRSA) and vancomycin-resistant *Enterococci* (VRE) [16, 17]. As mentioned above, LZD and DAP are also known to interact with WF, and therefore, pharmacists monitor the fluctuation of PT-INR carefully and provide prescription support [18].

2.1.3 Other agents

The administration of cardioprotective drugs such as angiotensin-converting enzyme inhibitors (ACEIs), angiotensin receptor blockers (ARBs), and/or beta-blockers is essential for patients awaiting HTx, and that of antiarrhythmic agents is an option to treat ventricular arrhythmias. Among these drugs, certain antiarrhythmic agents have the potential to cause drug–drug interactions, and pharmacists should pay careful attention to those.

Antiarrhythmic agents are categorized depending on their mechanism of cardiac action and certain types of arrhythmias, and the Vaughan Williams classification is the most widely recognized system. Vaugham Williams class Ib (mexiletine) and class III (AMD, sotalol) drugs are often administered to patients awaiting HTx. TDM is necessary for the optimal administration of these antiarrhythmic agents [19, 20]. Because AMD can interact with WF, pharmacists need to check side effects on the thyroid and lungs. Sotalol dosing is based on renal function, and a careful approach is recommended for initial dosing and up-titration.

2.2 Patient education

During hospitalization, patients and their families need to be educated that some foods and drinks in daily life may increase drug effects as mentioned above [7–9]. Especially, VK is a typical factor influencing the control of PT-INR in patients taking WF and is usually obtained from green vegetables and vegetable oils as well as VK supplements. In Japan, people also traditionally eat a large amount of boiled vegetables, and often eat *natto*, a traditional fermented food in Japan that produces VK in the intestinal flora. Japanese people tend to consume more VK-containing foods, and the therapeutic effectiveness of WF may be diminished by high VK intake. Therefore, HTRs are free to eat vegetables, but all HTRs are prohibited from eating *natto*, and *chlorella* and *green juice* are also sometimes prohibited throughout the dosing schedule of WF. Pharmacists explain the importance of dietary management to obtain stable PT-INR to the patients receiving VAD and their families/relatives during hospitalization [12]. Meanwhile, medical staffs cannot frequently check PT-INR and laboratory test values after discharge. To allow the patients to be aware of fluctuations in PT-INR values, pharmacists also need to educate them to monitor PT-INR by themselves using CoaguChek® and determine the WF dosage based on the results of the PT-INR scale.

A certain amount of variability can be seen among individual CoaguChek® devices, and therefore, we monitor PT-INR values calculated by blood sampling during patients' hospitalizations. Considering the difference between the CoaguChek® and PT-INR values, we are trying to obtain an optimal scale for WF adjustment.

HTx surgery is not scheduled, and there are restrictions on visiting rooms after the surgery for clean room management. Therefore, pharmacists must explain about post-transplant medication from the early stage during the HTx waiting period. In addition, pharmacists aim to remove patients' anxiety about pharmacotherapy associated with the change from anticoagulant therapy under heart failure to immunosuppressive therapy and also need to facilitate the introduction of self-managed immunosuppressive medication after transplantation.

3. Perioperative and postoperative HTx

3.1 Pharmaceutical management

3.1.1 Protocol preparation

The protocol for administration of antimicrobials and immunosuppressants during the perioperative period is prepared from the day before to the day of HTx. To create it, pharmacists check the recipient's conditions such as histories of side effects and allergy, laboratory values, preoperative bacterial infection status, viral antibody titer, and current prescriptions and then discuss the need for new or continuous prescriptions. In addition, pharmacists participate in medical staff meetings to confirm donor information including viral antibody titer and preoperative cardiac function and also confirm the timing when the recipient enters into an operating room and determine whether basiliximab should be administered. Basiliximab is not approved for the treatment of HTx in Japan, but a few reports have described the use of basiliximab as beneficial after HTx [21, 22]. Therefore, we usually prepare protocols in case we might use basiliximab for HTRs [23]. The protocol prepared for antibacterial and immunosuppressive therapies created by pharmacists based on this information is shared with cardiac surgeons, cardiologists, and RTCs after approval by the physician in charge.

3.1.2 Immunosuppressive agents

Perioperative immunosuppressive therapy basically consists of a combination of three drugs: calcineurin inhibitors (CNIs), mycophenolate mofetil (MMF), and steroids. Alternative immunosuppression strategies are needed for patients with renal impairment, fatal acute cellular rejection (AMR), antibody-mediated rejection (AMR), and infections. Herein, the immunosuppressive strategies are described by dividing it into three therapies: induction, maintenance, and response to rejection.

3.1.2.1 Induction therapy

Basiliximab is a chimeric mouse-human monoclonal antibody that binds to the receptor of interleukin 2 (IL-2), inhibiting the proliferation of T cells, and is approved for the suppression of acute rejection response after renal transplantation in Japan, but not for heart transplantation. Basiliximab has been widely used as an induction therapy in renal transplantation, although the incidence of adverse events, such as cytomegalovirus (CMV) infection, malignancies, or post-transplant lymphoproliferative disorders, is of concern [24].

At NCVC, the standard immunosuppression protocol for HTRs is the regular release tacrolimus (TAC)-based triple immunosuppression therapy. Usually, TAC and MMF are introduced for HTRs immediately after postoperative decannulation and passing the swallowing test. However, TAC has side effects such as nephrotoxicity and can exacerbate pre-HTx renal dysfunction of the HTR by increasing renal vasoconstriction caused by TAC. In such a patient, the introduction of induction therapy using basiliximab as well as two-week delayed start of administration of TAC is to be considered. To date, in our institute, the effect of induction therapy using basiliximab with delayed TAC administration on the clinical prognosis of HTRs has been verified as compared with that of a standard TAC-based triple immunosuppression therapy [23]. The former therapy might be feasible and safe for HTRs fulfilling certain inclusion criteria including renal function, sensitization for anti-human leukocyte antigen (HLA) antibody, and HTR- and donor-related risk factors, although a comprehensive evaluation of the clinical necessity of basiliximab-based induction therapy is necessary (see [23] for more detailed inclusion criteria). Basiliximab-based induction therapy is also applied to pediatric HTRs and the patients experiencing long-time aortic blockage.

3.1.2.2 Maintenance therapy

3.1.2.2.1 Calcineurin inhibitors (CNIs)

CNIs such as TAC and cyclosporine (CYA) exert their immunosuppressive effects by reducing interleukin-2 (IL-2) production and IL-2 receptor expression, leading to a reduction in T-cell activation. Briefly, TAC and CYA inhibit T-lymphocyte activation by binding to a member of the immunophilin family, FKBP12 and cyclosphilin, respectively. The complex formed by the drug-binding protein, calcium, calmodulin, and calcineurin inhibits calcineurin-mediated dephosphorylation and subsequent translocation of the nuclear factor (NF) of an activated T cell (NFAT) to the nucleus. NFAT initiates transcription of pro-inflammatory cytokines, including IL-2 and of its receptor. These CNIs also inhibit the activation of other transcription factors involved in IL-2 gene expression in T cells such as NF-kB. Thus, CNIs inhibit a variety of immune functions and have a narrow therapeutic index, meaning that lower exposure to a CNI induces organ rejection, whereas higher exposure induces serious infections and malignancies caused by overimmunosuppression. Therefore, pharmacists need to conduct TDM to adequately design dosage regimens of CNIs.

TAC and CYA are metabolized by the CYP3A subfamily, and many drug interactions with these CNIs reported in the solid organ transplant population are associated with intestinal and hepatic CYP3A. CYP3A is a most important drug metabolizing enzyme that has a wide substrate specificity, and a very large number of drugs are the substrates for this enzyme. Pharmacists routinely check newly prescribed medications in combination with CNIs, especially those on the list (**Table 1**), which are often used in HTRs at NCVC.

AMD is metabolized through the CYP3A metabolic pathway, and it has been reported that patients receiving AMD prior to transplant require a reduction of the TAC dose [25]. It is therefore necessary to check blood levels of both AMD and TAC carefully. Amlodipine, a substrate of CYP3A, is often used to control blood pressure during the perioperative period, and a careful control of the blood concentrations of TAC after the initiation of TAC is needed [26, 27]. Clotrimazole inhibits CYP3A function [28]. To date, oral clotrimazole lozenges have been used for prevention of opportunistic infections at NCVC, but we have experienced a need for dose adjustment of TAC by hospitalization when this drug is discontinued 6 months after HTx [29–31]. Herein, we have switched to oral amphotericin B for treatment, and since then, it has succeeded in maintaining stable pharmacokinetics of TAC [32]. HTRs with nontuberculous mycobacterial (NTM) disease take rifampicin (REP) and macrolides. REP induces the expression of various CYP subfamilies, whereas erythromycin and

Azole	Antimicrobial agents	Calcium channel blocker	Antiepileptic agent
Voriconazole	aminoglycosides	diltiazem	carbamazepine
ketoconazole	rifampicin	nifedipine	phenytoin
fluconazole	rifabutin	nicardipine	
itraconazole		verapamil	
clotrimazole		amlodipine	

Table 1.
A list of medications that pay particular attention to their interaction with TAC during waiting period for HTx, at HTx surgery and post-HTx at NCVC. TAC, tacrolimus; HTx, heart transplantation; NCVC, National Cerebral and Cardiovascular Center, Japan.

clarithromycin (CAM) among macrolides have a potential to inhibit CYP3A4 function and are metabolized by CYP3A4. The concomitant administration of these drugs can have a significant effect on the pharmacokinetics of TAC. For HTRs taking REP or CAM prior to HTx, pharmacists ask the specialists in advance to change from REP to rifabutin and from CAM to azithromycin to prevent worsening of NTM owing to immunosuppressive therapy and also consider the effect of concomitant drugs on the blood concentrations of TAC [33]. Even if the drugs are not used in combination with TAC, it should be noted that in patients taking drugs with a long half-life, such as AMD, before HTx, the drug may remain in the body for a long time post-HTx, thereby possibly affecting the pharmacokinetics of TAC.

Meanwhile, CYP3A5, as well as CYP3A4, is involved in TAC metabolism [34], and single nucleotide polymorphism in the *CYP3A5* gene, *CYP3A5*3* (6986A>G), is associated with alteration in its metabolic activity, thereby affecting the blood concentration of TAC [35]. The *CYP3A5* genotype is a factor to be considered for TAC dose adjustment. At NCVC, pharmacists determine the *CYP3A5* genotype with the consent of the recipient [35, 36]. As shown in the **Figure 1**, compared with the frequencies found by previous studies in the Japanese population, we have not found any significant difference in the frequencies of the genotypes between *CYP3A5*1/*1* or **1/*3* (CYP3A5 expresser) and *CYP3A5*3/*3* (CYP3A5 non-expresser) [37–39].

At NCVC, in the standard triple immunosuppressive therapy, TAC is generally initiated at a dose of 1 mg/day on the first or second postoperative day.

Thereafter, its dosage is adjusted to achieve an initial blood concentration range of 9–12 ng/mL within a week. Standard target trough levels of TAC to be maintained during the first year post-HTx are 9–12 ng/mL. Depending on the type of concomitant drug, the HTR's renal function, and the status of side effects, the dose of TAC is basically increased or decreased in one step with 0.2 or 0.5 mg as single dose, and in some case in two steps.

Meanwhile, as mentioned above, the total clearance of TAC in HTRs with *CYP3A*1/*1* or *CYP3A*1/*3* is considered to be higher than in those with *CYP3A*3/*3*. Therefore, in the former HTRs, it may be better to standardize two-step dose adjustment and also to set the starting dose to twice the standard levels, although this treatment strategy should be verified [26, 35].

3.1.2.2.2 MMF

MMF is an orally administered prodrug of mycophenolic acid (MPA), which blocks *de novo* biosynthesis of purine nucleotides and lymphocyte proliferation by

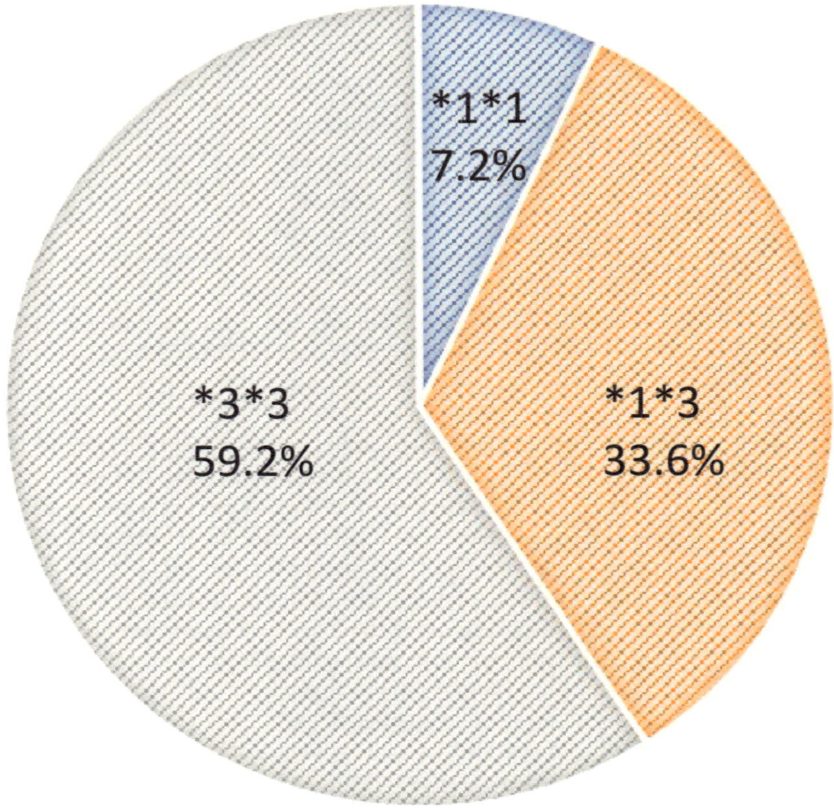

Figure 1.
Distribution of genetic polymorphisms of CYP3A5 in HTRs at NCVC.HTRs, heart transplant recipients; NCVC, National Cerebral and Cardiovascular Center, Japan.

suppressing the enzyme inosine monophosphate dehydrogenase [40]. Concerning MMF, the package insert clearly states that the dosage of MMF varies widely from 500 to 1500 mg per dose. Because the tolerated and effective doses vary from patient to patient, careful adjustment is necessary to achieve optimal therapeutic effects of MPA. In addition, patients with severe renal dysfunction need to be carefully taken care of because the blood levels of MPA can be high [41]. Immediately after HTx, the effects of heart failure are still present, and circulatory conditions are unstable. During this period, the appearance of side effects such as leukopenia should be noted. When the circulatory state has stabilized, pharmacists confirm pharmacokinetics and pharmacodynamics of MPA by area under the blood concentration-time curve (AUC) and make sure there is no rejection based on the myocardial biopsy results.

Diarrhea is one of the adverse effects observed during treatment with MMF [42, 43]. To alleviate it, Chinese herbal medicine *Hangeshashinto* is often used during cancer chemotherapy [44, 45], and it is also expected to be effective against diarrhea caused by treatment with MMF [46]. At NCVC, we additionally administer *Hangeshashinto* to patients treated with MMF, who are free from any suspected infection in the perioperative period or to post-HTx outpatients.

3.1.2.2.3 Steroids

Steroids have anti-inflammatory, immunosuppressive, and lympholytic effects by preventing the production of cytokines and vasoactive substances, including IL-1, IL-2, IL-6, tumor necrosis factor-α, chemokines, prostaglandins, major histocompatibility class II, and proteases. In HTx, methylprednisolone and prednisone are used frequently as part of the immunosuppressive regimen to prevent rejection. Intravenous methylprednisolone is administered at the initiation of the transplant procedure, and the dose is repeated until 3 weeks after the HTx. Thereafter, the steroid dose is gradually reduced until completion of 5 weeks post-HT, although methylprednisolone is switched to oral prednisolone if cardiac allograft rejection is not found at the myocardial biopsy after 3 weeks post-HTx.

Meanwhile, side effects are often a problem when using steroids, and pharmacists need to be aware of patient complaints and clinical findings. Delayed wound healing, diabetes, and gastric ulcer are often found in the postoperative acute phase, and osteoporosis, cataracts, hypertension, depression, and growth retardation are long-term problems.

At NCVC, HTRs are hospitalized for routine endomyocardial biopsies to assess graft rejection, coronary angiography, and coronary intravascular ultrasound with the development of cardiac allograft vasculopathy. If cardiac allograft rejection is not observed in the myocardial biopsy, the dose of steroid is tapered over 6–12 months before its discontinuation, except for HTRs with cardiac sarcoidosis who are treated with low-dose prednisolone. Meanwhile, if cardiac allograft rejection was detected in a regular myocardial biopsy after HTx, the patients are treated with augmented immunosuppression and intravenous steroids, and we consider the oral dose of steroid after the steroid pulse therapy.

We manage pediatric patients to decrease the dose of steroid or terminate steroid use as early as possible considering their healthy growth.

3.1.2.2.4 Everolimus (EVL)

Everolimus (EVL) is an inhibitor of the mammalian target of rapamycin (mTOR), a phosphatidylinositol 3-kinase-related kinase, and plays a central role in the regulation of many cellular functions including growth, proliferation, and survival [47]. EVL are usually introduced in HTRs during the maintenance phase after HTx and are often used by switching from or adding to MMF. Meanwhile, EVL can cause poor wound healing, and its initiation should be delayed up to about 2 months after surgery. The major reasons for the switching or adding are as follows: (1) post-transplant cardiac allograft vasculopathy (CAV) progression; (2) reduced renal function; and (3) malignant tumor complications, especially post-transplant lymphoma (PTLD). In an international consensus report, a target trough EVL concentration of 3–8 ng/mL was proposed [48], while paying attention to adverse events including hyperlipidemia, wound infection, acne-like skin lesions, and leukopenia. Meanwhile, EVL is a substrate of the CYP3A metabolic enzyme, and when used in combination with a CNI, the blood concentrations of the CNI need to be adjusted to 2/3 to 3/4 and sometimes 1/2, before concomitant use. Pharmacists herein prepare to renew the dosing regimens of EVL as well as CNI, which can contribute to reduce the burden on the physician. In the event of EVL introduction, the EVL protocol is prepared upon physician's request, and EVL blood concentration is monitored once or twice a week after EVL initiation, followed by myocardial biopsy approximately one month after EVL introduction. When preparing the EVL protocol, information on the rationale for the change of regimen and optimal blood concentration of EVL is collected from the physician, and then the change of regimen and the schedule of visiting the hospital for the collection of blood are explained to the patient. After the start of EVL administration, there are concerns about the occurrence of stomatitis. The pharmacists instruct the HTRs to maintain the mouth clean and to use dexamethasone ointment and azulene sulfonic acid as a treatment when stomatitis occurs. The blood concentration level of TAC and EVL is carefully monitored considering the competitive interaction with FK-binding protein.

3.1.2.3 Response to rejection

Rejection after HTx includes acute rejection immediately after surgery, acute cellular rejection (ACR) that may occur within a few weeks to 2 years post-HTx, and CAV after those. It is also classified into cellular rejection, antibody-related rejection (AMR), and mixed type according to the mechanism of onset. Among them, AMR has been paid attention to during maintenance immunosuppressive therapy after HTx.

For AMR, the following treatments can be considered: (1) plasmapheresis to remove antibodies from the circulation; (2) intravenous immunoglobulin therapy and anti-CD20 monoclonal antibody (rituximab) to suppress antibody production; (3) use of corticosteroids to suppress the inflammatory response; (4) change of immunosuppressive therapy (use of cyclophosphamide and change from CYA to TAC) and/or dose adjustment of immunosuppressive agents; and (5) use of antithymoglobulin to suppress helper T cells.

3.1.3 Prevention of infectious diseases

Because HTRs receive immunosuppressive therapy, sufficient prophylactic treatment against infections is necessary soon after HTx. Perioperative antibiotic therapy is selected based on microbiologic sensitivities. Prophylactic treatment for bacterial infections includes broad-spectrum drugs against Gram-positive and Gram-negative bacterium, such as LZD and doripenem. MRSA and fungal infections may also be problematic in patients bridged from VAD to HTx. Intravenous antifungals such as micafungin (MCFG) are administered for fungal infections. MCFG intravenous infusion is changed to AMPH B gargle after passing the drinking water test and continued for 6 months after HTx. To prevent opportunistic infection, HTRs receive anti-*Pneumocystis* prophylaxis with sulfamethoxazole/trimethoprim for life, and the dose is adjusted depending on the HTR's renal function. Cytomegalovirus (CMV)-seropositive HTRs are routinely administered CMV immunoglobulin immediately after the HTx, which is continued until 5 days post-HTx. In CMV-seronegative HTRs transplanted with organs from CMV-seropositive donors (CMV mismatch), anti-CMV drugs such as ganciclovir or its prodrug valganciclovir are administered prophylactically at half the therapeutic dosage within 10 days of HTx and are continued until 1 year after the HTx at NCVC. If the results of CMV antigenemia and real-time polymerase chain reaction tests are positive, an anti-CMV drug is initiated at a therapeutic dose (900 mg/day) in cases with clinical symptoms or as preemptive therapy in asymptomatic cases when CMV DNA exceeded the threshold set for active CMV infection. The dose of the anti-CMV drug is adjusted according to the patients' conditions such as renal function.

3.2 Patient education

After HTx, immunosuppressive therapy and prevention of opportunistic infections are in essence supported by the recipient's adherence to medication, and patient education is essential to ensure adherence and understanding of the need for lifelong pharmacotherapy. Patient education should start during the transplant waiting period and continue after HTx until the patient can self-manage by the time of discharge.

MMF is teratogenic and requires a contraceptive period of 6 weeks after discontinuation as well as during administration. Therefore, pharmacists need to educate potentially pregnant recipients on contraception.

If HTRs wish to give birth, the use of MMF and mizoribine is avoided, and it is switched to immunosuppressive therapy based on CNI and azathioprine use because MMF and mizoribine are known to be teratogenic. In addition, ACEIs and ARBs, which are administered as antihypertensive agents and cardiac protective agents, have also been reported to cause oligoamnios or increase the risk of teratogenicity. In such a case, we consider administering methyl-dopa as an antihypertensive agent as needed and changing to nifedipine after 20 weeks of gestation [49].

4. After discharge from HTx

4.1 Pharmaceutical management

HTRs who have passed the acute postoperative stage are treated in cooperation with hospitals near their homes, taking into consideration their return to society. In our institute, pharmacists provide continuous support for the dose adjustment of immunosuppressive drugs from our hospital to the collaborating hospital after discharge through fax and e-mail communication. However, there are sometimes inter-institutional differences in the results of immunosuppressant blood concentration owing to different measurement methods. Therefore, pharmacists need to confirm the measurement method with each collaborating hospital in advance to adjust the dose of immunosuppressant accordingly.

When patients are prescribed a new drug at a hospital or clinic, they are instructed to contact the RTC and ask for instructions on whether or not they can take the prescription medications. The RTC informs the physician and pharmacist about the new prescription drugs and the patient's condition, and then the pharmacist evaluates possible interactions between the new prescription drugs with the drug the patient is taking, especially immunosuppressive drugs. If interactions that affect the efficacy of the immunosuppressive drugs are expected, the pharmacist provides and shares the information with the physician. If the physician decides that the patient needs to continue taking the immunosuppressive drugs despite the interaction, the pharmacist recommends when to check their blood concentrations as needed.

4.2 Patient education

4.2.1 Patient education for therapy adherence

The main role of transplant pharmacists after discharge of the patient from the hospital is as follows: management of immunosuppressive therapy and infections during outpatient visits; guidance to improve medication adherence; and the development of protocols for dose adjustment and change of immunosuppressive agents as renal function deteriorates and CAV occurs. In particular, when changing the immunosuppressive agents, pharmacists have to explain the need to change the drug and the accompanying need for blood sampling to the patients and also instruct the patients to contact their local pharmacies to share the new protocols.

When patients return to society, they often have difficulties in taking their immunosuppressant medications on time owing the time and means of commuting to school or work. In such a case, pharmacists support the patients by shifting the time of taking the medication and also instruct them to pay attention to the time of blood collection before taking the medicine during outpatient visits.

CYA-associated side effects include hirsutism and gingival thickening. Hirsutism has cosmetic problems, especially for women and adolescents, and may reduce adherence to medication. In addition, gingival thickening, especially in infants, interferes with the subsequent development of teeth, and in some cases, repeated gingivectomy may be required. In this case, switching from CYA to TAC is a treatment option.

4.2.2 Diet and lifestyle

Diet and lifestyle are important from the perspective of CAV prevention, and nutritionists provide the patients with guidance about these points during hospitalization. In addition, hyperglycemia and hyperlipidemia have been reported as side effects of immunosuppressive drugs, and pharmacists provide guidance on diet and lifestyle precautions from the perspective of these side effects. To avoid and reduce interaction with immunosuppressive agents, pharmacists should explain what foods HTRs need to be aware of and why and instruct them to avoid their intake. Such foods and diet are dietary supplements, herbal medicines, herbal teas, and grapefruit juice [50]. Meanwhile, immunosuppressive agents are taken as time-release drugs and should be taken continuously at a set time. For this reason, pharmacists also make HTRs understand the importance to maintain a regular life rhythm.

5. Other relevant aspects

5.1 Individualized therapy

Although various factors such as concomitant medications, diet, and lifestyle can influence the pharmacokinetics of immunosuppressive agents and WF, genetic polymorphisms also need to be taken into consideration as variable factors affecting the pharmacokinetics of immunosuppressive drugs and WF during HTx waiting time and after HTx. Pharmacists need to collect and organize information about such variable factors that cause inter-individual or intra-individual fluctuations of these drugs in HTx patients and provide them to physicians. This contributes to not only individualized therapy, but also to reduce the burden on physicians and enable task sharing.

5.2 Certification of transplant pharmacists

In the United States, the Doctor of Pharmacy (Pharm.D.) degree was established in the 1950s, and the American Society of Hospital Pharmacists introduced a residency program in the 1960s that transformed the role of pharmacists in team medicine [51]. In organ transplantation, the specialty pharmacist system was accredited in 2018, and guidelines for pharmacist services and education have been developed [52].

The Canadian Hospital Pharmacists Association reported on the expertise of transplant pharmacists in 2018 [53].

6. Conclusions

Transplant pharmacists at each hospital have built up their own expertise and are participating in medical teams at each facility, playing a role in organ transplantation. Because transplantation medicine requires individualized medical care, there are many situations in which pharmacists can contribute. As a member of the medical team, transplant pharmacists are involved in anticoagulation and immunosuppressive therapy and provide prescription support, which not only reduces the burden on physicians, but also contributes to the promotion of effective and safe use of drugs. Transplant pharmacists as well as members of NST, infection control teams, or palliative care teams can contribute to healthcare economy and healthcare safety by taking the initiative of appropriate use of agents.

Meanwhile, it is hoped that an academic society-led transplant pharmacist will be established, and that specialized transplant pharmacists can provide individualized pharmacotherapy for antibiotics, anticoagulants, and immunosuppressive agents, which have a narrow range of treatment in the field of VAD and HTx treatment in Japan as well as other developed countries.

Conflict of interest

The authors declare no conflict of interest.

Author details

Megumi Ikura[1*], Kazuki Nakagita[1], Takaya Uno[1], Hiromi Takenaka[1], Sachi Matsuda[1], Miho Yoshii[1], Rikako Nagata[1], Ichiro Nakakura[1], Naoki Hayakawa[1], Tsutomu Nakamura[2], Kyoichi Wada[2] and Osamu Seguchi[3]

1 Department of Pharmacy, National Cerebral and Cardiovascular Center, Suita, Japan

2 Education and Research Center for Clinical Pharmacy, Faculty of Pharmacy, Osaka Medical and Pharmaceutical University, Takatsuki, Japan

3 Department of Transplant Medicine, National Cerebral and Cardiovascular Center, Suita, Japan

*Address all correspondence to: ikura.megumi48@ncvc.go.jp

References

[1] Rose EA, Gelijns AC, Moskowitz AJ, Heitjan DF, Stevenson LW, Dembitsky W, et al. Long-term use of a left ventricular assist device for end-stage heart failure. New England Journal of Medicine. 2001;**345**:1435-1443. DOI: 10.1056/NEJMoa012175

[2] Nakatani T, Sase K, Oshiyama H, Akiyama M, Horie M, Nawata K, et al. Japanese registry for mechanically assisted circulatory support: First report. Journal of Heart and Lung Transplant. 2017;**36**:1087-1096. DOI: 10.1016/j.healun.2017.08.002

[3] Seguchi O, Kuroda K, Kumai Y, Nakajima S, Yanase M, Wada K, et al. Clinical outcomes of patients with the HeartMate II left ventricular assist device: A single-center experience from Japan. Transplantation Proceedings. 2018;**50**:2726-2732. DOI: 10.1016/j.transproceed.2018.03.091

[4] Miller LW, Pagani FD, Russell SD, John R, Boyle AJ, Aaronson KD, et al. Use of a continuous-flow device in patients awaiting heart transplantation. New England Journal of Medicine. 2007;**357**:885-896. DOI: 10.1056/NEJMoa067758

[5] Slaughter MS, Rogers JG, Milano CA, Russell SD, Conte JV, Feldman D, et al. Advanced heart failure treated with continuous-flow left ventricular assist device. New England Journal of Medicine. 2009;**361**:2241-2251. DOI: 10.1056/NEJMoa0909938

[6] Hirsh J, Fuster V, Ansell J, Halperin JL, American Heart A, American College of Cardiology F. American Heart Association/American College of Cardiology Foundation guide to warfarin therapy. Circulation. 2003;**107**:1692-1711. DOI: 10.1161/01.CIR.0000063575.17904.4E

[7] Wells PS, Holbrook AM, Crowther NR, Hirsh J. Interactions of warfarin with drugs and food. Annals of Internal Medicine. 1994;**121**:676-683. DOI: 10.7326/0003-4819-121-9-199411010-00009

[8] Tan CSS, Lee SWH. Warfarin and food, herbal or dietary supplement interactions: A systematic review. British Journal of Clinical Pharmacololy. 2021;**87**:352-374. DOI: 10.1111/bcp.14404

[9] Holbrook AM, Pereira JA, Labiris R, McDonald H, Douketis JD, Crowther M, et al. Systematic overview of warfarin and its drug and food interactions. Archives of Internal Medicine. 2005;**165**:1095-1106. DOI: 10.1001/archinte.165.10.1095

[10] Calvo MS, Eyre DR, Gundberg CM. Molecular basis and clinical application of biological markers of bone turnover. Endocrine Reviews. 1996;**17**:333-368. DOI: 10.1210/edrv-17-4-333

[11] Rodriguez-Olleros Rodriguez C, Diaz CM. Vitamin K and bone health: A review on the effects of vitamin K deficiency and supplementation and the effect of non-vitamin K antagonist oral anticoagulants on different bone parameters. Journal of Osteoporosis. 2019;**2019**:2069176. DOI: 10.1155/2019/2069176

[12] Spielmann H, Seemann M, Friedrich N, Tigges-Limmer K, Albert W, Semmig-Konze S, et al. Self-management with the therapeutic regimen in patients with ventricular assist device (VAD) support - a scoping review. Heart & Lung. 2021;**50**:388-396. DOI: 10.1016/j.hrtlng.2021.01.019

[13] den Exter PL, Beeres S, Eikenboom J, Klok FA, Huisman MV. Anticoagulant treatment and bleeding complications in patients with left ventricular assist devices. Expert Review of Cardiovascular Therapy. 2020;**18**:363-372. DOI: 10.1080/14779072.2020.1773803

[14] Abdul-Aziz MH, Brady K, Cotta MO, Roberts JA. Therapeutic drug monitoring of antibiotics: Defining the therapeutic range. Therapeutic Drug Monitoring. 2022;**44**:19-31. DOI: 10.1097/FTD.0000000000000940

[15] Shinabarger D. Mechanism of action of the oxazolidinone antibacterial agents. Expert Opinion on Investigational Drugs. 1999;**8**:1195-1202. DOI: 10.1517/13543784.8.8.1195

[16] Safdar N, Andes D, Craig WA. In vivo pharmacodynamic activity of daptomycin. Antimicrobial Agents andChemotherapy. 2004;**48**:63-68. DOI: 10.1128/AAC.48.1.63-68.2004

[17] Silverman JA, Perlmutter NG, Shapiro HM. Correlation of daptomycin bactericidal activity and membrane depolarization in Staphylococcus aureus. Antimicrobial Agents and Chemotherapy. 2003;**47**:2538-2544. DOI: 10.1128/AAC.47.8.2538-2544.2003

[18] Kinoshita S, Wada K, Matsuda S, Kuwahara T, Sunami H, Sato T, et al. Interaction between warfarin and linezolid in patients with left ventricular assist system in Japan. Internal Medicine. 2016;**55**:719-724. DOI: 10.2169/internalmedicine.55.5756

[19] Jurgens G, Graudal NA, Kampmann JP. Therapeutic drug monitoring of antiarrhythmic drugs. Clinical Pharmacokinetics. 2003;**42**:647-663. DOI: 10.2165/00003088-200342070-00004

[20] Aonuma K, Shiga T, Atarashi H, Doki K, Echizen H, Hagiwara N, et al. Guidelines for therapeutic drug monitoring of cardiovascular drugs clinical use of blood drug concentration monitoring (JCS 2015)- digest version. Circulation Journal. 2017;**81**:581-612. DOI: 10.1253/circj.CJ-66-0138

[21] Chou NK, Wang SS, Chen YS, Yu HY, Chi NH, Wang CH, et al. Induction immunosuppression with basiliximab in heart transplantation. Transplantation Proceedings. 2008;**40**:2623-2625. DOI: 10.1016/j.transproceed.2008.07.113

[22] KittipibulV,TantrachotiP,OngcharitP, Ariyachaipanich A, Siwamogsatham S, Sritangsirikul S, et al. Low-dose basiliximab induction therapy in heart transplantation. Clinical Transplantation. 2017;**31**:e13132. DOI: 10.1111/ctr.13132

[23] Watanabe T, Yanase M, Seguchi O, Fujita T, Hamasaki T, Nakajima S, et al. Influence of induction therapy using basiliximab with delayed tacrolimus administration in heart transplant recipients - comparison with standard tacrolimus-based triple immunosuppression. Circulation Journal. 2020;**84**:2212-2223. DOI: 10.1253/circj.CJ-20-0164

[24] Chapman TM, Keating GM. Basiliximab: A review of its use as induction therapy in renal transplantation. Drugs. 2003;**63**: 2803-2835. DOI: 10.2165/00003495-200363240-00009

[25] Breslin NT, Salerno DM, Topkara VK, Latif F, Restaino S, Takeda K, et al. Prior amiodarone exposure reduces tacrolimus dosing requirements in heart transplant recipients. Progress in Transplantation. 2019;**29**:129-134. DOI: 10.1177/1526924819835840

[26] Zuo XC, Zhou YN, Zhang BK, Yang GP, Cheng ZN, Yuan H, et al. Effect of CYP3A5*3 polymorphism

on pharmacokinetic drug interaction between tacrolimus and amlodipine. Drug Metabolism and Pharmacokinetics. 2013;**28**:398-405. DOI: 10.2133/dmpk.dmpk-12-rg-148

[27] Rancic N, Dragojevic-Simic V, Vavic N, Kovacevic A, Segrt Z, Draskovic-Pavlovic B, et al. Tacrolimus concentration/dose ratio as a therapeutic drug monitoring strategy: The influence of gender and comedication. Vojnosanitetski Pregled. 2015;**72**:813-822. DOI: DOI

[28] Saad AH, DePestel DD, Carver PL. Factors influencing the magnitude and clinical significance of drug interactions between azole antifungals and select immunosuppressants. Pharmacotherapy. 2006;**26**:1730-1744. DOI: 10.1592/phco.26.12.1730

[29] Nakagita K, Wada K, Terada Y, Matsuda S, Terakawa N, Oita A, et al. Effect of fluconazole on the pharmacokinetics of everolimus and tacrolimus in a heart transplant recipient: Case report. International Journal of Clinical Pharmacology and Therapeutics. 2018;**56**:270-276. DOI: 10.5414/CP203209

[30] Uno T, Wada K, Matsuda S, Terada Y, Terakawa N, Oita A, et al. Effects of clotrimazole on tacrolimus pharmacokinetics in patients with heart transplants with different CYP3A5 genotypes. European Journal of Clinical Pharmacology. 2019;**75**:67-75. DOI: 10.1007/s00228-018-2558-6

[31] Uno T, Wada K, Hosomi K, Matsuda S, Ikura MM, Takenaka H, et al. Drug interactions between tacrolimus and clotrimazole troche: A data mining approach followed by a pharmacokinetic study. European Journal of Clinical Pharmacology. 2020;**76**:117-125. DOI: 10.1007/s00228-019-02770-6

[32] Ikura M, Nakamura T, Uno T, Nakagita K, Takenaka H, Matsuda S, et al. Discontinuation of oral amphotericin B therapy does not influence the pharmacokinetics of tacrolimus in heart transplant patients. International Journal of Clinical Pharmacology and Therapeutics. 2021;**59**:566-571. DOI: 10.5414/CP204005

[33] Takayoshi M, Wada K, Terada Y, Matsuda S, Nakagita K, Oita A, et al. Use of rifabutin to treat tuberculosis in a cardiac transplant recipient: A case report. International Journal of Clinical Pharmacology and Therapeutics. 2018;**56**:184-188. DOI: 10.5414/CP203137

[34] Iwasaki K. Metabolism of tacrolimus (FK506) and recent topics in clinical pharmacokinetics. Drug Metabolism and Pharmacokinetics. 2007;**22**:328-335. DOI: 10.2133/dmpk.22.328

[35] Uno T, Wada K, Matsuda S, Terada Y, Oita A, Kawase A, et al. Impact of the CYP3A5*1 allele on the pharmacokinetics of tacrolimus in Japanese heart transplant patients. European Journal of Drug Metabolism and Pharmacokinetics. 2018;**43**:665-673. DOI: 10.1007/s13318-018-0478-6

[36] Uno T, Wada K, Matsuda S, Terada Y, Oita A, Takada M, et al. Comparison of CYP3A5*3 genotyping assays for personalizing immunosuppressive therapy in heart transplant patients. International Journal of Clinical Pharmacology and Therapeutics. 2019;**57**:315-322. DOI: 10.5414/CP203381

[37] Hiratsuka M, Takekuma Y, Endo N, Narahara K, Hamdy SI, Kishikawa Y, et al. Allele and genotype frequencies of CYP2B6 and CYP3A5 in the Japanese population. European Journal of Clinical Pharmacology. 2002;**58**:417-421. DOI: 10.1007/s00228-002-0499-5

[38] Fukuen S, Fukuda T, Maune H, Ikenaga Y, Yamamoto I, Inaba T, et al. Novel detection assay by PCR-RFLP and frequency of the CYP3A5 SNPs, CYP3A5*3 and *6, in a Japanese population. Pharmacogenetics. 2002;**12**:331-334. DOI: 10.1097/00008571-200206000-00009

[39] Saeki M, Saito Y, Nakamura T, Murayama N, Kim SR, Ozawa S, et al. Single nucleotide polymorphisms and haplotype frequencies of CYP3A5 in a Japanese population. Human Mutation. 2003;**21**:653. DOI: 10.1002/humu.9147

[40] Ransom JT. Mechanism of action of mycophenolate mofetil. Therapeutic Drug Monitoring. 1995;**17**:681-684. DOI: 10.1097/00007691-199512000-00023

[41] van Gelder T. Mycophenolate blood level monitoring: Recent progress. American Journal of Transplantation. 2009;**9**:1495-1499. DOI: 10.1111/j.1600-6143.2009.02678.x

[42] Behrend M. Adverse gastrointestinal effects of mycophenolate mofetil: Aetiology, incidence and management. Drug Safety. 2001;**24**:645-663. DOI: 10.2165/00002018-200124090-00002

[43] Tielemans MM, van Boekel GAJ, van Gelder T, Tjwa ET, Hilbrands LB. Immunosuppressive drugs and the gastrointestinal tract in renal transplant patients. Transplantation Reviews. 2019;**33**:55-63. DOI: 10.1016/j.trre.2018.11.001

[44] Yamazaki K, Ariyoshi N, Miyauchi H, Ohira G, Kaneya N, Yamamoto K, et al. A randomized controlled, open-label early phase II trial comparing incidence of FOLFIRI.3-induced diarrhoea between Hangeshashinto and oral alkalization in Japanese patients with colorectal cancer. Journal of Clinical Pharmacy and Therapeutics. 2019;**44**:946-951. DOI: 10.1111/jcpt.13020

[45] Mori K, Kondo T, Kamiyama Y, Kano Y, Tominaga K. Preventive effect of Kampo medicine (Hangeshashin-to) against irinotecan-induced diarrhea in advanced non-small-cell lung cancer. Cancer Chemotherapy and Pharmacology. 2003;**51**:403-406. DOI: 10.1007/s00280-003-0585-0

[46] Watanabe M, Yuzawa K, Homma M, Ohkohchi N. Establishment of an animal model with side effects induced by mycophenolate mofetil and pharmacohistological analysis of them. Transplantation Proceedings. 2006;**38**:3323-3326. DOI: 10.1016/j.transproceed.2006.10.162

[47] Wullschleger S, Loewith R, Hall MN. TOR signaling in growth and metabolism. Cell. 2006;**124**:471-484. DOI: 10.1016/j.cell.2006.01.016

[48] Shipkova M, Hesselink DA, Holt DW, Billaud EM, van Gelder T, Kunicki PK, et al. Therapeutic drug monitoring of everolimus: A consensus report. Therapeutic Drug Monitoring. 2016;**38**:143-169. DOI: 10.1097/FTD.0000000000000260

[49] Defilippis EM, Kittleson MM. Pregnancy after heart transplantation. Journal of Cardiac Failure. 2021;**27**:176-184. DOI: 10.1016/j.cardfail.2020.07.011

[50] Abushammala I. Tacrolimus and herbs interactions: A review. Die Pharmazie. 2021;**76**:468-472. DOI: 10.1691/ph.2021.1684

[51] ASHP. Specialty Pharmacy Resource Guide: American Society of Health-System Pharmacist. Bethesda, MD, USA:

American Society of Health-System Pharmacists; 2015. Available from: https://www.ashp.org/-/media/assets/pharmacy-practice/resource-centers/specialty-pharmacy/specialty-pharmacy-resource-guide.ashx

[52] Maldonado AQ, Hall RC, Pilch NA, Ensor CR, Anders S, Gilarde JA, et al. ASHP guidelines on pharmacy services in solid organ transplantation. American Journal of Health-System Pharmacy. 2020;**77**:222-232. DOI: 10.1093/ajhp/zxz291

[53] Sam S, Guerin A, Rieutord A, Belaiche S, Bussieres JF. Roles and impacts of the transplant pharmacist: A systematic review. Canadian Journal of Hospital Pharmacy. 2018;**71**:324-337

Chapter 11

Limited Sampling Strategies to Monitoring Mycophenolic Acid Exposure in a Heterogeneous Population of Heart Transplant Recipients: A Pilot Study

Francesco Lo Re, Sandro Sponga, Jacopo Angelini, Chiara Nalli, Antonella Zucchetto, Ugolino Livi and Massimo Baraldo

Abstract

Mycophenolate mofetil (MMF) represents a cornerstone in heart transplant (HTx) treatment. The area under the 12-hour concentration-time curve ($AUC_{0\text{-}12h}$) of mycophenolic acid (MPA) -MMF's active drug- is associated with treatment outcome. Nonetheless, therapeutic drug monitoring (TDM) of MPA $AUC_{0\text{-}12h}$ is impractical to assess in clinical practice and Limited Sampling Strategies (LSSs) represent a consolidated tool to estimate $AUC_{0\text{-}12h}$. Two LSSs were previously generated in a selected cohort of HTx recipients treated with MMF and cyclosporine (CsA). This pilot study aimed to test these LSSs in a cohort of non-selected HTx recipients treated with MMF combined with CsA or tacrolimus (TAC). Complete PK profile was performed in 40 adults HTx recipients. MPA-$AUC_{0\text{-}12h}$ was estimated by two algorithms, LSS3 and LSS4, based on 3 and 4 time-points. The evaluation was made through linear regression and Bland-Altman analyses. Both LSS3 and LSS4 tended to underestimate the value of MPA-$AUC_{0\text{-}12h}$ (mean percentage prediction error, MPE%: −6.0%; and −4.8%, respectively). Nonetheless, high correlations (r: 0.92 and 0.94, respectively) and goodness of fit of linear regression models (R^2: 0.84 and 0.88, respectively) emerged for both LSSs. A study with a wider and more homogenous sample size should be performed to support these results.

Keywords: heart transplantation, immunosuppressive treatment, therapeutic drug monitoring, treatment efficacy, rejection prevention

1. Introduction

Mycophenolate Mofetil MMF (CellCept; Roche, Basel, Switzerland) is a widely prescribed drug as part of maintenance immunosuppressive regimen after heart transplant (HTx) [1]. It is frequently administered in association with calcineurin inhibitors (CNIs) like cyclosporine (CsA), tacrolimus (TAC), and prednisone.

MMF is a pro-drug that, after oral administration, is rapidly hydrolyzed to its active form, mycophenolic acid (MPA), by esterases mainly in the gastrointestinal wall, blood, and liver, but also in other tissues [2]. MPA is a selective, potent and reversible inhibitor of inosine-5′-monophosphate dehydrogenase (IMPDH), a key enzyme of the *de novo* purine synthesis. This block causes the arrest of the proliferation of T- and B-cells [2]. In addition to this major immunosuppressive mechanism, MPA could cause the alteration of lymphocyte and monocyte recruitment, adhesion, and penetration. Furthermore, exposure to MPA could result in the apoptosis of activated human T lymphocytes, and the reduction of cytokine production. Moreover, it has been evidenced an antiproliferative effect on monocytes, fibroblasts, endothelial cells, mesangial cells, and smooth muscle cells. Nonetheless, MPA could inhibit mesangial matrix expansion, and alter the cytoskeletal organization [3, 4]. Some of these effects, including the reduction of important lymphocyte cell surface antigens expression, are independent from IMPDH inhibition [5, 6].

Generally, MMF is prescribed at a fixed dose, but there are several pharmacokinetic (PK) factors that could affect its efficacy. After MMF administration, MPA shows non-linear absorption kinetics, and a complex inter-patient and intra-patients PK variability [7], that could be attributable to MPA enterohepatic circulation (EHC), graft function, genetic factors, changes in plasma protein binding, and drug–drug interactions. MPA time to reach the plasma maximum concentration (T_{max}) occurs after 1–2 hours after dosage [8].

MPA presents a higher bioavailability, ranging from 80.7–94% [8]. In blood, MPA widely binds serum albumin, from 97–99% in patients with normal renal and hepatic function. Consistently, it has been evidenced that hypoalbuminemia could increase MPA free fraction *in vitro* [9] and *in vivo* [10]. In particular, an increase of 2.2-fold of MPA free fraction emerged *in vitro* when MPA albumin was reduced from 41.4 g/L to 20.7 g/L, and a further increase of 41-fold when albumin was reduced to 0.07 g/L [9]. In a study including 42 adult kidney transplant recipients, a relationship between low serum albumin and an increased MPA free fraction was reported [10]. The authors identified a threshold of 31 g/L below of which MPA free fraction was considered to be significantly elevated, suggesting that the Therapeutic Drug Monitoring (TDM) of MPA free fraction could be recommended in patients with this clinical condition [10].

MPA is mainly metabolized in liver, kidney, and gastrointestinal tract by uridine 5′-diphospho-glucuronosyltransferases (UGTs). The major metabolite of MPA, 7-O-MPA-glucuronide (MPAG), is inactive but it is present in the plasma at higher concentrations than MPA. MPAG is excreted into the urine via active tubular secretion and into the bile by multi-drug resistance protein 2 (MRP-2), and at the gastrointestinal level MPAG could be de-conjugated back to MPA by gastrointestinal flora and then reabsorbed in the colon, resulting in a secondary plasma peak between 6 and 12 hours after oral administration. This may contribute to the 30–40% of MPA exposure. Severe renal impairment, liver disease, and hypoalbuminemia could affect MPA exposure [11]. The co-administration of CsA, by inhibiting the MRP-2 mainly in the gastrointestinal tract, causes a reduction of MPA EHC, resulting in an approximately 30–40% lower MPA exposure than when MMF is administered in combination with TAC [2, 8, 12]. Furthermore, it has been evidenced that CsA administration could affect MPA Clearance (Cl) [13]. Moreover, corticosteroids may reduce the exposure of MPA by inducing the expression of UGTs [8].

For these reasons, the execution of TDM could be an effective strategy to maximize the efficacy of the treatment also reduce the risk of toxicity. Several studies have suggested the importance of MPA TDM in renal and heart transplants recipients [14–16]. The best PK parameter correlating with the efficacy of treatment is represented by MPA's area under the plasma concentration-time curve from 0 to 12 hours (MPA AUC_{0-12h}) [11, 17] and several studies show that MPA plasma levels correlate to risk of rejection [18, 19]. The therapeutic range has been well determined in renal transplant recipients (30–60 mg × h/L) [20], and some authors suggested similar therapeutic thresholds on MPA-AUC_{0-12h} also in HTx [21, 22].

The entire MPA AUC_{0-12h} is difficult to calculate in clinical practice, due to its costly and laborious assessment. On the contrary, the single time-point measurement is the easiest for sampling, but it is not sufficiently predictive of patient outcome [20], taking also in consideration that MPA is characterized by >10-fold range variation in MPA AUC_{0-12h} dose-normalized among patients undergoing heart or renal transplantation [23, 24].

Limited Sampling Strategies (LSSs) represent the most relevant assessment in solid organ transplantation for dosage individualization, that could overcome this problem [20]. LSSs are algorithm-based strategies able to predict the entire AUC_{0-12h} without the necessity of sampling all the time-point concentrations after drug administration, but limiting the sampling to a reduced number of measurements, usually three time-points or even fewer. They can be developed by two main methods represented by multiple linear regression (MLR) or by with maximum a posteriori Bayesian estimation (MAP-BE).

MLR represents the simplest technique to develop an LSS. It requires statistical knowledge and the main strength of this approach is the adhesion to the sampling time.

On the other hand, developing an LSSs by maximum a posteriori Bayesian estimation (MAP-BE) is more complex because specialized PK modeling software knowledge is required.

From a methodological point of view, LSS should be generated on a cohort of patients (*training group*) and then validated in the second cohort of patients (*validation group*) to be used in clinical practice [25]. In the case of MLR LSSs, the relationship between the observed AUC_{0-12h} and the estimated blood concentration-time points must be determined in the *training group* through linear regression, considering AUC_{0-12h} as the dependent variable and the blood concentrations at each time point as the independent variables.

To exclude biased results, the LSS performance should be assessed in the *validation group* evaluating the mean prediction error or bias and the root mean squared prediction error or precision, as well as the median prediction error and the median absolute prediction error [26]. These same figures can be also calculated based on percentage prediction error, and expressed in percentages, to be more easily interpretable in the clinical contest as suggested by Baraldo et al. [25]. In both cases, the values of these parameters are inversely and proportionally linked to the LSS prediction. In the end, the correlation coefficient (r) and the coefficient of determination (R^2) between the estimated and the observed AUC_{0-12h} must be assessed.

Recently, Baraldo et al. reviewed the state of the art of MPA LSSs in HTx recipients [25]. In the last few years, the immunosuppression therapy after HTx has changed, with the massive use of TAC compared to CsA, in combination with MMF and corticosteroids.

This pilot study aimed to test, in a heterogeneous cohort of patients treated with MMF and CSA or TAC, two algorithms of LSSs previously generated by Baraldo et al. [27, 28] in a selected cohort of HTx recipients treated with MMF and CSA. These algorithms were selected due to their good performance [28] and given the hypothesis that the LSSs sampling time point schedule was able to determinate MPA $AUC_{0\text{-}12h}$ even when MMF was administrated combined with TAC.

If this pilot study reports positive results, the generation of new LSS in a population of HTx treated with MMF and TAC would not be required.

2. Methods

2.1 Study characteristics

This is a pilot observational, retrospective, cohort study. The study was performed at the University Hospital of Udine, in Italy. The study was approved by the Internal Review Board (I.R.B.) of the Commission for the Experimentation and Protection of Human Subjects of the Department of Medical Area of the University of Udine with the protocol number: 036/2020_IRB.

The study included 40 HTx recipients previously treated as per standard clinical practice with MMF and CsA or MMF and TAC, and prednisone, at the University Hospital of Udine, and routinely monitored for MPA quantification in the period starting from the 01st/01/2011 up to the 31st/12/2019. The patients included in the study were HTx recipients, aged 18 years old or more, and treated with MMF and either CsA or TAC and prednisone. Patients treated with immunosuppression drugs other than MMF, CsA and TAC, or with the absence of necessary information for the study in the clinical records or with the absence of informed consent for clinical, epidemiological research, training and study of pathologies were excluded from the study. All consecutive HTx recipients in the study period who met inclusion/exclusion criteria were included in the analysis.

All HTx recipients received a standard triple immunosuppressive therapy: MMF in combination with CsA or TAC and prednisone. The posology regimen of MMF varied from 1000 to 3500 mg/day, with a mean of 1785.5 mg/day ($\pm$ 553.4). While the mean CsA dose was 3.0 mg/kg/day ($\pm$ 1.3) p.o. in 2 divided doses, mean TAC dose was 0.1 mg/kg/day ($\pm$0.06). Patients treated with prokinetic drugs, resins or other drugs known to interfere with MPA PK, other than prednisone, were excluded from the analysis.

2.2 PK profiles of mycophenolate mofetil

A complete PK profile was available for the 40 HTx recipients included in the present analysis. Patients had been asked to take their usual morning dose of MMF after having a standard meal. Patients had not changed the therapeutic regimen for 30 days and had been at a steady state for MMF. Eight venous samples had been collected for the analysis of MPA plasma concentrations. For MPA assays, blood samples had been collected in EDTA tubes at 0 (pre-dose), 0.5, 1.25, 2, 4, 6, 8, and 12 hours after the morning dose. Separation of plasma was performed immediately in a centrifuge at 4°C. Plasma MPA concentration was measured using validated High Pressure Liquid Chromatography with UV Detector (HPLC/UV) method [23], that ensure to achieve an analytical precision and accuracy that fulfill the International Association of Therapeutic Drug Monitoring and Clinical Toxicology (IATDMCT) recommendations [20]. The laboratory reported the following parameters for the HPLC/UV method used for MPA quantification: limit of detection, 0.1 μg/mL; linearity, 0.1–40 μg/mL (R^2: 0.9988); intrabatch imprecision (CV), 3.15%, 1.55%, and 1.76%

at MPA plasma concentrations of 1.5, 5.0, 15.0 μg/mL, respectively; interbatch imprecision (CV), 3.41%, 3.21%, and 1.92% at MPA plasma concentrations of 1.5, 5.0, 15.0 μg/mL, respectively; overall inaccuracy (% Bias) of the procedure, ranged from 8.7% to 13.6%. MPA AUC_{0-12h} had been calculated by the linear trapezoidal rule.

2.3 Algorithms evaluation

The two algorithms used for MPA AUC_{0-12h} evaluation were the followings:

$$LSS3: MPA\ AUC_{0-12h} = 5.568 + 0.902 \times C_{1.25h} + 2.022 \times C_{2h} + 4.594 \times C_{6h}$$

$$LSS4: MPA\ AUC_{0-12h} = 3.800 + 1.015 \times C_{1.25h} + 1.819 \times C_{2h} + 1.566 \times C_{4h} + 3.479 \times C_{6h}$$

According to Sheiner and Beal, to assess the bias of the LSSs, we calculated Mean Percentage Prediction Error (MPE%) and the Median Percentage Prediction Error (MPPE%) [26]. To assess precision was calculated Root Mean Squared Percentage Prediction Error (RMSE%) and the Median Absolute Percentage Prediction Error (MAPE%) [26].

The MPE%, MPPE%, RMSE% and MAPE% were calculated as follows:

Bias:

$$MPE\% = mean\left(\frac{predicted\ AUC_{0-12h} - measured\ AUC_{0-12h}}{measured\ AUC_{0-12h}} \times 100\%\right) \quad (1)$$

$$MPPE\% = median\left(\frac{predicted\ AUC_{0-12h} - measured\ AUC_{0-12h}}{measured\ AUC_{0-12h}} \times 100\%\right) \quad (2)$$

Imprecision:

$$RMSE\% = \sqrt{mean\left(\frac{predicted\ AUC_{0-12h} - measured\ AUC_{0-12h}}{measured\ AUC_{0-12h}} \times 100\%\right)^2} \quad (3)$$

$$MAPE\% = median\left(\frac{|predicted\ AUC_{0-12h} - measured\ AUC_{0-12h}|}{measured\ AUC_{0-12h}} \times 100\%\right) \quad (4)$$

For bias, we set the limit of 15%, while for imprecision the limit was set at 20%. The percentage of estimated AUC_{0-12h} between 75–125% of the observed AUC_{0-12h} was also calculated.

To compare our results to an already validated algorithm, we tested one other LSS equation developed in HTx by Kaczmareck et al. [29]:

$$LSS_{Kazmareck}: MPA\ AUC_{0-12h} = 1.65 \times C_{0.5h} + 4.74 \times C_{2h}$$

2.4 Statistical consideration

Descriptive statistical analyses were conducted for all the study variables, reporting position and variability indexes (e.g., mean and standard deviation, SD) for quantitative variables. Differences between groups were evaluated using the Fisher's exact test for nominal variables and the Student's T-test for quantitative variables, and considering as statistically significant a p-value <0.05.

The two methods of LSS were validated by using both linear regression and Bland–Altman analysis, as recommended by the literature [26, 30]. All the analyses were performed with Medcalc Software version 19.7.2 ® (Med-Calc Software, Ostend, Belgium®). Pearson's linear correlation coefficient (*r*) was calculated using linear regression (considering the following categories for the absolute value |*r*|: <0.50 weak correlation, 0.50–0.80 moderate correlation; >0.80 strong correlation). The determination coefficient (R^2) was also reported to assess the goodness of fit of the linear models. Bland–Altman analysis was used to evaluate the agreement between the predicted AUC_{0-12h} and the measured AUC_{0-12h}.

3. Results

3.1 Patients characteristics

The main characteristics of study patients are reported in **Table 1**.

All patients were Caucasian and most of the analyzed patients shown normal renal and hepatic functionality. Patients treated to CsA- or TAC-based maintenance immunosuppression were comparable for most of the baseline characteristics, including age, body mass index (BMI), MMF administered dose, renal and hepatic function, except for sex, bilirubin, post transplantation time, MPA AUC_{0-12h} and MPA C_0. A number of 15 acute cell rejections occurred after a median time of 8.95 months from transplantation, especially in the patients group treated with MMF-CsA than in the MMF-TAC group (87% vs. 13%, respectively). According to the International Society for Heart and Lung Transplantation, the overall rejections were classified as follows: 8 GRADE 1R (55%), 5 GRADE 2R (33%) and 2 GRADE 3R (13%) [31]. No patients reported any episodes of diarrhea.

3.2 Method results

In the whole cohort of patients, a low tendency to underestimation of the value of MPA AUC_{0-12h} by both LSS3 and LSS4 emerged evaluating MPE% for mean values (−6.0% and − 4.8%, respectively) and MPPE% for median values (−3.8% and − 1.1%, respectively). The precision of LSS3 and LSS4 was acceptable, by evaluating RMSE% for mean values (19.6% and 16.2%, respectively) and MAPE% for median values (13.5% and 11.0%, respectively). The percentages of MPA AUC_{0-12h} predicted by LSS3 and LSS4 within the 25% of the MPA AUC_{0-12h} full value was 73% and 80%, for LSS3 and LSS4, respectively.

Linear regression and Bland–Altman analyses evidenced that both LSS3 and LSS4 methods can effectively predict the values of MPA AUC_{0-12h}. The value of *r* stated for both LSSs methods a strong correlation between the measured MPA AUC_{0-12h} and the AUC_{0-12h} predicted by both LSSs methods (*r*: 0.92 and 0.94 for LSS3 and LSS4, respectively). Finally, the R^2 (0.84; 0.88, for LSS3 and LSS4, respectively) indicates high goodness of fit of the regression line for both methods. The results are shown in **Figure 1a** and **b**. The Bland–Altman plots (**Figure 2a** and **b**) showed that the data were arranged almost totally within the range mean +/−1.96*SD. The visual inspection of the plots does not reveal any particular pattern, thus excluding other types of bias. This was also assessed by analyzing the linear dependence of the dots in the Bland Altman plot using linear regression, reporting the following results for LSS3 and LSS4 respectively (r = 0.51 and 0.55; R^2: 0.26 and 0.30). These results do not indicate linear dependence.

A subgroup analysis was also conducted stratifying the patients for the co- treatment.

	Total	MMF + CsA	MMF + TAC	*p*-value[a]
No. pts.	40	28	12	
Sex (No. males, % males)	30 (75%)	25 (89%)	5 (42%)	0.003
Age (years)	56.1 ± 12.1	58.4 ± 10.8	57.5 ± 13.7	0.10
MMF Dose (mg/day)	1785.7 ± 553.4	1785.7 ± 551.6	1791.7 ± 582.3	0.98
MMF Dose (mg/kg/day)	24.4 ± 8.1	23.1 ± 6.9	24.3 ± 4.6	0.22
Post-Transpl. time (months)	34.7 ± 52.5	45.1 ± 59.4	10.6 ± 14	0.01
BMI (Kg/m^2)	25.9 ± 5.4	26.5 ± 5.7	24.3 ± 4.6	0.21
ALT (IU/L)	26.5 ± 19.5	28.6 ± 20.9	25.9 ± 15.5	0.24
AST (IU/L)	22.9 ± 16.6	24.5 ± 18.6	19.0 ± 9.9	0.23
Bilirubin (mg/dL)	0.9 ± 0.7	1.1 ± 0.7	0.5 ± 0.2	<0.001
RBCs (x10^6/μL)	4.1 ± 0.6	4.2 ± 0.7	3.9 ± 0.5	0.08
Hb (g/dL)	12 ± 1.9	12.3 ± 1.9	11.4 ± 1.6	0.10
WBCs (x10^3/μL)	7.7 ± 2.8	8.1 ± 2.8	6.9 ± 2.8	0.25
Neutro (x10^3/μL)	5.7 ± 2.7	6.1 ± 2.8	5 ± 2.3	0.20
Lymph (x10^3/μL)	1.2 ± 0.6	1.2 ± 0.5	1.1 ± 0.5	0.73
Mono (x10^3/μL)	0.86 ± 1.3	0.9 ± 0.2	0.7 ± 0.2	0.41
Eos (x10^3/μL)	0.09 ± 0.08	0.09 ± 0.1	0.1 ± 0.1	0.84
Bas (x10^3/μL)	0.04 ± 0.03	0.04 ± 0	0.05 ± 0	0.74
CrCl (mL/min)[b]	62.0 ± 26.3	59.7 ± 25.4	67.4 ± 28.7	0.4
GFR (ml/min/1.73m^2)[c]	59.0 ± 23.4	56.4 ± 24.8	64.4 ± 19.9	0.3
MPA $AUC_{0\text{-}12h}$ (mg × h/L)	47.2 ± 24.7	36.4 ± 13.0	72.3 ± 27.6	0.001
MPA C_0 (ug/ml)	2.4 ± 2.0	1.6 ± 1.0	4.1 ± 2.6	<0.001
Prednisone (mg/day)	12.8 ± 9.4	11.9 ± 9.6	15.4 ± 8.8	0.24
Prednisone (mg/kg/day)	0.2 ± 0.1	0.2 ± 0.1	0.2 ± 0.2	0.10
CsA Dose(mg/day)	—	179.6 ± 75.4	—	
CsA Dose (mg/kg/day)	—	3.0 ± 1.3	—	
CsA C_0 (ng/mL)		177.1 ± 64.9		
TAC Dose (mg/day)	—	—	6.0 ± 5.0	
TAC Dose (mg/kg/day)	—	—	0.1 ± 0.06	
Tac C_0 (ng/mL)			10.6 ± 4.25	

[a]*p-values of 2-sided Fisher's exact test for nominal variables or T- test for quantitative variables.*
[b]*Evaluated by Cockcroft-Gault adjusted for body weight.*
[c]*Evaluated by CKD-EPI Equation.*
Data are reported as mean ± standard deviation, if not otherwise specified.
$AUC_{0\text{-}12h}$: Area under the plasma concentration-time curve from zero to 12 h; ALT: Alanine Aminotransferase; AST: Aspartate Aminotransferase; Bas: Basophils; BMI: Body Mass Index; C_0: pre-dose measurement; CsA: Cyclosporine; CrCl: Creatinine Clearance; Eos: Eosinophils; GFR: Glomerular Filtration Rate; Hb: Hemoglobin level; Lymph: Lymphocytes; Mono: Monocytes; MMF: Mycophenolate Mofetil; MPA: Mycophenolic Acid; Neutro: Neutrophils; RBCs: Red Blood Cells; TAC: Tacrolimus; WBCs: White Blood Cells.

Table 1.
Patients baseline demographical and clinical data, overall and according to the type of treatment.

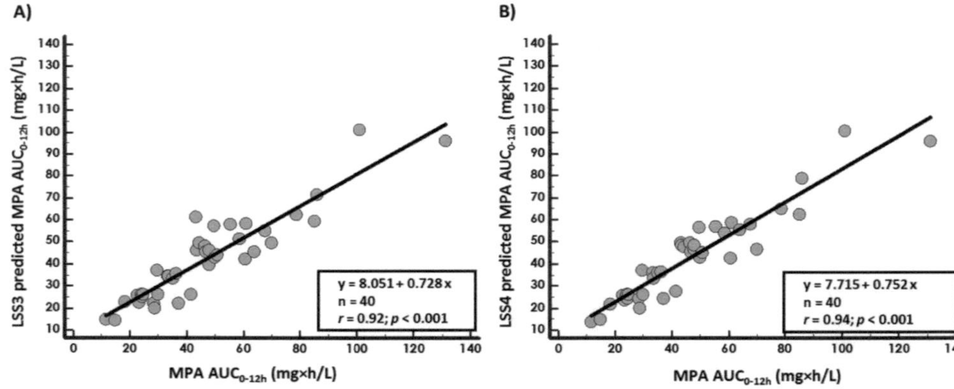

Figure 1.
Linear regression scatters plot of MPA $AUC_{0\text{-}12h}$ predicted versus MPA $AUC_{0\text{-}12h}$ measured, when MPA $AUC_{0\text{-}12h}$ predicted was calculated with LSS3 (A) and LSS4 (B) (n = 40 PK profile).

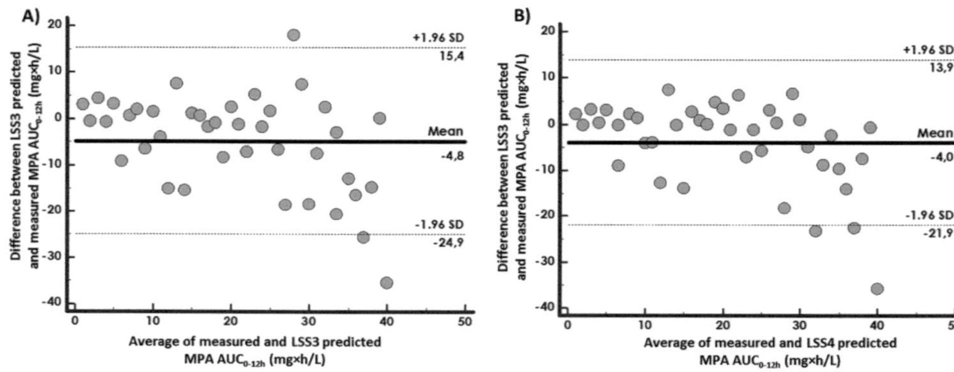

Figure 2.
Bland–Altman plots comparing MPA $AUC_{0\text{-}12h}$ predicted – MPA $AUC_{0\text{-}12h}$ measured and the average of MPA $AUC_{0\text{-}12h}$ predicted and MPA $AUC_{0\text{-}12h}$ measured, when MPA $AUC_{0\text{-}12h}$ predicted was calculated by LSS3 (A) and LSS4 (B) respectively (n = 40 PK profile).

Among 28 patients treated with MMF and CsA, the bias was acceptable, evaluating MPE% for mean values (−0.5% and − 0.3%) and MPPE% for median values (2.3% and 0.7%) for LSS3 and LSS4, respectively. Analogously, the precision was acceptable evaluating RMSE% (18.6% and 14.8%) and MAPE% (12.4% and 9.7%), for LSS3 and LSS4, respectively. The percentages of MPA $AUC_{0\text{-}12h}$ estimated by LSS3 and LSS4 within the 25% of the MPA $AUC_{0\text{-}12h}$ full value were 79% and 86%, respectively.

Finally, in the sub-group of 12 patients treated with MMF and TAC, these same features were the followings: MPE% = −18.9% and − 15.3%; MPPE% = −19.9% and − 14.0%; RMSE% = 21.7% and 19.2%; MAPE% = 19.0% and 14.0%, for LLS3 and LSS4, respectively.

The percentage of MPA $AUC_{0\text{-}12h}$ predicted within the 25% of the measured MPA $AUC_{0\text{-}12h}$ full value: 58% and 67%, for LSS3 and LSS4 respectively.

Despite the very low number of patients, also the linear regression analyses executed on the two subgroups of patients evidenced good results.

In the MMF and CsA group the results were the followings: r = 0.83 and 0.89; R^2 = 0.70 and 0.79, for LSS3 and LSS4 respectively; while in the MMF and TAC group

Population	Algorithm	MPE (%)	MPPE (%)	RMSE (%)	MAPE (%)	% within 75–125% of full $AUC_{0\text{-}12h}$	R^2
Overall (N = 40)	LSS3	−6.0	−3.8	19.6	13.5	73	0.84
	LSS4	−4.8	−1.1	16.2	11.0	80	0.88
MMF and CsA group (N = 28)	LSS3	−0.5	2.3	18.6	12.4	79	0.70
	LSS4	−0.3	0.7	14.8	9.7	86	0.79
MMF and TAC group (N = 12)	LSS3	−18.9	−19.9	21.7	19.0	58	0.87
	LSS4	−15.3	−14.0	19.2	14.0	67	0.86

$AUC_{0\text{-}12h}$: Area under the plasma concentration-time curve from zero to 12 h; CsA: Cyclosporine; LSS3: Limited Sampling Strategy based on 3 concentration sampling points; LSS4: Limited Sampling Strategy based on 4 concentration sampling points; MAPE%: Median Absolute Percentage Prediction Error; MMF: Mycophenolate Mofetil; MPA: Mycophenolic Acid; MPE%: Mean Percentage Prediction Error; MPPE%: Median Percentage Prediction Error; RMSE%: Root Mean Squared Percentage Prediction Error; R^2: coefficient of determination; TAC: Tacrolimus.

Table 2.
Predictive performance of LSS3 and LSS4 in the estimation of the observed MPA $AUC_{0\text{-}12h}$.

these were the results: r = 0.93 and 0.93; R^2 = 0.87 and 0.86, for LSS3 and LSS4 respectively. All these results are summarized on **Table 2.**

The analysis of Kaczamarek LSSs applied to our patient's data reports the following results: r = 0.70; R^2 = 0.49; MPE% = 11.4% and RMSE% = 66.1% in the overall population. By applying these LSSs in the TAC subgroup of patients, we evidenced the following results: r = 0.69; R^2 = 0.48; MPE% = −6.2% and RMSE% = 32.1%.

4. Discussion

The importance of MPA TDM for renal transplant patients is known, but its execution on HTx patients in clinical practice is still debated [17]. Specific large prospective randomized trials should be conducted, but the considerable inter- and intra-patient variability of MPA after organ transplantation suggest MPA TDM to optimize MPA exposure.

The systematic review regarding MPA TDM in HTx reported by Zuk et al. suggests that the relationship between MPA levels and the efficacy of the treatment in terms of allograft rejection in HTx patients is not defined, but LSS may be a better assessment strategy to prevent rejection than a single-time point model [32]. An LSS can be generated using two main methods: MAP-BE method and MLR analysis.

In the first case, any recorded patient sample is compared with data derived from the population PK study, and the covariates can be continually improved by updating the PK population data. The main advantage of the first approach is represented by the flexibility in the timing of the samples as recently demonstrated by Woillard et al. [22]. The main limit of this approach is represented by the employment of complex and specific software, requiring skilled professionals.

On the contrary, multiple regression analysis is simpler, but adherence to the sampling time is mandatory to apply the algorithms in clinical practice. To our knowledge, up to now, few LSSs were developed in HTx, and most of them were generated in patients treated with MMF and CsA [25]. Only three studies focused on LSSs in HTx recipients treated with MMF and TAC [29, 33, 34].

Xiang et al. [33] generated an LSS for the estimation of MMF dispersible tablets combined with TAC in 30 Chinese HTx patients. The comparison of MPA PK among MMF dispersible tablets and MMF did not show significant differences. The LSS with the best performance was the following: MPA $AUC_{0\text{-}12h} = 8.424 + 0.781 \times C_{0.5h} + 1.263 \times C_{2h} + 1.660 \times C_{4h} + 3.022 \times C_{6h}$ ($R^2 = 0.844$). The performance of this LSS can be considered comparable with our algorithms and both contain the C_{6h} sample timing point improving the MPA $AUC_{0\text{-}12h}$ estimation thanks to the inclusion of the typical secondary peak of MPA, minimizing the risk of MPA $AUC_{0\text{-}12h}$ underestimation. Nevertheless, this LSS was developed in Chinese patients so it could not properly fit the Caucasian population, although literature does not suggest this hypothesis [35]. Moreover, these LSSs were developed analyzing the plasma timing point by Liquid Chromatography with tandem mass spectrometry (LC/MS–MS), so they cannot be easily transferred in that laboratories which employ HPLC/UV methods.

Kaczmarek et al. [29] generated different LSSs in 28 HTx recipients treated with MMF and TAC. The best LSS was obtained using 4 sampling points: MPA-$AUC_{0\text{-}12\text{-}h} = 1.25 \times C_{1h} + 5.29 \times C_{4h} + 2.90 \times C_{8h} + 3.61 \times C_{10h}$ ($R^2 = 0.95$). The studied population is comparable to our population. Also, in this case, it can be seen that by sampling the timing point after several hours from MMF administration, a better MPA-$AUC_{0\text{-}12h}$ estimation can be achieved. These LSSs show an optimal performance, but it is based on a demanding sampling schedule that can be applied only on hospitalized patients, thus excluding the outpatient settings.

For this reason, authors proposed two different and more practical LSSs represented by: MPA $AUC_{0\text{-}12h} = 1.09 \times C_{0.5} + 1.19 \times C_{1h} + 3.60 \times C_{2h}$ ($R^2 = 0.84$) and MPA $AUC_{0\text{-}12h} = 1.65 \times C_{0.5h} + 4.74 \times C_{2h}$ ($R^2 = 0.75$). Due to the missing data about the C_{1h} in our population, we test the second LSS. The performance was not acceptable for the use in clinical practice as compared to our algorithms. This could be due to the absence of the C_{6h} sampling time point, resulting in MPA $AUC_{0\text{-}12h}$ underestimation.

Wada et al. [34] generated an LSS in 11 Chinese HTx recipients treated MMF and TAC approximately 9 months after transplantation. In this case, the author used the same analytical method, pharmacokinetic and statistical approaches.

They generated a 3-point model LSS based on C_{1h}, C_{2h} and C_{4h}: MPA $AUC_{0\text{-}12h} = 23.56 + 1.05 \times C_{1h} + 1.25 \times C_{2h} + 2.53 \times C_{4h}$ ($R^2 = 0.73$), with an MPE% of 2.73%. The results of Wada's study should be taken with caution because of the limited number of enrolled patients and the ethnic difference that could influence MPA PK.

On the other hand, Pawinski et al. proposed an accurate LSS in HTx patients treated with MMF (and CsA) [36] is based on 3 sampling time-points 2 hours after drug administration. The LSSs developed was the following: MPA $AUC_{0\text{-}12h} = 9.69 + 0.63 \times C_{0.5h} + 0.61 \times C_{1h} + 2.20 \times C_{2h}$. It showed a good performance ($R^2 = 0.84$), and for its sampling schedule it can be applied in the outpatient setting. Nevertheless, this LSS was generated on the patient in combination therapy with MMF and CsA. For this reason, this algorithm could be acceptable in patients co-treated with CsA because of its effect on reducing the typical MPA secondary peak, affecting MPA EHC [2]. Moreover, the authors developed an algorithm including the C_{6h} blood sample. It presented a similar R^2 and can be considered more predictive of the entire $AUC_{0\text{-}12h}$ because it can describe the typical MPA secondary peak that occurs approximately 6 to 12 hours after MMF oral dose administration, thus affecting global MPA exposure.

In our study the two evaluated LSSs reveal to be sufficiently precise and accurate for the estimation of the entire MPA $AUC_{0\text{-}12h}$ **Figure 1**. The major thesis that allows the application of these LSSs in this population is the presence of C_{6h} that offers the opportunity to estimate MPA PK accurately in both immunosuppressive regimens, even if it is not easy to apply in the outpatient setting.

This study has several limitations: 1) the whole study group was mainly composed by men, whereas, the small subgroup of patients treated with TAC included a high percentage of women. However, it has been demonstrated that MPA PK is not influenced by sex in solid organ recipients [8, 37], even if Tornatore et al. [38] showed differences in MPA and MPAG PK related to sex among stable renal transplant recipients receiving enteric-coated mycophenolate sodium combined with TAC.; 2) in this pilot study, the sample size of the MMF and TAC group was smaller than MMF and CsA group; 3) MMF and TAC group presented a higher C_0 and MPA $AUC_{0\text{-}12h}$. However, exposure to MPA when MMF is in combination therapy with CsA is approximately 30–40% lower than when given in monotherapy or with TAC [8, 39]; 4) the MMF and TAC group presented a lower level of bilirubin. Bilirubin could displace MPA from albumin binding sites, affecting MPA exposure [40]. However, this effect is limited to only patients presenting hyperbilirubinemia, and could be detected only when the free drug is measured [40]; 5) TDM was not planned to be executed at the same time for all enrolled patients but it was executed by clinical decision. This can be a source of bias, because it is known that the exposition of MPA $AUC_{0\text{-}12h}$ could vary extensively after HTx [11]; 6) furthermore, co-medications commonly used in clinical practice could alter MPA exposure [8, 11] . However, as shown in **Table 1**, the major clinical parameter, including age, BMI, liver and renal function between the two treatment groups were statistically comparable.

5. Conclusion

In this pilot study, two LSSs resulted to be sufficiently precise and accurate to predict MPA $AUC_{0\text{-}12h}$ in a heterogeneous cohort of HTx patients. This study confirmed that the two LSSs, generated in HTx recipients treated with MMF and CsA could be used also in patients treated with MMF and TAC, in particular on in hospitalized patients in the first period after HTx and in outpatients with suspected toxicity or at high risk of organ rejection with considerable social, healthcare and economic advantages.

These results suggest to confirm this hypothesis in a prospective study with a wider cohort of HTx recipients, treated mainly with MMF and TAC, and with a pre-planned TDM.

Acknowledgements

The authors thank the healthcare staff of the Clinical Pharmacology and Toxicology Institute “University Hospital Santa Maria della Misericordia”, Udine, Italy, for the collection of blood samples and the analyses performed.

Conflict of interest

The authors declare no conflict of interest.

The authors received no specific funding from any organization for this work.

Thanks

The authors thank Miss. Enza Pincente for the English revision of the Manuscript.

Nomenclature

$AUC_{0\text{-}12h}$	Area under the plasma concentration-time curve from zero to 12 h;
ALT	Alanine Aminotransferase;
AST	Aspartate Aminotransferase;
BMI	Body Mass Index;
C_0	pre-dose measurement;
Cl	Clearance;
CsA	Cyclosporine;
CrCl	Creatinine Clearance;
EDTA	Ethylenediaminetetraacetic acid;
EHC	enterohepatic circulation;
GFR	Glomerular Filtration Rate;
HPLC/UV	High Pressure Liquid Chromatography with UV Detector
IATDMCT	International Association of Therapeutic Drug Monitoring and Clinical Toxicology
IMPDH	inosine-5′-monophosphate dehydrogenase;
I.R.B.	Internal Review Board;
LC/MS–MS	Liquid Chromatography with tandem mass spectrometry;
LSS	Limited Sampling Strategy;
LSS3	Limited Sampling Strategy based on 3 concentration sampling point;
LSS4	Limited Sampling Strategy based on 4 concentration sampling point;
MAPE%	Median Absolute Percentage Predictive Error;
MPE%	Mean Percentage Prediction Error;
MMF	Mycophenolate Mofetil;
MRP-2	multi-drug resistance protein 2;
MPA	Mycophenolic Acid;
MPAG	7-O-MPA-glucuronide;
MPPE%	Median Percentage Predictive Error;
PK	Pharmacokinetics;
r	Pearson's linear correlation coefficient;
R^2	coefficient of determination;
RMSE%	Root Mean Squared Percentage Prediction Error
T_{max}	time to reach the plasma maximum concentration;
TAC	Tacrolimus;
TDM	Therapeutic Drug Monitoring;
UGTs	uridine 5′-diphospho-glucuronosyltransferases.

Author details

Francesco Lo Re[1], Sandro Sponga[2,3], Jacopo Angelini[1], Chiara Nalli[2], Antonella Zucchetto[4], Ugolino Livi[2,3] and Massimo Baraldo[1,3]*

1 Clinical Pharmacology Institute, "Azienda Sanitaria Universitaria Friuli Centrale (ASU FC)", Udine, Italy

2 Department of Cardiothoracic Surgery, "Azienda Sanitaria Universitaria Friuli Centrale (ASU FC)", Udine, Italy

3 Department of Medical Area (DAME), Udine University, Udine, Italy

4 Scientific Directorate, "Centro di Riferimento Oncologico di Aviano (CRO), IRCCS", Aviano (PN), Italy

*Address all correspondence to: massimo.baraldo@uniud.it

References

[1] Chambers DC, Cherikh WS, Harhay MO, Hayes DJ, Hsich E, Khush KK, et al. The international thoracic organ transplant registry of the International Society for Heart and Lung Transplantation: Thirty-sixth adult lung and heart-lung transplantation Report-2019; focus theme: Donor and recipient size match. The Journal of Heart and Lung Transplantation. 2019;**38**(10):1042-1055

[2] Staatz CE, Tett SE. Pharmacology and toxicology of mycophenolate in organ transplant recipients: An update. Archives of Toxicology. 2014;**88**(7):1351-1389. Available from: http://www.ncbi.nlm.nih.gov/pubmed/24792322

[3] Allison AC, Eugui EM. Mycophenolate mofetil and its mechanisms of action. Immunopharmacology. 2000;**47**(2–3):85-118

[4] Hackl A, Ehren R, Weber LT. Effect of mycophenolic acid in experimental, nontransplant glomerular diseases: New mechanisms beyond immune cells. Pediatric Nephrology. 2017;**32**(8):1315-1322

[5] Gummert JF, Barten MJ, Sherwood SW, van Gelder T, Morris RE. Pharmacodynamics of immunosuppression by mycophenolic acid: Inhibition of both lymphocyte proliferation and activation correlates with pharmacokinetics. The Journal of Pharmacology and Experimental Therapeutics. 1999;**291**(3):1100-1112

[6] Gummert JF, Barten MJ, van Gelder T, Billingham ME, Morris RE. Pharmacodynamics of mycophenolic acid in heart allograft recipients: Correlation of lymphocyte proliferation and activation with pharmacokinetics and graft histology. Transplantation. 2000;**70**(7):1038-1049

[7] de Winter BCM, Mathot RAA, Sombogaard F, Vulto AG, van Gelder T. Nonlinear relationship between mycophenolate mofetil dose and mycophenolic acid exposure: Implications for therapeutic drug monitoring. Clinical Journal of the American Society of Nephrology. 2011;**6**(3):656-663

[8] Staatz CE, Tett SE. Clinical pharmacokinetics and pharmacodynamics of mycophenolate in solid organ transplant recipients. Clinical Pharmacokinetics. 2007;**46**(1):13-58

[9] Nowak I, Shaw LM. Mycophenolic acid binding to human serum albumin: Characterization and relation to pharmacodynamics. Clinical Chemistry. 1995;**41**(7):1011-1017

[10] Atcheson BA, Taylor PJ, Kirkpatrick CMJ, Duffull SB, Mudge DW, Pillans PI, et al. Free mycophenolic acid should be monitored in renal transplant recipients with hypoalbuminemia. Therapeutic Drug Monitoring. 2004;**26**(3):284-286

[11] Kuypers DRJ, Le Meur Y, Cantarovich M, Tredger MJ, Tett SE, Cattaneo D, et al. Consensus report on therapeutic drug monitoring of mycophenolic acid in solid organ transplantation. Clinical Journal of the American Society of Nephrology. 2010;**5**(2):341-358

[12] Cattaneo D, Merlini S, Zenoni S, Baldelli S, Gotti E, Remuzzi G, et al. Influence of Co-medication with Sirolimus or cyclosporine on mycophenolic acid pharmacokinetics in kidney transplantation. American

Journal of Transplantation. 2005;**5**(12): 2937-2944. Available from: http://doi.wiley.com/10.1111/j.1600-6143.2005.01107.x

[13] Yau W-P, Vathsala A, Lou H-X, Zhou S, Chan E. Mechanism-based enterohepatic circulation model of mycophenolic acid and its glucuronide metabolite: Assessment of impact of cyclosporine dose in Asian renal transplant patients. Journal of Clinical Pharmacology. 2009;**49**(6):684-699

[14] van Gelder T, Hilbrands LB, Vanrenterghem Y, Weimar W, de Fijter JW, Squifflet JP, et al. A randomized double-blind, multicenter plasma concentration controlled study of the safety and efficacy of oral mycophenolate mofetil for the prevention of acute rejection after kidney transplantation. Transplantation. 1999;**68**(2):261-266

[15] Hale MD, Nicholls AJ, Bullingham RE, Hené R, Hoitsma A, Squifflet JP, et al. The pharmacokinetic-pharmacodynamic relationship for mycophenolate mofetil in renal transplantation. Clinical Pharmacology and Therapeutics. 1998;**64**(6):672-683

[16] DeNofrio D, Loh E, Kao A, Korecka M, Pickering FW, Craig KA, et al. Mycophenolic acid concentrations are associated with cardiac allograft rejection. The Journal of Heart and Lung Transplantation. 2000;**19**(11):1071-1076

[17] Kiang TKL, Ensom MHH. Therapeutic drug monitoring of mycophenolate in adult solid organ transplant patients: An update. Expert Opinion on Drug Metabolism & Toxicology. 2016;**12**(5):545-553

[18] Yamani MH, Starling RC, Goormastic M, Van Lente F, Smedira N, McCarthy P, et al. The impact of routine mycophenolate mofetil drug monitoring on the treatment of cardiac allograft rejection. Transplantation. 2000 Jun;**69**(11):2326-2330

[19] Hesse CJ, Vantrimpont P, van Riemsdijk-van Overbeeke IC, van Gelder T, Balk AH, Weimar W. The value of routine monitoring of mycophenolic acid plasma levels after clinical heart transplantation. Transplantation Proceedings. 2001;**33**(3):2163-2164

[20] Bergan S, Brunet M, Hesselink DA, Johnson-Davis KL, Kunicki PK, Lemaitre F, et al. Personalized therapy for mycophenolate: Consensus report by the International Association of Therapeutic Drug Monitoring and Clinical Toxicology. Therapeutic Drug Monitoring. 2021;**43**(2):150-200. Available from: https://journals.lww.com/10.1097/FTD.0000000000000871

[21] Figurski MJ, Pawiński T, Goldberg LR, DeNofrio D, Nawrocki A, Taylor DO, et al. Pharmacokinetic monitoring of mycophenolic acid in heart transplant patients: Correlation the side-effects and rejections with pharmacokinetic parameters. Annals of Transplantation. 2012;**17**(1):68-78

[22] Woillard J-B, Saint-Marcoux F, Monchaud C, Youdarène R, Pouche L, Marquet P. Mycophenolic mofetil optimized pharmacokinetic modelling, and exposure-effect associations in adult heart transplant recipients. Pharmacological Research. 2015;**99**: 308-315. Available from: https://www.sciencedirect.com/science/article/pii/S1043661815001450

[23] Shaw LM, Korecka M, van Breeman R, Nowak I, Brayman KL. Analysis, pharmacokinetics and therapeutic drug monitoring of mycophenolic acid. Clinical Biochemistry. 1998;**31**(5): 323-328

[24] Shaw LM, Kaplan B, DeNofrio D, Korecka M, Brayman KL. Pharmacokinetics and concentration-control investigations of mycophenolic acid in adults after transplantation. Therapeutic Drug Monitoring. 2000; **22**(1):14-19

[25] Baraldo M, Sponga S, Livi U. Therapeutic drug monitoring of Micophenolate Mofetil in cardiac transplant patients by limited sampling strategy: An update. In: Rescigno G, Firstenberg MS, editors. Topics in Heart Failure Management [Internet]. Rijeka: IntechOpen; 2018. Available from: https://www.intechopen.com/books/topics-in-heart-failure-management/therapeutic-drug-monitoring-of-mico phenolate-mofetil-in-cardiac-transplant-patients-by-limited-sampl

[26] Sheiner LB, Beal SL. Some suggestions for measuring predictive performance. Journal of Pharmacokinetics and Biopharmaceutics. 1981;**9**(4):503-512

[27] Baraldo M, Isola M, Feruglio MT, Francesconi A, Franceschi L, Tursi V, et al. Therapeutic mycophenolic acid monitoring by means of limited sampling strategy in orthotopic heart transplant patients. Transplantation Proceedings. 2005;**37**(5):2240-2243

[28] Baraldo M, Cojutti PG, Isola M, Feruglio MT, Tursi V, Livi U, et al. Validation of limited sampling strategy for estimation of mycophenolic acid exposure during the first year after heart transplantation. Transplantation Proceedings. 2009;**41**(10): 4277-4284

[29] Kaczmarek I, Bigdeli AK, Vogeser M, Mueller T, Beiras-Fernandez A, Kaczmarek P, et al. Defining algorithms for efficient therapeutic drug monitoring of mycophenolate mofetil in heart transplant recipients. Therapeutic Drug Monitoring. 2008;**30**(4):419–427

[30] Bland JM, Altman DG. Statistical methods for assessing agreement between two methods of clinical measurement. Lancet (London, England). 1986;**1**(8476):307-310

[31] Billingham M, Kobashigawa JA. The revised ISHLT heart biopsy grading scale. The Journal of Heart and Lung Transplantation: the Official Publication of the International Society for Heart Transplantation. 2005;**24**:1709

[32] Zuk DM, Pearson GJ. Monitoring of mycophenolate mofetil in orthotopic heart transplant recipients–a systematic review. Transplantation Reviews (Orlando, Fla.). 2009;**23**(3):171-177

[33] Xiang H, Zhou H, Zhang J, Sun Y, Wang Y, Han Y, et al. Limited sampling strategy for estimation of mycophenolic acid exposure in adult chinese heart transplant recipients. Frontiers in Pharmacology. 2021;**12**:652333

[34] Wada K, Takada M, Kotake T, Ochi H, Morishita H, Komamura K, et al. Limited sampling strategy for mycophenolic acid in Japanese heart transplant recipients. Circulation Journal. 2007;**71**(7):1022-1028

[35] Ling J, Shi J, Jiang Q, Jiao Z. Population pharmacokinetics of mycophenolic acid and its main glucuronide metabolite: A comparison between healthy Chinese and Caucasian subjects receiving mycophenolate mofetil. European Journal of Clinical Pharmacology. 2015;**71**(1):95-106

[36] Pawinski T, Kunicki PK, Sobieszczanska-Malek M, Gralak B, Szlaska I. A limited sampling strategy for estimating mycophenolic acid area under the curve in adult heart transplant

patients treated with concomitant cyclosporine. Journal of Clinical Pharmacy and Therapeutics. 2009;**34**(1): 89-101

[37] Pescovitz MD, Guasch A, Gaston R, Rajagopalan P, Tomlanovich S, Weinstein S, et al. Equivalent pharmacokinetics of mycophenolate Mofetil in African-American and Caucasian male and female stable renal allograft recipients. American Journal of Transplantation. 2003;**3**(12):1581-1586. DOI: 10.1046/j.1600-6135.2003.00243.x

[38] Tornatore KM, Meaney CJ, Wilding GE, Chang SS, Gundroo A, Cooper LM, et al. Influence of sex and race on mycophenolic acid pharmacokinetics in stable African American and Caucasian renal transplant recipients. Clinical Pharmacokinetics. 2015;**54**(4):423-434

[39] van Gelder T, Klupp J, Barten MJ, Christians U, Morris RE. Comparison of the effects of tacrolimus and cyclosporine on the pharmacokinetics of mycophenolic acid. Therapeutic Drug Monitoring. 2001;**23**(2):119-128

[40] Shaw LM, Figurski M, Milone MC, Trofe J, Bloom RD. Therapeutic drug monitoring of mycophenolic acid. Clinical Journal of the American Society of Nephrology. 2007;**2**(5):1062 LP-1061072. Available from: http://cjasn.asnjournals.org/content/2/5/1062.abstract

Section 6

Cardiac Allograft Vasculopathy

Chapter 12

Diagnostic Intravascular Imaging Modalities for Cardiac Allograft Vasculopathy

Yasumasa Tsukamoto, Takuya Watanabe, Hiroki Mochizuki, Masaya Shimojima, Tasuku Hada, Satsuki Fukushima, Tomoyuki Fujita and Osamu Seguchi

Abstract

Cardiac allograft vasculopathy (CAV) is one of the major factors limiting long-term survival after heart transplantation (HTX). Typically, concentric vascular thickening and fibrosis with marked intimal proliferation are found in CAV. Most of HTX patients often remain free from symptoms of typical angina. Therefore, surveillance diagnostic exams are often performed. The gold standard of diagnosing CAV is coronary angiography (CAG). However, CAG can often be a less sensitive modality for the detection of diffuse concentric lesions. Intravascular ultrasound (IVUS) is helpful for direct imaging of vessel walls and provides useful information about coronary intimal thickening; however, it is difficult to evaluate plaque morphology in detail. Optimal coherence tomography (OCT), which delivers high resolution of 10 μm, can provide more details on plaque morphology than conventional imaging modalities. Recently, OCT imaging revealed new insight in CAV such as the development of atherosclerotic lesions and complicated coronary lesions. We review the pathogenesis, clinical features, diagnosis of CAV, with a particular focus on diagnostic intravascular imaging modalities.

Keywords: cardiac allograft vasculopathy, heart transplantation, intravascular imaging, coronary angiography, intravascular ultrasound, optical coherence tomography

1. Introduction

Orthotopic heart transplantation (HTX) has become a well-established treatment option for patients with end-stage heart failure. But HTX brings following various comorbidities, including rejection, hematologic and other malignancies, infectious diseases, renal failure, and cardiac allograft vasculopathy (CAV).

CAV remains one of the most significant causes of morbidity and mortality after HTX, with almost half of survival recipients have CAV by 10 years post-transplant [1]. Concentric coronary intima thickening is usually found in CAV, but its pathophysiology has not been well known. The early detection of CAV is paramount, but can be difficult, because most of HTX recipients are free from symptoms of typical angina, and the

IntechOpen

clinical presentation of CAV can be insidiously, secondary to the denervation of the cardiac graft. Coronary angiography (CAG) has been performed as the gold standard in routine CAV surveillance. However, the analysis of CAV by CAG has limitations, because the early detection of diffuse CAV lesions is difficult. Intravascular imaging such as intravascular ultrasound (IVUS) and optimal coherence tomography (OCT), which has been used for the evaluation of common coronary artery diseases in recent years, has made it possible to accurately evaluate the thickness and structure of the coronary arterial wall. These modalities have contributed to not only early detection of the CAV, but also provide new insights in CAV. We review the pathogenesis, clinical features, diagnosis of CAV, with a particular focus on diagnostic imaging modalities.

2. Pathophysiology

Typical CAV affects the coronary arteries diffusely. Histopathologically, CAV is characterized by concentric thickening of the vessel wall due to intima and smooth muscle hypertrophy, affecting the large and small coronary arteries (**Figure 1**). On the other hand, the pathophysiology and molecular basis of CAV also include contributions from the mechanism of atherosclerosis. The exact etiology of CAV remains well unknown, but both immunological and nonimmunological mechanisms are thought to contribute to the development of CAV [2].

The immunological mechanism may contribute to the development of CAV. It is thought that both cellular and humoral immune responses of recipients are directed against grafts. The immune response of recipients can be triggered via direct or indirect pathways. In the direct pathway, recipient T cells are activated after recognition of the allogeneic major histocompatibility complex (MHC) on the surface of donor endothelial cells by recipient dendritic cells. The indirect pathway is triggered when recipient antigen-presenting cells, mainly dendritic cells, present MHC-derived donor antigens from cardiac grafts [3]. It leads to the production of donor-specific antibodies (DSA) and inflammatory cytokines and damage to the endothelium due to B cell and T cell activation [4]. Antibodies such as anti-human leukocyte antigen (HLA) and anti-endothelial antibody also activate the complement system, which may be involved in vascular endothelial cell injury in the graft and contribute to CAV and rejection [5].

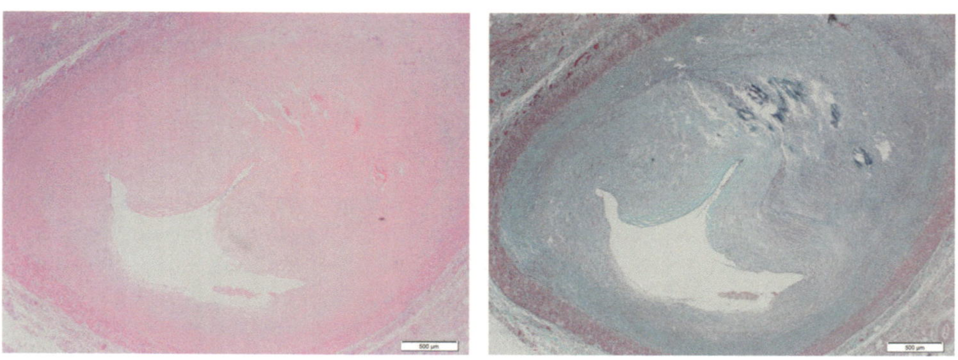

Figure 1.
Histopathological image of cardiac allograft vasculopathy. H&E (left) and Masson-trichrome (right) stain of the left anterior descending artery demonstrating fibromuscular intimal hyperplasia in a HTX recipient with cardiac allograft vasculopathy.

Damaged endothelial cells present MHC class II antigen, which activates CD4+ T cells. In addition to DSA, many non-HLA antibodies are expressed in endothelial cells and may be involved in the development of CAV [6, 7]. Many of these mediators in the immunological pathway have been demonstrated to predict the development of CAV.

The nonimmunological mechanisms include donor and peri-transplant factors, traditional risk factors for coronary atherosclerosis, and particular infections such as cytomegalovirus (CMV) infection. Donor-related factors such as older age, donor-derived coronary artery disease, higher body mass index, hypertension, diabetes mellitus, cigarette use are associated with increased risks of CAV [8–10]. Physiologic changes at the donor caused by brain death can trigger the production of proinflammatory cytokines leading to the endothelial injury [11, 12]. Systemic activation of matrix metalloproteinases in donors with intracerebral hemorrhage can contribute to the migration of smooth muscle cells from the coronary media into the intima [13]. Ischemia–reperfusion injury at the time of transplantation also plays a significant role in endothelial dysfunction and the pathophysiology of CAV [14]. Traditional cardiovascular risk factors are also associated with the development of CAV. Risk factors for coronary atherosclerosis include hypertension, dyslipidemia, glucose intolerance (diabetes), obesity, renal insufficiency [15]. It should be noted that commonly used immunosuppressive agents such as steroids, calcineurin inhibitors, and mTOR inhibitors may lead to exacerbation of these metabolic abnormalities. CMV infection may also affect the development of CAV [16].

3. Epidemiology

According to the International Society of Heart and Lung Transplantation (ISHLT) registry in 2019, the incidence of CAV is declining with each era [17]. Regardless of disease severity, CAV is detected in 7.7% of recipients by 1 year, 29.0% by 5 years, and 46.8% by 10 years after HTX. CAV is less likely to develop in female recipients than in males. CAV is the fourth leading cause of death for recipients more than 3 years after HTX. In addition, graft failure, which is another major cause of death after HTX, may reflect undiagnosed CAV. CAV remains to be associated with lower survival; however, survival in patients with CAV has improved in the most recent era.

4. Clinical features

As a result of denervation after cardiac transplantation, HTX recipients with CAV may often not notice symptoms of typical angina associated with myocardial ischemia or infarction. Therefore, most of recipients remain asymptomatic or have unspecific symptoms. However, the clinical presentation can be insidiously, and severe cardiac ischemia and/or myocardial infarction due to CAV can cause the development of heart failure, electrical instability, or sudden death [18].

5. Diagnosis

Due to the morbidity and mortality associated with CAV, diagnosis of CAV is important. CAV may present insidiously without significant symptoms in post-HTX patients. Therefore, surveillance testing is important for early detection of CAV in

CAV grade	Severity	Coronary angiographic findings	Allograft dysfunction
CAV0	Not significant	No detectable angiographic lesion	Absent
CAV1	Mild	Angiographic LM <50% or primary vessel with maximum lesion of <70% or any branch stenosis <70% (including diffuse narrowing)	Absent
CAV2	Moderate	Angiographic LM <50% or a single primary vessel ≥70% or isolated branch stenosis ≥70% in branches of 2 systems	Absent
CAV3	Severe	Angiographic LM ≥50% or two or more primary vessels ≥70% stenosis or isolated branch stenosis ≥70% in all 3 systems	Left ventricular ejection fraction ≤45% with CAV1 or CAV2 or evidence of restrictive physiology*

**Restrictive cardiac allograft physiology is defined as symptomatic heart failure with echocardiographic E to A velocity ratio > 2, shortened isovolumetric relaxation time (<60 ms), shortened deceleration time (<150 ms), or restrictive hemodynamic values (Right Atrial Pressure > 12 mmHg, Pulmonary Capillary Wedge Pressure > 25 mmHg, Cardiac Index <2 l/min/m^2).*
Abbreviations: ISHLT International Society of Heart and Lung Transplantation, CAV cardiac allograft vasculopathy, LM left main.
Adapted with permission from Mehra et al. [19]

Table 1.
ISHLT nomenclature for cardiac allograft vasculopathy.

patients after HTX. Coronary angiography (CAG) is recommended by the ISHLT for diagnosing and grading CAV (**Table 1**) [19]. CAG has been the gold standard test for CAV monitoring and diagnosis. However, CAG can often be a less sensitive modality for the detection of diffuse concentric lesions because CAG can only provide information about the vessel lumen [20]. Intracoronary imaging has enabled examination of the vessel wall and detection of early intimal thickening of CAV. Intravascular ultrasound (IVUS) is helpful for direct imaging of vessel walls and provides useful information about coronary intimal thickening. Therefore, IVUS is utilized in many institutions in addition to CAG for the evaluation of CAV. Optimal coherence tomography (OCT) can deliver higher resolution and provide more details on plaque morphology than conventional imaging modalities.

Transcatheter procedures carry the risks associated with invasive examinations. These risks include bleeding, thromboembolism, contrast-induced nephropathy, vascular injury, infection, death from invasive procedures. **Table 2** summarizes the intravascular detection approaches of CAV after HTX.

5.1 Coronary angiography (CAG)

CAG has been the gold standard test and recommended by the ISHLT for definitive diagnosis and surveillance of CAV. It is commonly performed at one month after HTX and then annually or biannually. Less frequent CAG may be considered if recipients are free from CAV at 3–5 years after HTX [21]. The ISHLT recommended classification of CAV is mainly based on CAG results. By the classification, CAV can be separated into not significant (CAV0), mild (CAV1), intermediate (CAV2), and severe (CAV3) (**Table 1**) [19]. The prognostic significance of CAG was validated in HTX recipients. In a large multicenter study, 50% of recipients with severe CAV died or underwent retransplantation within 5 years after HTX [22]. Another retrospective analysis

Imaging Modality	Information	Advantages	Disadvantages
CAG	Coronary luminal stenosis	Widely available Prognostic Current gold standard for CAV screening Angiographic CAV prognostic of outcomes	Inability to assess arterial wall Low sensitivity for detecting early CAV Significant interobserver variability in grading Microvasculature not assessed Lumen patency can be preserved due to remodeling
IVUS	Luminal stenosis Arterial wall Quantification of intimal thickening Plaque characterization	High spatial resolution with good tissue penetration Prognostic More sensitive than angiography Virtual histology IVUS allows assessment of plaque components	More invasive than CAG Costly Requires technical expertise Difficult to match sites exactly for intimal measurements Catheter too large for smaller vessels
OCT	Luminal stenosis Arterial wall Quantification of intimal thickening Plaque characterization	10-fold greater resolution over IVUS Some prognostic data Detects intimal thickening earlier than IVUS Defines more detailed plaque characteristics and microstructures Low interobserver variability	More invasive than CAG Costly Requires technical expertise Additional contrast exposure Poorer tissue penetration than IVUS Unclear whether higher resolution has a beneficial outcome over IVUS
FFR	Fractional flow reserve	Evaluation of micro- and macrovascular function Some prognostic data	More invasive than CAG Costly Requires technical skills

Table 2.
Summary of intravascular imaging modalities for cardiac allograft vasculopathy.

showed no difference in outcome between HTX recipients with CAV0 and CAV1; however, CAV2 and CAV3 were associated with an increased risk of adverse events [23]. Rapidly progressive CAV and the development of CAV in the first year after HTX are associated with major adverse cardiac events [24].

One of the key limitations of CAG is the insensitivity to early detection of diffuse concentric lesions due to its inability to visualize beyond the arterial lumen. Studies comparing CAG and IVUS showed that the sensitivity and the negative predictive value (NPV) for detecting CAV were 43–44% and 27–57%, respectively [25]. A histopathological study of explanted allografts revealed that 75% had significant intimal hyperplasia with CAV, despite normal CAG results [26]. CAG is also limited for the detection of microvascular lesions. The limitations of CAG have necessitated the development of other diagnostic modalities for evaluation of vessel walls and microvascular lesions. Frequent CAG, an invasive angiography surveillance, subsequently increases the risk of treatment complications, patient discomfort, radiation, and nephrotoxicity.

5.2 Intravascular ultrasound (IVUS)

IVUS is becoming to be regarded as the new gold standard for surveillance of CAV since it can provide excellent visualization of vessel walls and lumens [20]. IVUS can provide cross-sectional imaging of vessel walls and lumens with high penetrance and assessment of coronary plaque volume. The maximal intimal thickness (MIT) measured by IVUS provides a detailed description of plaque burden.

IVUS began to be used in the early 1990s as an imaging modality of validating CAG in HTX recipients.

A number of studies on IVUS findings revealed detailed pathophysiology of CAV progression. A study on IVUS examinations showed that the majority of recipients 1 or more years after HTX have coronary intimal thickening, although not apparent on CAG [27]. IVUS findings also showed that the most rapid progression of intimal thickening occurs in the first year after HTX, followed by a gradual progression over time [28]. Based on previous studies, it should be defined as clinically significant CAV when the width of the intima layer exceeds 0.3 mm or when the total width of the intimal and medial layer exceeds 0.5 mm [29].

There are many reports on the association between IVUS findings and the prognosis of HTX recipients. HTX recipients with severe intima thickening confirmed by IVUS were reported to have a higher incidence of cardiac events [30]. A multicenter study demonstrated that rapidly progressing CAV, defined as an increase in MIT $\geq$ 0.5 mm from baseline in the first year after HTX, is associated with not only the development of angiographic CAV but also death, graft loss, and cardiovascular events within 5 years [31]. Another study also showed that rapidly progressive CAV is a powerful predictor of all-cause mortality, myocardial infarction, and angiographic abnormalities [32]. An increase of 0.35 mm in MIT at 5 years after HTX was reported to be associated with an increased risk of significant adverse cardiovascular events [33].

IVUS technology is advancing, with higher-resolution images, 3D images, and mechanical retractions of IVUS catheters enabling more accurate assessment of coronary arteries. Recent clinical trials have performed volumetric analysis with IVUS, where the percentage of atheroma volume more accurately reflects the burden of the disease and has less variability in its measurements. According to pilot data from Cleveland Clinic, the percentage of atheroma volume was reported to increase by an average of 3.1% in the first year in HTX recipients, while in the nontransplanted population increased by 1% [19]. According to a serial 3D volumetric IVUS study, paradoxical vessel remodeling, which is defined as an increase in the intimal volume with a decrease in the overall volume of the vessel, of the proximal left anterior descending artery (LAD) segment at 1 year is a major determinant of mortality or retransplantation [34]. Interestingly, this study demonstrated that intimal thickening was more pronounced in proximal LAD while vascular remodeling was observed throughout the vessel. This is different from the increase in blood vessel size that compensates for luminal stenosis in native coronary artery disease. A recent study of serial volumetric IVUS by our group suggests that preexisting donor-transmitted atherosclerosis correlates with the worsening change in CAV several years after HTX [35].

Virtual histology IVUS (VH-IVUS) technology is based on spectral analysis of IVUS high-frequency ultrasound signals. With VH-IVUS, different plaque morphologies can be categorized into four types (for example, fibrous, fibrofatty, calcified, and necrotic core) and subsequently quantified. A study evaluating CAV with VH-IVUS showed that fibrotic plaques are the most common plaque component, while calcification and lipid plaques are less frequently observed [36]. Another study reported a significant association between inflammatory plaques and histories of previous rejection [37]. A study examining posttransplant duration and plaque morphology revealed a significant correlation between posttransplant duration and plaque components with VH-IVUS. The study also found that necrotic core and calcium increased with time after transplantation, and both fibrous and fibrofatty components decreased at follow-up [38].

Although IVUS can provide data on changes in intimal thickness and vascular remodeling, there are still certain limitations in assessing CAV. Due to the relatively large diameter of the IVUS catheter, it can only be used in coronary arteries with sufficient lumen. Therefore, it is not possible to assess small vascular disease that may develop even in the early stages of CAV. There is evidence that the measurement of intimal thickness does not necessarily correlate with pathological findings in coronary microvascular lesions, which suggests discordant progression of CAV [39]. Drawbacks of IVUS include the cost of catheters, the expertise needed to interpret images, and the increased risk of potential complications such as coronary artery spasm and dissection, thrombosis, increased contrast doses, and vascular access due to the use of anticoagulants.

5.3 Optical coherence tomography (OCT)

Optical coherence tomography (OCT) is a novel intravascular imaging modality employing long-wavelength light, usually near-infrared light, which penetrates the coronary vessel wall. OCT was initially used noninvasively for retinal imaging. Since the development of smaller OCT catheters, their application to coronary arteries has increased. And OCT is now widely applied in the assessment of native coronary atherosclerosis. The use of OCT for CAV assessment has a relatively short history, and it is not included in CAV surveillance recommendations. However, it can provide key insights into the pathogenesis of CAV, and various studies have been conducted.

OCT can provide images of vessel walls constructed with extremely high spatial resolution of 10 μm, which is 10-fold greater than that with IVUS (**Figure 2**). Therefore, OCT can provide information such as intimal thickness, intima-media interface display, plaque characteristics, and detection of slight intimal hyperplasia. Considering the nature of CAV and excellent precision and accuracy of OCT, it can be an ideal modality for evaluation of CAV.

An early study comparing OCT and IVUS in non-HTX cadaveric coronary arteries revealed that histologically measured intima-media thickness was more highly correlated with OCT than IVUS [40]. An initial study comparing OCT and IVUS in seven posttransplant patients suggested that OCT, compared with IVUS, could be more sensitive for early detection of CAV, because intimal hyperplasia thickness $\leq$ 150 μm was under the resolution of IVUS and therefore could be diagnosed only with OCT [41]. Another study described that the assessment of CAV by OCT had a good correlation with IVUS measurements, but OCT could provide lower interobserver variability and better plaque characterization than IVUS [42].

High-resolution OCT images can identify plaque features and microstructures, such as fibrous plaque, fibrocalcific plaque, fibroatheroma, fibrous cap, intimal vasculature, and thrombus, providing a more detailed pathophysiological assessment of the coronary arteries (**Figure 3**) [43]. Therefore, a study using OCT clarified the difference in pathophysiology between CAV and native CAD [44]. The study showed that coronary lesions in HTX patients were more homogeneous than in non-HTX patients, involving the entire coronary vascular tree and having a higher number of microvessels. HTX patients with prior high-grade cellular rejection had similar intima areas, smaller external elastic lamia areas, smaller lumen areas, and higher prevalence of macrophages than non-HTX patients.

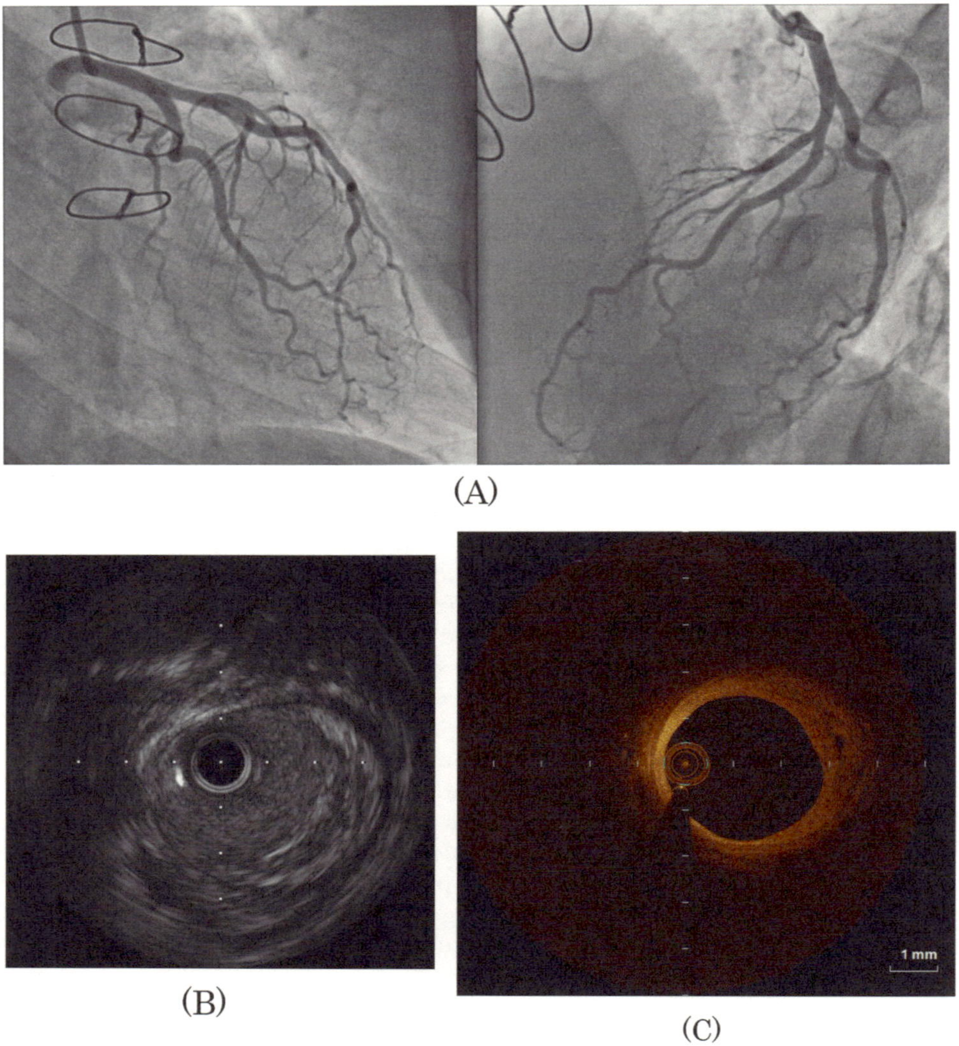

Figure 2.
Coronary angiography, intravascular ultrasound, and optical coherence tomography in cardiac allograft vasculopathy. The proximal left anterior descending (LAD) is almost angiografically normal (A), but intravascular ultrasound provides a coronary plaque image in the corresponding region (B). Optical coherence tomography provides more details on plaque morphology (C).

Analysis of plaque characteristics by OCT gives new insight into CAV that the pathogenesis is more complex than the previously reported diffuse intimal hyperplasia. The OCTCAV study suggested that in addition to post-HTX intimal hyperplasia, traditional atherosclerosis, such as lipid-rich or calcified atherosclerotic plaques, may also be a factor associated with CAV and graft failure [45]. Another study demonstrated that findings typical of atherosclerosis, such as lipid-rich pools, calcifications, and eccentric plaques, were found in CAV lesions, with a significant increase in prevalence with longer post-HTX periods [46]. In addition, the study revealed that vulnerable and complex lesions with thin-cap fibroatheromas, macrophages, microchannels, intraluminal thrombus, intimal lacerations, and layered complex plaque

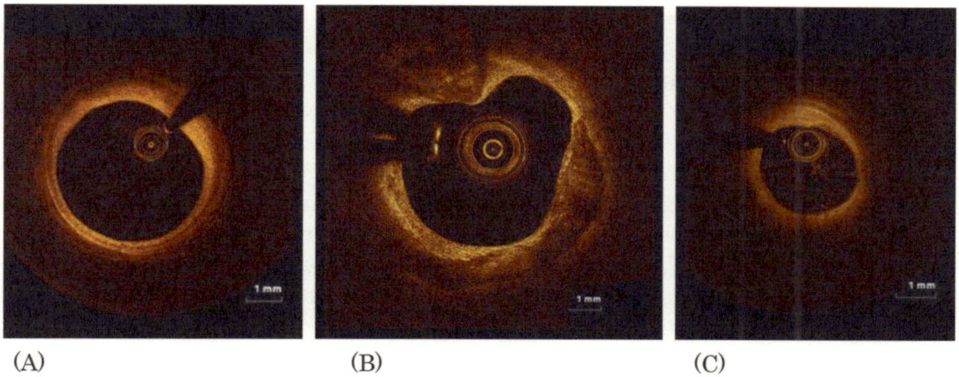

Figure 3.
Plaque morphology classified by OCT. (A) Fibrous plaque. (B) Fibrocalcific plaque. (C) Fibroatheroma.

also increased over time. At follow-up, the characteristics of plaque vulnerability evaluated by OCT correlated with changes in plaque volume 1 year later [47]. These findings regarding impacts of plaque vulnerability on the progression of CAV may suggest the importance of further aggressive treatment for previously known coronary risk factors such as dyslipidemia, diabetes, and hypertension.

Layered fibrotic plaque (LFP) is one of the microstructures that can be detected by OCT, defined as homogeneous, signal-rich tissue but predominantly with a signal intensity lower than surrounding or deeper layers of intimal tissue and with a clearly layered structure. A study characterizing the CAV phenotypes in multivessel OCT on the progression of CAV revealed that LFP was the most prevalent plaque component [48]. LFP was strongly associated with nonfatal CAV progression and suggested to be associated with the gradual progression of CAV caused by thrombus formation in vessel walls. The authors also demonstrated early changes in the coronary artery microstructure after HTX using serial OCT scans [49]. The study described that early CAV formation during the first year after HTX was characterized by a marked intimal layer thickening strongly associated with LFP progression. In contrast, the degree of lipid plaque and calcification remained stable. From these, the authors conclude that the formation of LFP plays an important role in the mechanism of CAV.

Neovascularization is also one of the microstructures of CAV, which is difficult to detect with previous imaging modalities, and OCT has provided new insights into its prevalence, distribution, and association with clinical events [50]. A study evaluating vasa vasorum (VV) by OCT in a small number of HTX recipients revealed that plaque volume of coronary artery was correlated with VV lumen volume [51]. Another study demonstrated that OCT could visualize microchannels considered to represent neovascularization, and OCT-identified microchannels increased sharply within the first year and were correlated with intimal volume and coronary risks [52]. Another study evaluating VV by OCT and the change in plaque volume by serial IVUS tests showed a significant association between the VV volume and the progression of plaque volume [53]. Another recent study also showed the significant association of OCT-detected neovessels within the intima with CAV [54]. These findings suggest that neovascularization may be a potential predictor and possible therapeutic target to attenuate CAV.

Since OCT can detect small structural changes in coronary arteries, it may be useful for elucidating the pathophysiology of CAV. The association between rejection and OCT findings has been evaluated in several studies [55–57]. A retrospective study comparing

OCT findings in pediatric and adult HTX recipients suggested age- and time-dependent differences in the prevalence of absolute and relative intimal hyperplasia [58].

A complete washout of the coronary vessels is needed, usually with a significant volume of contrast medium, to obtain high-quality OCT images. HTX recipients are often exposed to multiple risk factors for renal dysfunction, including immunosuppressive agent nephrotoxicity, hypertension, and diabetes, resulting in chronic kidney disease. Patients with moderate to severe renal failure should be concerned about the additional use of iodinated contrast. It has been reported that saline or low-molecular-weight dextran can provide similar OCT image quality as iodinated contrast, and these techniques have the potential to extend OCT to patients with renal dysfunction [59, 60].

As noted, OCT is very useful for evaluating CAV; however, it has some limitations. First, tissue penetration obtained in OCT imaging is 1.5–3 mm and lower than IVUS, which means whole vascular morphology, particularly in cases of large vessels and significant remodeling, cannot be evaluated. Second, although many studies have been conducted, it has been still unknown how the earlier detection and more accurate surveillance of CAV affect management and that will lead to significant improvement in outcomes. Procedural complications of OCT include coronary artery dissection, coronary artery spasm, and contrast-associated nephropathy.

5.4 Fractional flow reserve (FFR)

Fractional flow reserve (FFR) is not an imaging modality; however, it is a physiological assessment of coronary artery stenosis that can be performed at the same time as CAG and can accurately determine the hemodynamic severity of coronary artery disease. FFR can be quantified by measuring the intracoronary pressure using a pressure guide wire in the condition of coronary vasodilator-induced maximal myocardial hyperemia. FFR has become one of the major procedures for assessing the need for coronary intervention.

In a study comparing FFR and IVUS findings in angiographic CAV-free HTX recipients, FFR correlated with IVUS-detected plaque burden and was abnormal in a significant proportion of asymptomatic recipients [61]. A study evaluating serial changes in FFR by the same group showed that FFR correlated with anatomical changes and worsened in the first year after heart transplantation [62]. Another study showed that invasive measures of coronary physiology determined early after heart transplantation were significant predictors of late death or retransplantation [63].

Currently, FFR is generally considered to be the most accurate diagnostic method in the diagnosis of myocardial ischemia in patients with coronary artery stenosis; however, the therapeutic consequences based on hemodynamic parameters are not sufficient in CAV.

6. Conclusions

CAV remains a significant obstacle to long-term survival of HTX recipients. Current guidelines of ISHLT recommend conventional CAG as the gold standard for CAV diagnosis and grading because of its cost-effectiveness, wide availability, and low rate of complications. The intravascular imaging modalities have provided better visualization of the coronary arteries, enabling early detection of CAV and detailed pathological assessment. OCT, which provides high-resolution images, has revealed new insights into the complex pathophysiology of CAV. However, the clinical value of detailed CAV assessments by IVUS or OCT remains often uncertain, because no randomized trials based on IVUS or OCT have been conducted. Therefore, further studies are needed to determine the clinical relevance of each parameter and the impact of early detection of CAV on the outcome of HTX recipients.

Conflict of interest

The authors declare no conflict of interest.

Author details

Yasumasa Tsukamoto[1*], Takuya Watanabe[1], Hiroki Mochizuki[1], Masaya Shimojima[1], Tasuku Hada[1], Satsuki Fukushima[2], Tomoyuki Fujita[2] and Osamu Seguchi[1]

1 Department of Transplantation, National Cerebral and Cardiovascular Center, Suita, Japan

2 Department of Adult Cardiac Surgery, National Cerebral and Cardiovascular Center, Suita, Japan

*Address all correspondence to: tsukkan@gmail.com

References

[1] Khush KK, Cherikh WS, Chambers DC, Goldfarb S, Hayes D, Kucheryavaya AY, et al. The international thoracic organ transplant registry of the International Society for Heart and Lung Transplantation: Thirty-fifth adult heart transplantation Report-2018; focus theme: Multiorgan transplantation. The Journal of Heart and Lung Transplantation. 2018;**37**:1155-1168

[2] Schmauss D, Weis M. Cardiac allograft vasculopathy: Recent developments. Circulation. 2008;**117**:2131-2141

[3] Rogers NJ, Lechler RI. Allorecognition. American Journal of Transplantation. 2001;**1**:97-102

[4] Kaczmarek I, Deutsch MA, Kauke T, Beiras-Fernandez A, Schmoeckel M, Vicol C, et al. Donor-specific HLA alloantibodies: Long-term impact on cardiac allograft vasculopathy and mortality after heart transplant. Experimental and Clinical Transplantation. 2008;**6**:229-235

[5] Wehner J, Morrell CN, Reynolds T, Rodriguez ER, Baldwin WM 3rd. Antibody and complement in transplant vasculopathy. Circulation Research. 2007;**100**:191-203

[6] Yousufuddin M, Haji S, Starling RC, Tuzcu EM, Ratliff NB, Cook DJ, et al. Cardiac angiotensin II receptors as predictors of transplant coronary artery disease following heart transplantation. European Heart Journal. 2004;**25**:377-385

[7] Kauke T, Kaczmarek I, Dick A, Schmoeckel M, Deutsch MA, Beiras-Fernandez A, et al. Anti-MICA antibodies are related to adverse outcome in heart transplant recipients. The Journal of Heart and Lung Transplantation. 2009;**28**:305-311

[8] Roig E, Almenar L, Crespo-Leiro M, Segovia J, Mirabet S, Delgado J, et al. Muniz J and rest of the participants of the Spanish heart transplantation R. heart transplantation using allografts from older donors: Multicenter study results. The Journal of Heart and Lung Transplantation. 2015;**34**:790-796

[9] Kransdorf EP, Loghmanpour NA, Kanwar MK, Temkit MH, Stehlik J. Prediction model for cardiac allograft vasculopathy: Comparison of three multivariable methods. Clinical Transplantation. 2017;**31**(4). DOI: 10.1111/ctr.12925

[10] Langstraat M, Musters KJS, Manintveld O, Masetti M, Potena L. Coronary artery disease in heart transplantation: New concepts for an old disease. Transplant International. 2018;**31**:787-827

[11] Mehra MR, Uber PA, Ventura HO, Scott RL, Park MH. The impact of mode of donor brain death on cardiac allograft vasculopathy: An intravascular ultrasound study. Journal of the American College of Cardiology. 2004;**43**:806-810

[12] Lee F, Nair V, Chih S. Cardiac allograft vasculopathy: Insights on pathogenesis and therapy. Clinical Transplantation. 2020;**34**:e13794

[13] Yamani MH, Starling RC, Cook DJ, Tuzcu EM, Abdo A, Paul P, et al. Donor spontaneous intracerebral hemorrhage is associated with systemic activation of matrix metalloproteinase-2 and matrix metalloproteinase-9 and subsequent development of coronary vasculopathy in the heart transplant recipient. Circulation. 2003;**108**:1724-1728

[14] Rahmani M, Cruz RP, Granville DJ, McManus BM. Allograft vasculopathy

versus atherosclerosis. Circulation Research. 2006;**99**:801-815

[15] Nikolova AP, Kobashigawa JA. Cardiac allograft vasculopathy: The enduring enemy of cardiac transplantation. Transplantation. 2019;**103**:1338-1348

[16] Delgado JF, Reyne AG, de Dios S, Lopez-Medrano F, Jurado A, Juan RS, et al. Influence of cytomegalovirus infection in the development of cardiac allograft vasculopathy after heart transplantation. The Journal of Heart and Lung Transplantation. 2015;**34**:1112-1119

[17] Khush KK, Cherikh WS, Chambers DC, Harhay MO, Hayes D Jr, Hsich E, et al. The international thoracic organ transplant registry of the International Society for Heart and Lung Transplantation: Thirty-sixth adult heart transplantation report - 2019; focus theme: Donor and recipient size match. The Journal of Heart and Lung Transplantation. 2019;**38**:1056-1066

[18] Lee MS, Tadwalkar RV, Fearon WF, Kirtane AJ, Patel AJ, Patel CB, et al. Cardiac allograft vasculopathy: A review. Catheterization and Cardiovascular Interventions. 2018;**92**:E527-E536

[19] Mehra MR, Crespo-Leiro MG, Dipchand A, Ensminger SM, Hiemann NE, Kobashigawa JA, et al. International Society for Heart and Lung Transplantation working formulation of a standardized nomenclature for cardiac allograft vasculopathy-2010. The Journal of Heart and Lung Transplantation. 2010;**29**:717-727

[20] Olymbios M, Kwiecinski J, Berman DS, Kobashigawa JA. Imaging in heart transplant patients. JACC: Cardiovascular Imaging. 2018;**11**:1514-1530

[21] Costanzo MR, Dipchand A, Starling R, Anderson A, Chan M, Desai S, et al. International Society of H and Lung Transplantation G. the International Society of Heart and Lung Transplantation Guidelines for the care of heart transplant recipients. The Journal of Heart and Lung Transplantation. 2010;**29**:914-956

[22] Costanzo MR, Naftel DC, Pritzker MR, Heilman JK 3rd, Boehmer JP, Brozena SC, et al. Heart transplant coronary artery disease detected by coronary angiography: A multiinstitutional study of preoperative donor and recipient risk factors. Cardiac transplant research database. The Journal of Heart and Lung Transplantation. 1998;**17**:744-753

[23] Prada-Delgado O, Estevez-Loureiro R, Paniagua-Martin MJ, Lopez-Sainz A, Crespo-Leiro MG. Prevalence and prognostic value of cardiac allograft vasculopathy 1 year after heart transplantation according to the ISHLT recommended nomenclature. The Journal of Heart and Lung Transplantation. 2012;**31**:332-333

[24] Mehra MR. Contemporary concepts in prevention and treatment of cardiac allograft vasculopathy. American Journal of Transplantation. 2006;**6**:1248-1256

[25] Pollack A, Nazif T, Mancini D, Weisz G. Detection and imaging of cardiac allograft vasculopathy. JACC: Cardiovascular Imaging. 2013;**6**:613-623

[26] Johnson DE, Alderman EL, Schroeder JS, Gao SZ, Hunt S, DeCampli WM, et al. Transplant coronary artery disease: Histopathologic correlations with angiographic morphology. Journal of the American College of Cardiology. 1991;**17**:449-457

[27] St Goar FG, Pinto FJ, Alderman EL, Valantine HA, Schroeder JS, Gao SZ, et al. Intracoronary ultrasound in cardiac

transplant recipients. In vivo evidence of "angiographically silent" intimal thickening. Circulation. 1992;**85**:979-987

[28] Tsutsui H, Ziada KM, Schoenhagen P, Iyisoy A, Magyar WA, Crowe TD, et al. Lumen loss in transplant coronary artery disease is a biphasic process involving early intimal thickening and late constrictive remodeling: Results from a 5-year serial intravascular ultrasound study. Circulation. 2001;**104**:653-657

[29] Rickenbacher PR, Pinto FJ, Lewis NP, Hunt SA, Alderman EL, Schroeder JS, et al. Prognostic importance of intimal thickness as measured by intracoronary ultrasound after cardiac transplantation. Circulation. 1995;**92**:3445-3452

[30] Mehra MR, Ventura HO, Stapleton DD, Smart FW, Collins TC, Ramee SR. Presence of severe intimal thickening by intravascular ultrasonography predicts cardiac events in cardiac allograft vasculopathy. The Journal of Heart and Lung Transplantation. 1995;**14**:632-639

[31] Kobashigawa JA, Tobis JM, Starling RC, Tuzcu EM, Smith AL, Valantine HA, et al. Multicenter intravascular ultrasound validation study among heart transplant recipients: Outcomes after five years. Journal of the American College of Cardiology. 2005;**45**:1532-1537

[32] Tuzcu EM, Kapadia SR, Sachar R, Ziada KM, Crowe TD, Feng J, et al. Intravascular ultrasound evidence of angiographically silent progression in coronary atherosclerosis predicts long-term morbidity and mortality after cardiac transplantation. Journal of the American College of Cardiology. 2005;**45**:1538-1542

[33] Potena L, Masetti M, Sabatino M, Bacchi-Reggiani ML, Pece V, Prestinenzi P, et al. Interplay of coronary angiography and intravascular ultrasound in predicting long-term outcomes after heart transplantation. The Journal of Heart and Lung Transplantation. 2015;**34**:1146-1153

[34] Okada K, Kitahara H, Yang HM, Tanaka S, Kobayashi Y, Kimura T, et al. Paradoxical vessel Remodeling of the proximal segment of the left anterior descending artery predicts long-term mortality after heart transplantation. JACC: Heart Failure. 2015;**3**:942-952

[35] Watanabe T, Seguchi O, Yanase M, Fujita T, Murata Y, Sato T, et al. Donor-transmitted atherosclerosis associated with worsening cardiac allograft vasculopathy after heart transplantation: Serial volumetric intravascular ultrasound analysis. Transplantation. 2017;**101**:1310-1319

[36] Torres HJ, Merello L, Ramos SA, Aninat MA, Becerra LE, Mora AD, et al. Prevalence of cardiac allograft vasculopathy assessed with coronary angiography versus coronary vascular ultrasound and virtual histology. Transplantation Proceedings. 2011;**43**:2318-2321

[37] Raichlin E, Bae JH, Kushwaha SS, Lennon RJ, Prasad A, Rihal CS, et al. Inflammatory burden of cardiac allograft coronary atherosclerotic plaque is associated with early recurrent cellular rejection and predicts a higher risk of vasculopathy progression. Journal of the American College of Cardiology. 2009;**53**:1279-1286

[38] Hernandez JM, de Prada JA, Burgos V, Sainz Laso F, Valls MF, Vilchez FG, et al. Virtual histology intravascular ultrasound assessment of cardiac allograft vasculopathy from 1 to 20 years after heart transplantation. The Journal of Heart and Lung Transplantation. 2009;**28**:156-162

[39] Clausell N, Butany J, Molossi S, Lonn E, Gladstone P, Rabinovitch M, et al. Abnormalities in intramyocardial arteries detected in cardiac transplant biopsy specimens and lack of correlation with abnormal intracoronary ultrasound or endothelial dysfunction in large epicardial coronary arteries. Journal of the American College of Cardiology. 1995;**26**:110-119

[40] Kume T, Akasaka T, Kawamoto T, Watanabe N, Toyota E, Neishi Y, et al. Assessment of coronary intima--media thickness by optical coherence tomography: Comparison with intravascular ultrasound. Circulation Journal. 2005;**69**:903-907

[41] Hou J, Lv H, Jia H, Zhang S, Xing L, Liu H, et al. OCT assessment of allograft vasculopathy in heart transplant recipients. JACC: Cardiovascular Imaging. 2012;**5**:662-663

[42] Garrido IP, García-Lara J, Pinar E, Pastor-Pérez F, Sánchez-Mas J, Valdés-Chavarri M, et al. Optical coherence tomography and highly sensitivity troponin T for evaluating cardiac allograft vasculopathy. The American Journal of Cardiology. 2012;**110**:655-661

[43] Tearney GJ, Regar E, Akasaka T, Adriaenssens T, Barlis P, Bezerra HG, et al. Consensus standards for acquisition, measurement, and reporting of intravascular optical coherence tomography studies: A report from the international working Group for Intravascular Optical Coherence Tomography Standardization and Validation. Journal of the American College of Cardiology. 2012;**59**:1058-1072

[44] Shan P, Dong L, Maehara A, Nazif TM, Ali ZA, Rabbani LE, et al. Comparison between cardiac allograft vasculopathy and native coronary atherosclerosis by optical coherence tomography. The American Journal of Cardiology. 2016;**117**:1361-1368

[45] Khandhar SJ, Yamamoto H, Teuteberg JJ, Shullo MA, Bezerra HG, Costa MA, et al. Optical coherence tomography for characterization of cardiac allograft vasculopathy after heart transplantation (OCTCAV study). The Journal of Heart and Lung Transplantation. 2013;**32**:596-602

[46] Cassar A, Matsuo Y, Herrmann J, Li J, Lennon RJ, Gulati R, et al. Coronary atherosclerosis with vulnerable plaque and complicated lesions in transplant recipients: New insight into cardiac allograft vasculopathy by optical coherence tomography. European Heart Journal. 2013;**34**:2610-2617

[47] Park KH, Sun T, Liu Z, Yang SW, Lennon RJ, Lerman LO, et al. Relationship between markers of plaque vulnerability in optical coherence tomography and atherosclerotic progression in adult patients with heart transplantation. The Journal of Heart and Lung Transplantation. 2017;**36**:185-192

[48] Clemmensen TS, Holm NR, Eiskjær H, Løgstrup BB, Christiansen EH, Dijkstra J, et al. Layered fibrotic plaques are the predominant component in cardiac allograft vasculopathy: Systematic findings and risk stratification by OCT. JACC: Cardiovascular Imaging. 2017;**10**:773-784

[49] Clemmensen TS, Holm NR, Eiskjær H, Jakobsen L, Berg K, Neghabat O, et al. Detection of early changes in the coronary artery microstructure after heart transplantation: A prospective optical coherence tomography study. The Journal of Heart and Lung Transplantation. 2018;**37**:486-495

[50] Acharya D, Loyaga-Rendon RY, Chatterjee A, Rajapreyar I, Lee K. Optical coherence tomography in cardiac allograft vasculopathy: State-of-the-art review. Circulation. Heart Failure. 2021;**14**:e008416

[51] Aoki T, Rodriguez-Porcel M, Matsuo Y, Cassar A, Kwon TG, Franchi F, et al. Evaluation of coronary adventitial vasa vasorum using 3D optical coherence tomography--animal and human studies. Atherosclerosis. 2015;**239**:203-208

[52] Ichibori Y, Ohtani T, Nakatani D, Tachibana K, Yamaguchi O, Toda K, et al. Optical coherence tomography and intravascular ultrasound evaluation of cardiac allograft vasculopathy with and without intimal neovascularization. European Heart Journal Cardiovascular Imaging. 2016;**17**:51-58

[53] Park KH, Kwon TG, Matsuzawa Y, Sun T, Liu Z, Lennon RJ, et al. Association between the vasa vasorum and the atherosclerotic changes in cardiac allograft vasculopathy: Volumetric analysis. European Heart Journal Cardiovascular Imaging. 2016;**17**:272-279

[54] Chahal DS, Parikh R, Yoo D, Aje T, Ramani G, Srivastava MC. Association of Intimal Neovessels Noted by optical coherence tomography with cardiac allograft vasculopathy. Cureus. 2020; **12**:e7454

[55] Clemmensen TS, Koefoed-Nielsen P, Jensen LA, Poulsen SH, Holm NR, Løgstrup BB, et al. Donor-specific antibodies are associated with micro- and macrovascular coronary disease, restrictive myocardial damage, and poor outcome in heart-transplanted patients. Clinical Transplantation. 2017;**31**(9). DOI: 10.1111/ctr.13033

[56] Pazdernik M, Bedanova H, Chen Z, Kautzner J, Melenovsky V, Malek I, et al. Donor specific anti-HLA antibodies and cardiac allograft vasculopathy: A prospective study using highly automated 3-D optical coherence tomography analysis. Transplant Immunology. 2021;**65**:101340

[57] Dong L, Maehara A, Nazif TM, Pollack AT, Saito S, Rabbani LE, et al. Optical coherence tomographic evaluation of transplant coronary artery vasculopathy with correlation to cellular rejection. Circulation. Cardiovascular Interventions. 2014;**7**:199-206

[58] Orban M, Ulrich S, Dischl D, von Samson-Himmelstjerna P, Schramm R, Tippmann K, et al. Cardiac allograft vasculopathy: Differences of absolute and relative intimal hyperplasia in children versus adults in optical coherence tomography. International Journal of Cardiology. 2021;**328**:227-234

[59] Gupta A, Chhikara S, Vijayvergiya R, Seth A, Mahesh NK, Akasaka T, et al. Saline as an alternative to radio-contrast for optical coherence tomography guided percutaneous coronary intervention: A prospective comparison. Cardiovascular Revascularization Medicine. 2021;**34**:86-91. DOI: 10.1016/j.carrev.2021.01.010

[60] Frick K, Michael TT, Alomar M, Mohammed A, Rangan BV, Abdullah S, et al. Low molecular weight dextran provides similar optical coherence tomography coronary imaging compared to radiographic contrast media. Catheterization and Cardiovascular Interventions. 2014;**84**:727-731

[61] Fearon WF, Nakamura M, Lee DP, Rezaee M, Vagelos RH, Hunt SA, et al. Simultaneous assessment of fractional and coronary flow reserves in cardiac transplant recipients: Physiologic investigation for transplant Arteriopathy (PITA study). Circulation. 2003;**108**:1605-1610

[62] Fearon WF, Hirohata A, Nakamura M, Luikart H, Lee DP, Vagelos RH, et al. Discordant changes in epicardial and microvascular coronary physiology after cardiac transplantation: Physiologic investigation for transplant Arteriopathy II (PITA II) study. The Journal of Heart and Lung Transplantation. 2006;**25**:765-771

[63] Yang HM, Khush K, Luikart H, Okada K, Lim HS, Kobayashi Y, et al. Invasive assessment of coronary physiology predicts late mortality after heart transplantation. Circulation. 2016;**133**:1945-1950

Section 7

Gene Therapy

Chapter 13

Gene Therapy for Cardiac Transplantation

Michelle Mendiola Pla, Yuting Chiang, Jun-Neng Roan and Dawn E. Bowles

Abstract

Gene therapy is an advanced treatment approach that alters the genetic composition of cells to confer therapeutic protein or RNA expression to the target organ. It has been successfully introduced into clinical practice for the treatment of various diseases. Cardiac transplantation stands to benefit from applications of gene therapy to prevent the onset of post-transplantation complications, such as primary graft dysfunction, cardiac allograft vasculopathy, and rejection. Additionally, gene therapy can be used to minimize or potentially eliminate the need for immunosuppression post-transplantation. Several animal models and delivery strategies have been developed over the years with the goal of achieving robust gene expression in the heart. However, a method for doing this has yet to be successfully translated into clinical practice. The recent advances in *ex vivo* perfusion for organ preservation provide potential ways to overcome several barriers to achieving gene therapy for cardiac transplantation into clinical practice. Optimizing the selection of the gene-carrying vector for gene delivery and selection of the therapeutic gene to be conferred is also crucial for being able to implement gene therapy in cardiac transplantation. Here, we discuss the history and current state of research on gene therapy for cardiac transplantation.

Keywords: gene therapy, cardiac transplantation, gene delivery, viral vectors, non-viral vectors

1. Introduction

Cardiac transplantation is the gold standard therapy for end-stage heart failure. The perfection of surgical interventions, development of modern immunosuppressive therapies, and implementation of rigorous transplant care protocols have contributed to better outcomes over the last several years [1, 2]. However, cardiac transplantation is limited by the number of available donor hearts, primary graft dysfunction (PGD), rejection of the heart, as well as by the side effects caused by immunosuppression therapy [3]. Gene therapy is an advanced treatment intervention that can potentially bridge the gap to overcome these common post-transplantation complications. The success of commercially available gene therapy interventions, such as Zolgensma for spinal muscular atrophy and Luxturna for Leber congenital amaurosis, demonstrates that gene therapy provides a viable treatment option for people who would otherwise suffer from diseases that have traditionally been thought of as impossible to treat.

Gene therapy works by altering the genetic composition of cells to confer therapeutic protein or RNA expression to the target organ. To date, it has been commercially used to treat spinal muscular atrophy, Duchenne muscular dystrophy, and for various types of ocular disorders [4]. There are currently many gene therapy clinical trials underway and growing in number (clinicaltrials.gov). Gene therapy based interventions have been studied for various cardiovascular diseases, such as coronary artery disease (CAD), heart failure (HF), and myocardial ischemia (MI) [5]. However, no intervention has yet been able to attain robust or long-term transgene expression in the heart in clinical practice. One promising intervention for HF was the AAV1-SERCA2a therapeutic which was evaluated in human clinical trials (CUPID, AGENT-HF, SERCA-LVAD). The trials, unfortunately, failed to demonstrate that the intervention led to a statistically significant difference in the primary endpoint of time to recurrent HF and secondary endpoint of time to first terminal events [6–8].

The heart is a complex target for gene therapy interventions due to its location in the body, the mechanical force of blood flow, endothelial barriers, cellular barriers, and the body's immune response [9]. A cardiac graft being treated prior to transplantation is uniquely amenable to gene therapy as most of these traditional barriers of gene delivery to the heart can be overcome. Through gene therapy, a cardiac allograft can be engineered to express selected therapeutic genes that could prevent the onset of post-transplantation complications and potentially minimize or eliminate the need for traditional systemic immunosuppression medications [10, 11]. Gene therapy for heart transplantation, though attractive, has not been translated clinically.

There are major challenges that need to be overcome for gene therapy to be able to be applied for cardiac transplantation. One of them is that, despite major advances in the understanding of transplant immunology, there remains an incomplete understanding of the mechanisms of both rejection and tolerance. This includes the understanding of the details of regulatory cytokine networks, MHC-antigen interactions during the rejection process, and a complete understanding of co-stimulatory factors and their functions [12]. Another challenge is that most current gene delivery mechanisms confer a transient, low level of gene expression [13]. With the current understanding of gene therapy in the context, it also is unclear what is the optimal dose of the therapeutic transgene needed to confer an appreciable clinical effect. However, recent investigations describe methods of robust and global gene delivery to cardiac grafts that offer promise to overcome this challenge. Similarly, viral vector delivery systems pose risks to the host and allograft via eliciting undesired immune reactions, off-target gene delivery, and genome integration. With the recent success and clinical adoption of *ex vivo* normothermic perfusion, the possibility of gene delivery that is isolated to the cardiac graft is feasible and promising for translation into clinical practice. Ex vivo normothermic perfusion also provides the optimal environment for viral vectors to be able to attach and enter cardiac cells for efficient transduction. With the advances that have been made to address these challenges, it will not be long before we witness the successful application of gene therapy to cardiac transplantation.

To achieve a successful gene therapy intervention for cardiac transplantation, several components need to be addressed: disease or indication and therapeutic target, use of an appropriate animal to test the therapeutic, selection of the vector for gene delivery, and method for vector delivery. Here we review select post-transplantation complications and potential targets where gene therapy can be implemented to prevent them. We will also review translational animal models that have been developed for investigating gene therapeutic targets. Finally, we will discuss the different viral and non-viral vectors that can be used for gene delivery, the selection of promoters, and the different modalities that have been investigated for the delivery of vectors to cardiac grafts.

2. Disease and therapeutic targets for cardiac transplantation

There are various insults that a cardiac graft experiences prior to, during, and after transplantation. Early damage to the cardiac graft can happen during the brain or cardiac death of the donor, organ procurement, organ preservation time, the implantation procedure, or as a result of reperfusion injury. These points of insult to the cardiac graft can trigger both innate and adaptive immune responses that result in injury. Common complications that occur following transplantation include primary graft dysfunction (PGD), coronary allograft vasculopathy (CAV), and rejection.

2.1 Primary graft dysfunction

PGD is a leading cause of early mortality post-transplantation [14]. The diagnosis of PGD occurs in the first 24 hours following heart transplantation. It presents as severe ventricular dysfunction of the cardiac graft in the immediate post-transplant period, resulting in low cardiac output and hypotension despite the presence of adequate filling pressures [15]. Either the left, right, or both ventricles can be involved, and the severity of the dysfunction can range from mild to moderate to severe depending on the extent of circulatory support that is needed to maintain hemodynamic stability [16].

Numerous causative factors, starting from donor death to weaning the heart from cardiopulmonary bypass in the recipient, have been identified that contribute to the cause of PGD [17]. These factors relate to ischemic and ischemic-reperfusion injury of the cardiac graft. Additionally, the onset of systemic inflammatory response syndrome and the development of vasoplegic syndrome in the recipient have also been identified as significant causes [18]. Finally, the use of extended criteria donors, such as donation after cardiac death (DCD), has also been identified as a significant risk factor for PGD [19].

The treatment of PGD is primarily through supportive care. It is typically initially managed with the use of inotropic support using catecholamines and phosphodiesterase inhibitors. The next escalation in care is typically the use of an intra-aortic balloon pump, followed by the initiation of advanced mechanical support using extracorporeal membranous oxygenation.

2.2 Cardiac allograft Vasculopathy

Cardiac allograft vasculopathy (CAV) is a major cause of late heart graft failure [20]. It is characterized by diffuse and concentric narrowing of large epicardial and small intramyocardial arteries due to intimal fibromuscular hyperplasia, atherosclerosis, and vasculitis. As a result, the transplant recipient develops pathological changes within the donor blood vessels leading to a spectrum of diseases ranging from MI to HF. CAV is often unable to be diagnosed by coronary angiography and requires intravascular ultrasound for diagnosis.

The main driver of CAV is believed to be the immune system of the host. The intimal thickening seen in CAV results from an accumulation of smooth muscle cells (SMC) accompanied by the infiltration of T cells and macrophages which further contribute to intimal expansion [21, 22]. Yet CAV lesions characteristically stop at the suture line between the donor and the recipient. The endothelial lining of the vessels remains intact in CAV lesions suggesting that SMC injury may result from sterile inflammation as is seen during cold and warm ischemia effects and ischemia–reperfusion injuries [23].

Current treatments are based on vascular risk factor management and the use of statins and mTOR inhibitors (sirolimus and everolimus) to reduce the development of the disease. Percutaneous revascularization is used to treat focal obstructive coronary stenosis but repeat revascularization rates are high due to restenosis and disease progression [24]. However, patients who go on to develop allograft dysfunction require re-transplantation [25, 26].

2.3 Rejection and immunosuppression

Cardiac allograft rejection is among the most common causes of death in heart transplant recipients [1]. Acute rejection is categorized into hyperacute rejection acute cellular rejection (ACR), and antibody mediated rejection (AMR). Currently, recipients undergo routine screening for rejection with endomyocardial biopsies obtained by a bioptome. Hyperacute rejection is due to the presence of preformed host antibodies against the graft and portends an inevitable immediate immune rejection resulting in death [27]. ACR and AMR take longer to manifest and are thus amenable to potential gene therapy intervention and we will focus our discussion on these forms of rejection. To prevent rejection of the cardiac allograft, patients are treated with systemic multidrug immunotherapies. Multidrug immunosuppressive regimens currently used in human transplant recipients are associated with an increased risk of malignancy and opportunistic infections, a metabolic syndrome characterized by insulin resistance and dyslipidemia, and drug-specific toxicity [11].

2.4 Potential targets for gene therapy

An understanding of the different insults that the cardiac graft experiences during the different steps of transplantation helps to identify potential targets for gene therapy for cardiac transplantation. The cardiac graft endothelium is vulnerable to ischemic reperfusion injury. In this setting, leukocytes adhere to the activated endothelium. The complement system becomes activated, neutrophils migrate into the cardiac graft, subsequently followed by natural killer cells and macrophage infiltration. These early non-specific inflammatory reactions are then followed by alloimmune reactions that result in massive graft infiltration by dendritic cells, T-cells, B-cells, and macrophages. Donor-derived dendritic cells leave the cardiac graft and migrate to recipient lymph nodes and the spleen. There they present donor antigen to recipient T cells directly and trigger acute rejection.

2.4.1 Inflammatory targets

Many candidate genes that interfere with one of these inflammatory mechanisms have been investigated in the context of cardiac transplantation. One such gene is endothelial nitric oxide synthase (eNOS). eNOS produces nitric oxide which is vasoprotective. Delivery of eNOS into the donor heart attenuated ischemic reperfusion injury, leukocyte infiltration, and cardiac graft rejection in a rabbit model [28]. Similarly, superoxide dismutase (SOD) gene delivery into a donor heart attenuated ischemic reperfusion injury after organ preservation and transplantation in a rabbit model [29]. SOD functions as a free radical scavenger that neutralizes reactive oxygen species generated during ischemic reperfusion injuries. Another target, nuclear factor-kappa B (NFkB), is a transcription factor involved in the up-regulation of pro-inflammatory gene products. One possible therapeutic intervention is to block NFkB in endothelial cells to attenuate ischemia–reperfusion injury in the myocardium. Sakaguchi et al. blocked NFkB by using double-stranded oligodeoxynucleotides with a specific affinity for NFkB (NFkB decoy group) to transduce rat hearts utilizing HVJ envelope [30]. The hearts were then preserved for 16 hours in hypothermic preservation solution before being heterotopically transplanted into a recipient rat. What they found is that the intervention attenuated ischemic reperfusion injury after prolonged heart preservation in hypothermic solution. Another protein that is up-regulated during inflammation and serves as a potential target for gene therapy is heat shock protein-70 (HSP-70). It has an essential role in protein folding and translocation and as chaperones for intracellular proteins. HSP-70 has particularly been shown to be associated with protection against ischemia–reperfusion injury. Jayakumar et al. infused rat hearts using 1 mL of the gene vector solution then incubated the hearts on ice for 10 minutes before heterotopically transplanting them into a recipient rat [31]. 4 days after the intervention, the hearts were perfused on a Langendorff apparatus for 45 minutes followed by reperfusion for 1 hour. They found that post-ischemic recovery of mechanical function was greater in the treatment arm versus control, recovery of coronary flow was greater as well. The conclusion was that HSP-70 gene transduction protects both the mechanical and endothelial function of the cardiac graft.

2.4.2 Rejection targets

The most direct and immediate barrier to the success of cardiac transplantation is the recipient immune response. Currently, the most effective clinical therapy is lifetime immunosuppressive therapy. Knowledge about the immune response in transplantation has grown tremendously in recent years such that gene therapy can be used to intervene on different targets of the immune response. Both cell and antibody mediated effector mechanisms are responsible for acute rejection [32]. A strategy to protect the cardiac graft from recipient immune responses is through the delivery of genes that confer proteins to the graft that modulate host immune responses. These would include cytokines or soluble ligands. Qin et al. utilized a retrovirus and a plasmid delivery system to transfer genes that encode transforming growth factor beta-1 (TGF-β and interleukin 10 (IL-10) to a mouse myoblast and non-vascularized cardiac graft [33]. Grafts transduced with either of these genes had significantly prolonged survival when compared with the vector alone (39 days with IL-10 vs. 26 days with TGF-β vs. 12 days with vector alone). The therapeutic effect of transduced IL-10 and TGF-β1 has been demonstrated in follow-up investigations using different types of vectors [34–36].

Another point of gene intervention would be at the point of T-cell costimulatory activation. Cytotoxic T lymphocyte antigen-4 (CTLA-4) is a protein that modulates T-cell costimulatory activation. It becomes upregulated on T-cells upon T-cell activation. Gene delivery of a soluble CTLA-4 immunoglobulin fusion protein (CTLA4Ig) into the donor heart was associated with detectable CTLA4Ig serum levels 120 days after transplantation as well as long-term cardiac graft survival, >100 days in a rat model [37]. However, the expression of CTLA4Ig did enter systemic circulation causing some systemic immunosuppression in the rats. Another similar target is the programmed death-1 (PD-1) gene. It is expressed on activated T-cells, B-cells, and myeloid cells. When PD-1 binds one of its ligands, PD-L1 or PD-L2, it leads to the inhibition of activated T-cells. PD-L1 and PD-1 play an important role in both acute and chronic rejection of transplanted hearts in animal studies [38–40]. In rejecting human transplanted hearts, PD-L1 expression is decreased relative to PD-1 expression [41]. Gene delivery of soluble PDL1Ig fusion protein into the donor heart moderately prolonged cardiac graft survival in rats [42].

2.4.3 Cardiac ischemic disease targets

An additional example of gene therapy applied to treat cardiac disease involves targeting angiogenic gene therapy that facilitates neovascularization to augment blood flow in ischemic myocardium. These include vascular endothelial growth factor (VEGF), fibroblast growth factor (FGF), and hepatocyte growth factor (HGF). In particular, these targets have been assessed for treating ischemic disease caused by MI or congestive heart failure. Rosengart et al. delivered 4×10^8 to 4×10^{10} particle units of an adenoviral vector encoding the VEGF gene to individuals undergoing bypass graft surgery and as the sole therapy to the experimental group via mini-thoracotomy. The intervention demonstrated no adverse events and there was symptomatic improvement in both groups [43].

The Angiogenic Gene Therapy (AGENT) clinical trials were the first randomized control trial studies investigating the benefits of stimulating coronary angiogenesis with gene therapy using FGF-4 [44]. FGF-4 was delivered using adenovirus administered by infusion into the coronary arteries of patients with chronic stable angina. AGENT evaluated incremental doses of 3×10^8 to 1×10^{11} particle units. The overall improvement in exercise treadmill time was similar for those in the treatment and the control arms. However, post-hoc analysis showed that when baseline neutralizing antibody titer was controlled for, patients with titers less than 1:100, 44% had increased their exercise treadmill time by more than 30%. In patients with titers greater than 1:100, only 7% had increased their exercise treadmill time by more than 30%. AGENT 2 investigated whether FGF-4 improved myocardial perfusion compared with placebo. A significant decrease in ischemic defect size was observed in the treatment arm (21% relative decrease) that was not observed in the placebo group. AGENT 3 and 4 were planned to determine the efficacy and safety of FGF-4 in the larger population, however, an interim review of the data demonstrated no differences in exercise treadmill time and therefore recruitment was stopped.

HGF as a therapeutic target has been evaluated in numerous studies. In the context of therapy for MI, Jin et al. investigated the long-term effects of HGF in a rat MI model [45]. Utilizing an adenoviral vector for delivery of HGR, the vector was injected directly into the infarct border zone immediately after permanent coronary ligation. 10 weeks post-intervention, there was no significant difference in the left ventricular ejection fraction, but capillary density was significantly higher in the treatment groups, whereas arteriole density was unchanged. Masahiro et al. describe the use of recombinant HGF delivered by HVJ envelope for prolonged cardiac graft preservation in rats during hypothermic storage [46]. The rationale for this choice is that HGF functions as an antiapoptotic factor in the heart. They concluded that the administration of HGF prevented myocardial apoptosis and improved cardiac function after prolonged myocardial preservation in hypothermic solution.

3. Animal models

Selection of an appropriate animal model for heart transplantation is critical to be able to translate a potential gene therapy intervention from the laboratory bench to the patient bedside. Numerous small animal models using rodents have been described where the heart is transplanted either heterotopically or orthotopically in the recipient animal. Similarly, there have been numerous large animal models described using pigs, sheep, and non-human primates (NHP). We will discuss examples of different types of small and large animal models in heart transplantation and in what instances an investigator may choose one over the other.

3.1 Heterotopic heart transplantation

Heterotopic heart transplantation (HHT) is when the transplanted heart is placed in an ectopic position inside of the recipient without the removal of the recipient's native heart. Intra-abdominal HHT is primarily used to investigate transplantation biology and is also suitable for studying unloading induced changes in the heart [47]. The heart of a donor animal is explanted and subsequently transplanted into the abdomen of a recipient animal. To accomplish this the donor ascending aorta is anastomosed to the recipient infrarenal aorta and the donor pulmonary aorta is anastomosed to the recipient inferior vena cava. The result of this configuration is that the graft beats with reduced left ventricular filling while coronary perfusion is preserved. It offers several advantages over orthotopic transplantation in research applications such as technical simplicity, better accessibility for biopsies, and survival of the recipient even in cases of graft rejection [48].

The first heterotopic abdominal heart transplantation was published using rats by Abbott et al. [49] in 1964 and subsequently modified by Ono et al. [50]. The technique of the latter has been widely adopted as the standard HHT rodent model. Heterotopic heart transplantation in mice is more challenging than in rats, however, testing mechanistic hypotheses is more practical in mice given the greater diversity of genetic modifications available in mice. The advantage of using a small animal model is that they are less costly when compared to the cost of a large animal. A larger number of small animals can be used to assess and describe the effects of a therapeutic transgene. It also allows for several transgenes to be tested in parallel to study the differences in efficacy between them. The main challenge in using small animals is that the micro-surgical implantation technique is very challenging given their smaller size. Another aspect that makes this surgery more challenging to do in smaller animals is that they have a lower tolerance for blood loss. Because of this, it is especially important that there be minimal blood loss during the procedure and that the anastomoses be hemostatic at the time of procedure completion.

The advantage of large animals is that the results of the gene therapy intervention are able to be translated more quickly into clinical practice than are the results obtained from small animal studies. However, large animals are very costly to acquire and maintain in comparison to small models. In the setting of small primates, Minanov et al. positioned NHP hearts into the iliac fossa of primate recipients [51]. More recently this transplant configuration has been used to investigate interventions in xenotransplantation using a porcine heart transplanted into a baboon [52–54]. Porcine to porcine heart transplantation is also used in the research setting to investigate the immune system effects of cardiac transplantation as well as gene therapy interventions (**Figure 1**) [55–57]. This surgical research model is also amenable for modeling post-cardiac transplantation complications, such as CAV and rejection, without subjecting the animal to a high risk of morbidity or mortality [55, 58]. The recent success of a porcine to human xenotransplantation using genetically modified pigs to minimize rejection by the human immune system of the xenograft stresses the importance of the selection of the appropriate animal model. After procuring the heart, the xenograft was preserved utilizing an *ex vivo* perfusion device until the time of implantation. The experiments leading up to this milestone utilized the heterotopic heart transplantation model to establish the longevity of the graft against rejection [53, 59].

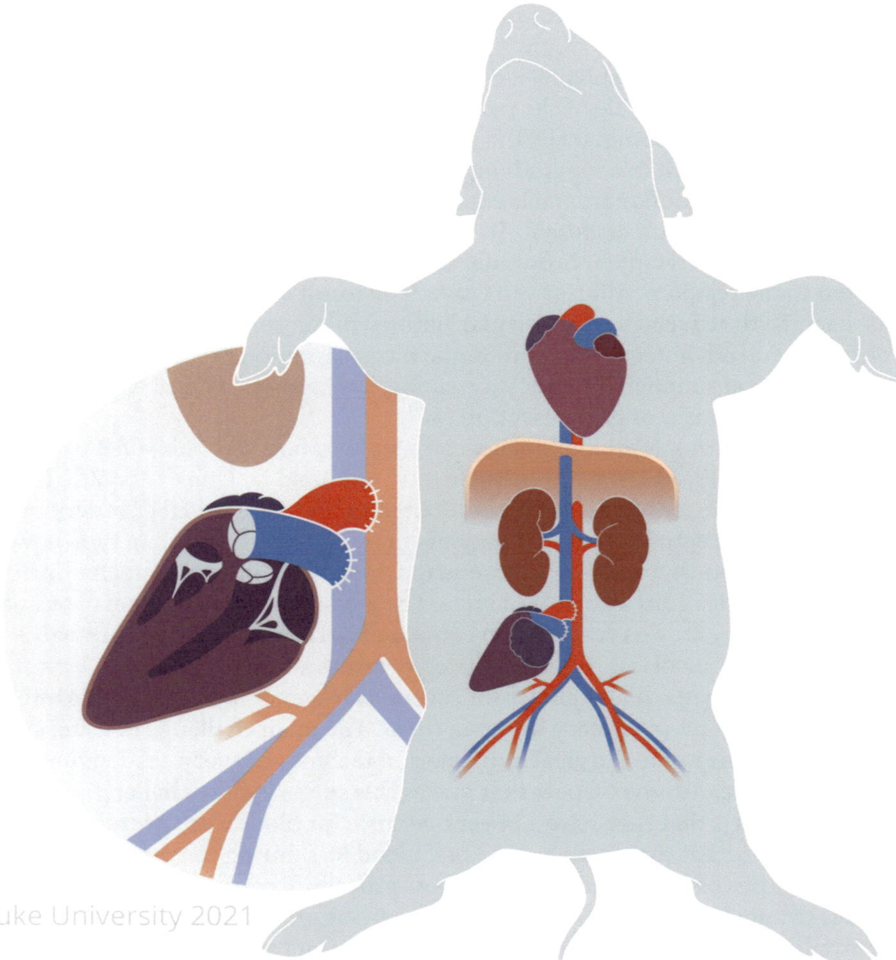

Figure 1.
Heterotopic heart transplantation in the intra-abdominal position in a large animal porcine model. The donor aorta is anastomosed to the recipient infrarenal aorta and the donor pulmonary artery is anastomosed to the recipient inferior vena cava.

3.2 Orthotopic heart transplantation

Orthotopic heart transplantation is when the transplanted heart is placed in the position of the recipient's native heart. As such, the cardiac graft takes over providing the cardiovascular support of the recipient. This transplant configuration in research is most useful to investigate the cardiac graft's overall ability to support the recipient following an administration of a new intervention. The pros of this design are that it most closely reflects clinical practice so one can investigate beyond the immunopathologic changes the heart undergoes after transplantation. This approach allows the investigator to determine whether an intervention permits the transplanted heart to perform its intended function to support the recipient's cardiovascular system. This has been successfully described in porcine to porcine models, as well as in pig to baboon xenotransplantation models [60–62].

4. Vectors for gene delivery

Vectors for gene delivery comprise viral and non-viral vectors. Viral vectors are the more efficient of the two but are also associated with more side effects than non-viral vectors. Each type of viral vector confers different gene expression characteristics, such as the length of time for transgene expression and the intensity of transgene expression (**Table 1**). Additionally, when constructing the optimal vector for cardiac gene delivery consideration must be given to the selection of promoter. Constitutively active promoters, such as CMV or RSV promoters, confer broad tissue tropism and strong expression. However, cardiac-specific promoters, such as myosin heavy chain promoter, myosin light chain promoter, and troponin T promoter have been used to restrict transgene expression in the heart [63]. While the cardiac-specific promoters focus gene delivery to cardiac tissue, they confer weaker expression when compared with constitutively active promoters (**Table 2**).

Viral vector	Genetic material	Capacity	Transduction ability	Peak gene expression	Main advantages	Characteristics
Adenovirus	dsDNA	4.5–36 kb	Transduces both dividing and non-dividing cells.	1–7 days	Efficiently delivers genes to most tissues.	Short-term but highly efficient gene delivery. Can elicit a strong inflammatory response.
Adeno-associated virus	ssDNA	4.7 kb	Transduces both dividing and non-dividing cells.	2–4 weeks	Low immunogenicity. Broad but specific tropism.	Long-term gene expression. Low immunogenicity.
Lentivirus	RNA	8 kb	Transduces both dividing and non-dividing cells.	4–6 days	Can carry multiple transgenes. Persistent gene transfer in dividing cells.	Persistent gene expression in dividing cells. Low but potential risk of mutagenesis.

Table 1.
Summary of common viral vectors used in gene therapy.

Reference	Transduced gene	Therapeutic mechanism	Transduction method	Key findings/conclusions
Iwata et al. [28]	eNOS	Attenuation of ischemia–reperfusion injury	Lipid/DNA complex via intra-op coronary infusion	Allogeneic rabbit heart transplant model demonstrated that intramyocardial neutrophil and T-cell populations were halved in eNOS transduced hearts. NF-kB activation in microvascular endothelial cells and cardiomyocytes was significantly reduced.
Abunasra et al. [29]	SOD	Attenuation of ischemia–reperfusion injury	Ad via *ex vivo* perfusion	Heterotopic heart transplant model in rats demonstrated positive immunoreactivity for SOD and 86.8% +/− recovery of pre-ischemic left ventricular pressure.
Jayakumar et al. [31]	HSP-70	Attenuation of ischemia–reperfusion injury	HVJ envelope via *ex vivo* perfusion	Heterotopic heart transplant model in rats demonstrated greater post-ischemic recovery of mechanical function and greater recovery of coronary flow in HSP-70 treated mice.
Sakaguchi et al. [30]	NF-kB decoy	Attenuation of ischemia–reperfusion injury	HVJ envelope via *ex vivo* coronary infusion	Heterotopic heart transplant model in rats demonstrated introduction of NF-kB decoy into the nuclei of endothelial cells and cardiomyocytes. After 1 hour of reperfusion the NF-kB decoy group showed significantly higher degrees of recovery of left ventricular function.
Guillot et al. [37]	CTLA4Ig	Attenuation of T-cell costimulatory pathway	Ad via intramyocardial injection	Heterotopic heart transplant model in rats demonstrated indefinite graft survival (>100 days) and could be detected in the graft at least 1 year after gene transfer. Evident suppression of antibody production against donor alloantigens up to at least 120 days after gene transfer.
Dudler et al. [42]	PD-L1Ig	Attenuation of T-cell costimulatory pathway	Ad via *ex vivo* coronary infusion	Heterotopic heart transplant model in rats demonstrated a prolonged median survival time (17 days vs. 11 days). Also demonstrated a decreased number of CD4 cells and monocytes/macrophages infiltrating the graft.
Grines et al. [44]	FGF	Angiogenic therapy	Ad via intracoronary infusion	Randomized controlled trial that enrolled patients with chronic stable angina demonstrated improved exercise time on a treadmill for those treated with intervention and had a baseline time < or equal to 10 minutes. Intervention decreased the ischemic defect size. Larger efficacy studies failed to demonstrate significant differences in exercise time on a treadmill so the trial was stopped.
Rosengart et al. [43]	VEGF	Angiogenic therapy	Ad via intramyocardial injection	Phase I clinical study that enrolled patients with clinically significant coronary artery disease. There were no systemic or cardiac related adverse events related to vector administration. Coronary angiography and stress sestamibi scan showed improvement in the treated area. All patients reported improvement in angina class after therapy.

Reference	Transduced gene	Therapeutic mechanism	Transduction method	Key findings/conclusions
Jin et al. [45]	HGF	Angiogenic therapy	Ad via intramyocardial injection	Myocardial infarction model in rats demonstrated no significant difference in the left ventricular ejection fraction. It did observe increased capillary density in the treatment group.
Ryugo et al. [46]	HGF	Angiogenic therapy/ Antiapoptosis	HVJ via cold static storage	Cardiac grafts procured from rats demonstrated that HGF treated hearts had a significantly higher recovery rate of left ventricular developed pressure. c-MET/ HGF receptor expression was stronger in the treatment group.

Table 2.
Summary of investigations of gene therapy for cardiac transplantation.

4.1 Adenoviral vectors

Adenovirus (Ad) vectors have high transduction efficiency. They are able to transduce both quiescent and dividing cells and maintain epichromosomal persistence in the host cell [64]. Ad vectors also have a broad tropism profile and large packaging capacity (4.5-36 kb). They offer efficient transduction of cardiomyocytes. However, gene expression is transient, peaking 1–7 days after delivery and then diminishing until it ceases at about 2–3 weeks after transduction [65]. They carry double-stranded DNA. Their main disadvantage is the widely pre-existing viral immunity among the general population. Since Ad is strongly immunogenic it causes undesired immune responses in treated subjects [66]. In order to overcome this and improve their capacity, Ad vectors have undergone several generations of engineering.

The first generation of Ad vectors was designed by removing the E1A gene which makes it so the recombinant Ad is unable to replicate within the host cell [67]. With the deletion of this gene, complementary cell lines, such as HEK293, had to be designed to express E1A and E1B in order to produce the viral vector. The main disadvantages of the first generation of Ad were that de novo expression of Ad proteins could activate the host immune response and there was still the possibility of spontaneous homologous recombination between the vector and engineered E1 region from HEK293 that could generate replication-competent adenovirus [68].

In the second generation of Ad vectors, further early gene regions (E2a, E2b, or E4) of the vector were deleted to permit additional space for the transgenes. As in the first generation, the deleted genes needed to be complemented by engineered production cell lines. However, the deletion of these genes led to inefficient complementation of E2/4 with engineered cell lines thus negatively affecting viral vector amplification, resulting in lower titers. Another disadvantage was that the native Ad late genes that were still retained within the viral genome could trigger host immunogenicity and cellular toxicity [69].

Finally, the third generation of Ad vectors have all Ad viral sequences deleted except for the inverted terminal repeat sequences and packaging signal. As such, these are referred to as "gutless" or "high capacity" Ad vectors (HCAd). The production of HCAds in cell culture requires an adenoviral helper virus similar to the first-generation Ad vectors. Compared with the previous Ad vector generations, HCAds have reduced immunogenicity, prolonged transduction in the host cell, and a significantly larger transgene capacity [64]. Their large transgene capacity makes it so that multiple transgenes could be delivered. The main disadvantage of HCAds is the challenge of ensuring that the helper virus is eliminated from the final vector preparation.

4.2 Adeno-associated viral vectors

Adeno-associated viral (AAV) vectors were discovered as a contaminant of Ad preparations in 1965 [70]. They lack essential genes needed for replication and expression of their own genome. They are not known to cause any human diseases. AAV vector was first used in humans in 1995 to deliver the cystic fibrosis transmembrane regulator (CFTR) gene into a patient with cystic fibrosis using the AAV2 capsid [71]. Today, recombinant AAVs are the leading vectors for the delivery of gene therapies. The first recombinant AAV gene therapy product, Glybera, was approved by the European Medicines Agency to treat lipoprotein lipase deficiency in 2012. Five years later, Luxturna was approved as the first recombinant AAV gene therapy product in the United States [72, 73].

AAVs carry single-stranded DNA (ssDNA). However, the efficiency of AAVs are limited by ssDNA in that it needs to be converted to double-stranded DNA (dsDNA) prior to expression. This step is circumvented through the use of self-complementary vectors which package an inverted repeat genome that can fold into dsDNA without the requirement for DNA synthesis or base-pairing between multiple vector genomes [74]. Transgene expression peaks at around 2–4 weeks after delivery. AAVs can carry transgenes up to 4.7 kb in size.

There are 13 natural AAV serotypes. These have been isolated from laboratory Ad stocks and mostly from human or non-human primate origin [75]. Engineering or recombinant AAV capsids confer the vector the capability to transduce multiple tissue types. Recombinant AAVs are composed of the same capsid sequence and structure as found in wild-type AAVs. Recombinant AAVs encapsidate genomes that are devoid of all AAV protein-coding sequences and that have therapeutic genes designed in their place. The complete removal of viral coding sequences maximizes the packaging capacity of these AAVs and contributes to their low immunogenicity and cytotoxicity [73].

Capsid development approaches are based on rational design and directed evolution. The rational design was among the first approaches to improve vector capsids. This entailed adding peptide sequences onto the surface of the capsid to direct the tropism of the vector and deter immunological recognition [76]. While rational design allowed for the early development of specialized AAVs, a major limitation of that approach is that there oftentimes is insufficient knowledge regarding AAV cell surface binding, internalization, trafficking, uncoating, and gene expression. The basis of directed evolution is in the simulation of natural evolution. Capsid libraries are placed under selective pressure to yield genetic variants with specific biological properties and advantageous characteristics. This way directed evolution of the capsid does not require a prior understanding of the molecular mechanisms involved in the selection criteria [73].

Cell-type specific transgene expression, however, is conferred at the level of gene transcription by the promoters used in AAV vectors. The serotype AAV9 has been shown to have the highest cardiac gene transduction efficacy in mice and rats with either systemic or direct cardiac injection [77, 78]. Meanwhile, the serotype AAV6 has proven to be a more effective vector when injected into the myocardium of pigs and non-human primates [79, 80]. Piacentino et al. described a recombinant AAV serotype engineered via rational design, termed SASTG, which has extremely high-level cardiac transduction and tropism [81]. A challenge for AAV-mediated gene therapy is overcoming the negative effect that innate immunity has on transgene expression. Yet adaptive immunity to the capsid and the foreign transgene is the main factor for decreased efficacy. Notwithstanding, recombinant AAVs are accepted as the least immunogenic when compared to other viral vectors. Patients that have been exposed to AAV serotypes that gene therapy is based on will have a high chance of forming antibodies against the vector capsid [82]. One plausible way of removing these anti-AAV antibodies from the bloodstream is by using plasmapheresis [83]. Another described pre-treatment is the use of IgG-cleaving endopeptidases which reduce IgG antibodies from the serum [84]. Besides removing the neutralizing antibodies, investigators have also utilized rational design and directed evolution to develop AAV capsids that evade neutralizing antibodies [85–88].

4.3 Lentivirus

Lentiviral vectors constitute a genus of the retrovirus family. They permit long-term transgene expression by integrating the delivered genes into the host genome and can carry transgenes up to 8 kb in size [89]. They can deliver single-stranded RNA to both dividing and non-dividing cells and display robust transduction efficiency [90]. A unique advantage of lentiviral vectors is the ability to express multiple genes from a single vector [91, 92]. Transgene expression peaks after 4–6 days. The immune response to lentiviral vectors is low but concerns remain about potential insertional mutagenesis and off-target gene expression [93]. They have a preference for targeting the coding regions of genes, carrying the risk of insertional oncogenesis [94]. Additionally, the vector lacks tropism for the heart, making it unideal for heart-specific delivery through *in vivo* delivery, however, may have a role in *ex vivo* delivery [95, 96].

4.4 Non-viral vectors

Naked nucleic acids allow for the delivery of large genes in high quantities. These include DNAs, mRNAs, micro RNAs, and siRNAs. However, the lack of protection from endonuclease degradation makes them unreliable with low cellular internalization of the transgene [97]. Additionally, naked nucleic acids have an uncondensed shape and polyanionic charge that does not allow for their efficient uptake into cells. The half-life of plasmid DNA is about 10 minutes following systemic injection into mice [98].

Nanoparticles have been developed to interact with nucleic acids to protect them from degradation and condense them into nano-sized complexes that can be internalized by cells. Two main types of nanoparticles being used in investigations are lipid-based and cationic polymer-based. Another modification that is being used to improve the uptake of naked nucleic acids by cells is through chemical modification to mRNA to reduce the activation of the immune system and improve the stability of the RNA. These modified mRNAs are attractive agents for short-term gene delivery to the myocardium [99].

4.5 Hemagglutinating virus of Japan envelope vector

Wild-type hemagglutinating virus of Japan (HVJ) was discovered in 1953 and is a member of the paramyxovirus family. The envelope of HVJ is composed of a lipid bilayer and two integral membrane glycoproteins, F and HN, that project from the viral surface [100, 101]. HVJ envelope vector is constructed by incorporation of plasmid DNA into inactivated HVJ-containing liposomes [102]. During the preparation of the envelope vector, HN and F are retained but all the genome inside of HVJ is removed. It has high efficacy to induce a molecule into a target cell by the strong action of fusing cells on its membrane. Additionally, the removal of all the virus genomes confers low immunogenicity to the vector and eliminates replication and viral gene expression in cells. It is in essence a "viral, non-viral hybrid vector" [101]. HVJ can be used to deliver DNA, RNA, and oligonucleotides efficiently both *in vitro* and *in vivo*. The genetic material is entrapped within the HVJ liposomes and directly introduced into the cellular cytoplasm by means of the fusion activity of HVJ and not by endocytosis.

5. Methods for delivery of vectors for cardiac gene therapy

Gene delivery to any organ is a challenging feat. Gene delivery to the whole cardiac allograft is an especially challenging task given numerous obstacles. *In vivo* physiologic barriers include the heart's location in the body, the mechanical force of blood flow, endothelial barriers, cellular barriers, and the body's immune response [9]. Additional barriers involve the limited spread of the vectors from the site of vector exposure to achieve widespread transgene expression as well as the lack of an effective procedure for delivering the vectors without causing significant injury to the cardiac tissue that also maximizes the exposure time to cardiac tissue to the vector.

5.1 Intramyocardial injection

Direct intramyocardial injection of the vector into the myocardium is one such technique for vector delivery. It is easy to perform the injections and could theoretically be performed during graft procurement or after cardiac transplantation. Guzman et al. described the use of this technique for the delivery of adenovirus injected through a 25-gauge needle into the cardiac apex [103]. The intramyocardial injection has also been described in a clinical trial where subjects underwent a thoracotomy with the injection of vascular endothelial growth factor-2 naked deoxyribonucleic acid. They found that the procedure is well tolerated and reported few major adverse cardiac events at 1 year [104]. The major limitation of this technique for cardiac transplantation is that it only allows for limited focal delivery and the inability to target deeper muscular structures of the heart, such as the septum. Additionally, it is challenging to keep all of the injected material inside of the myocardium, leading to leakage from the needle holes and causing injury to the heart [105].

5.2 Intracoronary infusion

Intracoronary infusion of the vector is another described technique. By this method, the vectors are infused directly into the coronary arteries and reach the target cells for transduction by transit through the coronary arterial tree. Intracoronary infusion can be achieved by several methods: coronary catheterization prior to procurement, *in vivo* coronary infusion through the cardioplegia catheter prior to explantation, and *ex vivo* coronary infusion.

Catheterization of the coronary arteries for delivery and infusion through the cardioplegia catheter at the time of the graft procurement allows for a more dispersed and homogenous distribution of transgene delivery than is achieved through intramyocardial injections. Generally, transgene expression is able to be observed along with the distribution of the coronary arteries [2]. Several disadvantages exist with these delivery techniques. One is the negative effect pre-existing coronary artery disease has on the ability of vectors to reach their cellular target. Another is that since the infusion of the vector is based on a single bolus delivery when using a catheter-based approach, there is a large amount of vector that is lost to the systemic circulation resulting in poor transduction efficacy of the heart and a significant amount of off-target transduction. Finally, transduction efficacy is hampered by the presence of circulating neutralizing antibodies in the recipient against viral vectors. Vector particles containing proteins that are similar to antigens that humans are exposed to following natural infection may be neutralized by antibodies upon injection in some humans because of pre-existing immunity [106].

5.3 Complete heart isolation by cardiopulmonary bypass

Administration of the vectors during cardiopulmonary bypass featuring complete heart isolation and continuous cardiac perfusion addresses the issues associated with the catheter-based intracoronary infusion. The technique for achieving this was described by Katz et al. using separate pumps for the systemic and cardiac circuits permitting continuous isolated arrested heart perfusion [8]. This allows for the vectors to be recirculated through the coronary circulation of the heart, allowing for additional opportunities for the vectors to attach to cells and achieve entry. However, cardioplegia arrest requires for the heart and circulation to be maintained at a cold temperature (4°C) which is not favorable for vector attachment and entry into the target cells [107].

5.4 *Ex vivo* perfusion

The procedure for cardiac transplantation offers a unique opportunity for gene delivery that does not exist for other indications for therapeutic intervention for heart disease. The cardiac graft is removed from the recipient and preserved for a period of time *ex vivo* until it is implanted into the recipient. During this time the heart can be treated in isolation, obviating the need for additional procedures on the donor or recipient and minimizing or potentially eliminating the risk of off-target transduction by the gene delivering vector. With the recent FDA approval of *ex vivo* perfusion devices for organ preservation during transplantation, the ability to deliver vectors via *ex vivo* coronary perfusion seems plausible for introducing gene therapy interventions to the cardiac allograft that confer global transgene expression to the whole graft. Currently, there are two methods of ex vivo heart perfusion: hypothermic (4°C) and normothermic (>32°C). Hypothermic ex vivo perfusion involves pumping a cold crystalloid solution into the coronary arteries of the arrested heart to deliver oxygen and nutrients while removing toxic metabolites [108]. Normothermic ex vivo perfusion maintains the donor heart in a warm, contractile, near physiologic state during transport from the donor to the recipient. The donor heart is arrested prior to being placed on the perfusion device and then prepared by cannulation of the aorta and pulmonary artery and ligation of the superior vena cava and inferior vena cava. The circuit is primed with 1–1.2 L of donor blood mixed with a crystalloid perfusate solution. The cannulated heart is reanimated by pumping oxygenated blood mixed with the perfusate solution that enters the aorta to perfuse the coronary arteries. The coronary sinus effluent then crosses the tricuspid valve and gets pumped by the right ventricle into the cannulated pulmonary artery [109].

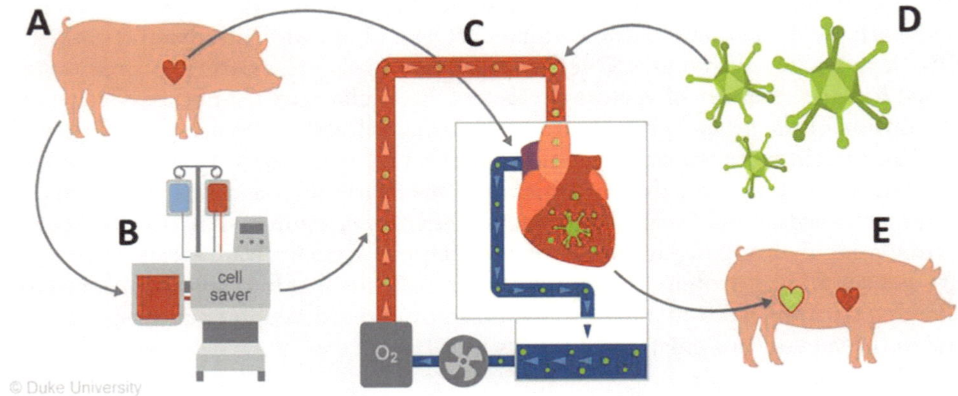

Figure 2.
Schematic for delivery of viral vectors to a cardiac allograft using normothermic, sanguinous ex vivo perfusion. The heart and blood are collected from the donor (a). The blood is then washed to remove any vector neutralizing components from the donor serum (B). The cardiac graft is perfused on the ex vivo perfusion device (C) and the viral vectors are added to the perfusion circuit to transduce cardiac graft (D). After completion of the perfusion/transduction period, the cardiac allograft is transplanted into the recipient pig in the heterotopic, intra-abdominal position.

Gene delivery to a whole cardiac graft has been described in both small and large animal models utilizing *ex vivo* perfusion methods. Kypson et al. described a successful adenovirus-mediated transfer of the marker genes LacZ and Luciferase that was accomplished by flushing the rat heart before performing implantation of the heart into the recipient rat [110]. Similarly, utilizing a pig model Bishawi et al. described a successful adenovirus-mediated transfer of the marker gene Luciferase that was accomplished by utilizing the Organ Care System™ ex vivo perfusion device (TransMedics, Inc) [56]. The porcine heart was perfused ex vivo with normothermic, sanguinous perfusate containing the adenoviral-luciferase vector for two hours prior to implantation into the recipient pig (**Figure 2**).

There are several advantages that make ex vivo normothermic, sanguinous perfusion the ideal platform for translating gene therapy into clinical practice. The ability to recirculate the perfusate through the coronary arteries multiple times over a prolonged period of time optimizes the chances the delivery vectors attach to the target cells and enter. Normothermic perfusion provides a favorable environment for viral vectors to be able to efficiently transduce cells, enabling receptor-mediated vector entry and optimizing the downstream processes of transductions [107]. The main obstacle to overcome with this vector delivery modality is the use of whole blood from the donor to make the circulating perfusate. The presence of preformed antibodies to different viral vectors could effectively neutralize the ability of the viral vectors to achieve cellular attachment. One successful intervention to overcome this is the addition of a blood washing step prior to adding the donor blood to the perfusion device and this way remove any neutralizing blood components [56].

6. Conclusion

Gene therapy for cardiac transplantation promises to transform clinical practice in the near future with cardiac grafts that are more robust and lasting than ever.

However, in order to achieve its widespread adoption, there are various factors that need to be taken into consideration for how to achieve successful vector delivery and transgene expression to the cardiac graft. Here, we discussed several considerations such as choice of vector, choice of the therapeutic gene, and choice of vector delivery mechanism. Just as important is the selection of the appropriate animal model for determining the efficacy and therapeutic effect of a gene therapy construct. The successful translation of gene therapy interventions for cardiac transplantation can potentially minimize or eliminate the incidence of post-transplantation complications and the need for systemic immunosuppression therapy.

Author details

Michelle Mendiola Pla[1], Yuting Chiang[2], Jun-Neng Roan[3] and Dawn E. Bowles[1*]

1 Duke University, Durham, NC, USA

2 Columbia University, New York, NY, USA

3 National Cheng Kung University, Tainan, Taiwan

*Address all correspondence to: dawn.bowles@duke.edu

References

[1] Stehlik J, Kobashigawa J, Hunt SA, Reichenspurner H, Kirklin JK. Honoring 50 Years of Clinical Heart Transplantation in Circulation: In-Depth State-of-the-Art Review. Circulation. 2018;**137**(1):71-87

[2] Li Y, Guo S, Liu G, Yuan Y, Wang W, Zheng Z, et al. Three preservation solutions for cold storage of heart allografts: A systematic review and meta-analysis. Artificial Organs. 2016;**40**(5):489-496

[3] Tonsho M, Michel S, Ahmed Z, Alessandrini A, Madsen JC. Heart transplantation: challenges facing the field. Cold Spring Harbor Perspectives in Medicine. 2014;**4**(5):a015636

[4] Mendell JR, Al-Zaidy SA, Rodino-Klapac LR, Goodspeed K, Gray SJ, Kay CN, et al. Current clinical applications of in vivo gene therapy with AAVs. Molecular Therapy. 2021;**29**(2):464-488

[5] Gaffney MM, Hynes SO, Barry F, O'Brien T. Cardiovascular gene therapy: Current status and therapeutic potential. British Journal of Pharmacology. 2007;**152**(2):175-188

[6] Hulot JS, Ishikawa K, Hajjar RJ. Gene therapy for the treatment of heart failure: Promise postponed. European Heart Journal. 2016;**37**(21):1651-1658

[7] Hulot JS, Salem JE, Redheuil A, Collet JP, Varnous S, Jourdain P, et al. Effect of intracoronary administration of AAV1/SERCA2a on ventricular remodelling in patients with advanced systolic heart failure: Results from the AGENT-HF randomized phase 2 trial. European Journal of Heart Failure. 2017;**19**(11):1534-1541

[8] Katz MG, Fargnoli AS, Yarnall C, Perez A, Isidro A, Hajjar RJ, et al. Technique of complete heart isolation with continuous cardiac perfusion during cardiopulmonary bypass: new opportunities for gene therapy. The Journal of Extra-Corporeal Technology. 2018;**50**(3):193-198

[9] Sahoo S, Kariya T, Ishikawa K. Targeted delivery of therapeutic agents to the heart. Nature Reviews. Cardiology. 2021;**18**(6):389-399

[10] Giannoukakis N, Thomson A, Robbins P. Gene therapy in transplantation. Gene Therapy. 1999;**6**(9):1499-1511

[11] Vassalli G, Roehrich M-E, Vogt P, Pedrazzini GB, Siclari F, Moccetti T, et al. Modalities and future prospects of gene therapy in heart transplantation. European Journal of Cardio-Thoracic Surgery. 2009;**35**(6):1036-1044

[12] Moore DJ, Markmann JF, Deng S. Avenues for immunomodulation and graft protection by gene therapy in transplantation. Transplant International. 2006;**19**(6):435-445

[13] Katz MG, Fargnoli AS, Kendle AP, Hajjar RJ, Bridges CR. Gene therapy in cardiac surgery: clinical trials, challenges, and perspectives. The Annals of Thoracic Surgery. 2016;**101**(6):2407-2416

[14] Singh SSA, Dalzell JR, Berry C, Al-Attar N. Primary graft dysfunction after heart transplantation: A thorn amongst the roses. Heart Failure Reviews. 2019;**24**(5):805-820

[15] Iyer A, Kumarasinghe G, Hicks M, Watson A, Gao L, Doyle A, et al. Primary graft failure after heart transplantation. J Transplant. 2011;**2011**:175768

[16] Kobashigawa J, Zuckermann A, Macdonald P, Leprince P, Esmailian F, Luu M, et al. Report from a consensus conference on primary graft dysfunction after cardiac transplantation. The Journal of Heart and Lung Transplantation. 2014;**33**(4):327-340

[17] Chew HC, Kumarasinghe G, Iyer A, Hicks M, Gao L, Doyle A, et al. Primary graft dysfunction after heart transplantation. Current Transplantation Reports. 2014;**1**(4):257-265

[18] Patarroyo M, Simbaqueba C, Shrestha K, Starling RC, Smedira N, Tang WH, et al. Pre-operative risk factors and clinical outcomes associated with vasoplegia in recipients of orthotopic heart transplantation in the contemporary era. The Journal of Heart and Lung Transplantation. 2012;**31**(3):282-287

[19] White CW, Messer SJ, Large SR, Conway J, Kim DH, Kutsogiannis DJ, et al. transplantation of hearts donated after circulatory death. Front Cardiovasc Med. 2018;**5**:8

[20] Pober JS, Jane-Wit D, Qin L, Tellides G. Interacting mechanisms in the pathogenesis of cardiac allograft vasculopathy. Arteriosclerosis, Thrombosis, and Vascular Biology. 2014;**34**(8):1609-1614

[21] Salomon RN, Hughes CC, Schoen FJ, Payne DD, Pober JS, Libby P. Human coronary transplantation-associated arteriosclerosis. Evidence for a chronic immune reaction to activated graft endothelial cells. The American Journal of Pathology. 1991;**138**(4):791-798

[22] Van Loosdregt J, Van Oosterhout MFM, Bruggink AH, Van Wichen DF, Van Kuik J, De Koning E, et al. The chemokine and chemokine receptor profile of infiltrating cells in the wall of arteries with cardiac allograft vasculopathy is indicative of a memory T–Helper 1 Response. Circulation. 2006;**114**(15):1599-1607

[23] Frye CC, Bery AI, Kreisel D, Kulkarni HS. Sterile inflammation in thoracic transplantation. Cellular and Molecular Life Sciences. 2021;**78**(2):581-601

[24] Lee MS, Lluri G, Finch W, Park KW. Role of percutaneous coronary intervention in the treatment of cardiac allograft vasculopathy. The American Journal of Cardiology. 2018;**121**(9):1051-1055

[25] Tremblay-Gravel M, Racine N, de Denus S, Ducharme A, Pelletier GB, Giraldeau G, et al. Changes in outcomes of cardiac allograft vasculopathy over 30 years following heart transplantation. JACC Heart Fail. 2017;**5**(12):891-901

[26] Khush KK, Cherikh WS, Chambers DC, Goldfarb S, Hayes D Jr, Kucheryavaya AY, et al. The International Thoracic Organ Transplant Registry of the International Society for Heart and Lung Transplantation: Thirty-fifth Adult Heart Transplantation Report-2018; Focus Theme: Multiorgan Transplantation. The Journal of Heart and Lung Transplantation. 2018;**37**(10):1155-1168

[27] Suarez-Pierre A, Kilic A. Surgical considerations for cardiac allograft rejection. Cardiovascular Pathology. 2019;**42**:59-63

[28] Iwata A, Sai S, Nitta Y, Chen M, de Fries-Hallstrand R, Dalesandro J, et al. Liposome-mediated gene transfection of endothelial nitric oxide synthase reduces endothelial activation and leukocyte infiltration in transplanted hearts. Circulation. 2001;**103**(22):2753-2759

[29] Abunasra HJ, Smolenski RT, Yap J, Sheppard M, O'Brien T, Yacoub MH. Multigene adenoviral therapy for the attenuation of ischemia-reperfusion

injury after preservation for cardiac transplantation. The Journal of Thoracic and Cardiovascular Surgery. 2003;**125**(5):998-1006

[30] Sakaguchi T, Sawa Y, Fukushima N, Nishimura M, Ichikawa H, Kaneda Y, et al. A novel strategy of decoy transfection against nuclear factor-κB in myocardial preservation. The Annals of Thoracic Surgery. 2001;**71**(2):624-629

[31] Jayakumar J, Suzuki K, Khan M, Smolenski RT, Farrell A, Latif N, et al. Gene therapy for myocardial protection. Circulation. 2000;**102**(suppl_3):Iii-302-IiIii-6

[32] Hayry P. Molecular pathology of acute and chronic rejection. Transplantation Proceedings. 1994;**26**(6):3280-3284

[33] Qin L, Chavin KD, Ding Y, Favaro JP, Woodward JE, Lin J, et al. Multiple vectors effectively achieve gene transfer in a murine cardiac transplantation model. Immunosuppression with TGF-beta 1 or vIL-10. Transplantation. 1995;**59**(6):809-816

[34] Vassalli G, Fleury S, Li J, Goy J-J, Kappenberger L, Von Segesser LK. Gene transfer of cytoprotective and immunomodulatory molecules for prevention of cardiac allograft rejection. European Journal of Cardio-Thoracic Surgery. 2003;**24**(5):794-806

[35] Fujisawa K, Saito S, Okada Y, Fujiwara T, Yagi T, Iwagaki H, et al. Suppression of Allogeneic Response by Viral IL-10 Gene Transfer. Cell Transplantation. 2003;**12**(4):379-387

[36] Cheng J, Xia SS, Xie S, Tang LG, Shi XF. Transforming Growth Factor β1–Modified Donor Cell Transfusion Induced Allo-Heart Tolerance. Transplantation Proceedings. 2005;**37**(5):2360-2364

[37] Guillot C, Mathieu P, Coathalem H, Le Mauff B, Castro MG, Tesson L, et al. Tolerance to cardiac allografts via local and systemic mechanisms after adenovirus-mediated CTLA4Ig expression. Journal of Immunology. 2000;**164**(10):5258-5268

[38] Wang W, Carper K, Malone F, Latchman Y, Perkins J, Fu Y, et al. PD-L1/PD-1 Signal Deficiency Promotes Allogeneic Immune Responses and Accelerates Heart Allograft Rejection. Transplantation. 2008;**86**(6):836-844

[39] Özkaynak E, Wang L, Goodearl A, McDonald K, Qin S, O'Keefe T, et al. Programmed Death-1 Targeting Can Promote Allograft Survival. The Journal of Immunology. 2002;**169**(11):6546-6553

[40] Koga N, Suzuki J-I, Kosuge H, Haraguchi G, Onai Y, Futamatsu H, et al. Blockade of the interaction between PD-1 and PD-L1 accelerates graft arterial disease in cardiac allografts. Arteriosclerosis, Thrombosis, and Vascular Biology. 2004;**24**(11):2057-2062

[41] Bishawi M, Bowles D, Pla MM, Oakes F, Chiang Y, Schroder J, et al. PD-1 and PD-L1 expression in cardiac transplantation. Cardiovascular Pathology. 2021;**54**:107331

[42] Dudler J, Li J, Pagnotta M, Pascual M, von Segesser LK, Vassalli G. Gene transfer of programmed death ligand-1. Ig prolongs cardiac allograft survival. Transplantation. 2006;**82**(12):1733-1737

[43] Rosengart TK, Lee LY, Patel SR, Sanborn TA, Parikh M, Bergman GW, et al. Angiogenesis Gene Therapy. Circulation. 1999;**100**(5):468-474

[44] Grines CL. The AGENT clinical trials programme. European Heart Journal Supplements. 2004;**6**(suppl_E):E18-E23

[45] Jin YN, Inubushi M, Masamoto K, Odaka K, Aoki I, Tsuji AB, et al. Long-term effects of hepatocyte growth factor gene therapy in rat myocardial infarct model. Gene Therapy. 2012;**19**(8):836-843

[46] Ryugo M, Sawa Y, Ono M, Fukushima N, Aleshin AN, Mizuno S, et al. Myocardial Protective Effect of Human Recombinant Hepatocyte Growth Factor for Prolonged Heart Graft Preservation in Rats. Transplantation. 2004;**78**(8):1153-1158

[47] Westhofen S, Jelinek M, Dreher L, Biermann D, Martin J, Vitzhum H, et al. The heterotopic heart transplantation in mice as a small animal model to study mechanical unloading – Establishment of the procedure, perioperative management and postoperative scoring. PLoS One. 2019;**14**(4):e0214513

[48] Kadner A, Chen RH, Adams DH. Heterotopic heart transplantation: experimental development and clinical experience. European Journal of Cardio-Thoracic Surgery. 2000;**17**(4):474-481

[49] Abbott CP, Lindsey ES, Creech O Jr, Dewitt CW. A technique for heart transplantation in the rat. Archives of Surgery. 1964;**89**:645-652

[50] Ono K, Lindsey ES. Improved technique of heart transplantation in rats. The Journal of Thoracic and Cardiovascular Surgery. 1969;**57**(2):225-229

[51] Minanov OP, Kwiatkowski P, Popilskis S, Michler RE. Modified technique for heterotopic heart transplantation in small primates. The Annals of Thoracic Surgery. 1997;**63**(1):258-260

[52] Adams DH, Chen RH, Kadner A, Naficy S. Technique for heterotopic pig heart xenotransplantation in primates. The Annals of Thoracic Surgery. 1999;**68**(1):265-268

[53] Goerlich CE, DiChiacchio L, Zhang T, Singh AK, Lewis B, Tatarov I, et al. Heterotopic Porcine Cardiac Xenotransplantation in the Intra-Abdominal Position in a Non-Human Primate Model. Scientific Reports. 2020;**10**(1):10709

[54] Iwase H, Ekser B, Satyananda V, Bhama J, Hara H, Ezzelarab M, et al. Pig-to-baboon heterotopic heart transplantation--exploratory preliminary experience with pigs transgenic for human thrombomodulin and comparison of three costimulation blockade-based regimens. Xenotransplantation. 2015;**22**(3):211-220

[55] Madsen JC, Sachs DH, Fallon JT, Weissman NJ. Cardiac allograft vasculopathy in partially inbred miniature swine. I. Time course, pathology, and dependence on immune mechanisms. The Journal of Thoracic and Cardiovascular Surgery. 1996;**111**(6):1230-1239

[56] Bishawi M, Roan JN, Milano CA, Daneshmand MA, Schroder JN, Chiang Y, et al. A normothermic ex vivo organ perfusion delivery method for cardiac transplantation gene therapy. Scientific Reports. 2019;**9**(1):8029

[57] Au-Mendiola Pla M, Au-Evans A, Au-Lee FH, Au-Chiang Y, Au-Bishawi M, Au-Vekstein A, et al. A Porcine Heterotopic Heart Transplantation Protocol for Delivery of Therapeutics to a Cardiac Allograft. JoVE. 2022;**180**:e63114

[58] Amano J, Akashima T, Terasaki T, Wada Y, Ito-Amano M, Suzuki J, et al. Characteristics of cardiac allograft vasculopathy induced by immunomodulation in the miniature Swine. Annals of Thoracic and Cardiovascular Surgery. 2015;**21**(1):45-52

[59] Singh AK, Chan JL, Dichiacchio L, Hardy NL, Corcoran PC, Lewis BGT, et al. Cardiac xenografts show reduced survival in the absence of transgenic human thrombomodulin expression in donor pigs. Xenotransplantation. 2019;**26**(2):e12465

[60] Ali AA, White P, Xiang B, Lin HY, Tsui SS, Ashley E, et al. Hearts from DCD donors display acceptable biventricular function after heart transplantation in pigs. American Journal of Transplantation. 2011;**11**(8):1621-1632

[61] Langin M, Reichart B, Steen S, Sjoberg T, Paskevicius A, Liao Q, et al. Cold non-ischemic heart preservation with continuous perfusion prevents early graft failure in orthotopic pig-to-baboon xenotransplantation. Xenotransplantation. 2021;**28**(1):e12636

[62] Fukushima N, Bouchart F, Gundry SR, Nehlsen-Cannarella S, Gusewitch G, Chang L, et al. The role of anti-pig antibody in pig-to-baboon cardiac xenotransplant rejection. Transplantation. 1994;**57**(6):923-928

[63] Pacak CA, Sakai Y, Thattaliyath BD, Mah CS, Byrne BJ. Tissue specific promoters improve specificity of AAV9 mediated transgene expression following intra-vascular gene delivery in neonatal mice. Genet Vaccines Ther. 2008;**6**:13

[64] Bulcha JT, Wang Y, Ma H, Tai PWL, Gao G. Viral vector platforms within the gene therapy landscape. Signal Transduction and Targeted Therapy. 2021;**6**(1):53

[65] Chu D, Sullivan CC, Weitzman MD, Du L, Wolf PL, Jamieson SW, et al. Direct comparison of efficiency and stability of gene transfer into the mammalian heart using adeno-associated virus versus adenovirus vectors. The Journal of Thoracic and Cardiovascular Surgery. 2003;**126**(3):671-679

[66] Crystal RG. Adenovirus: the first effective in vivo gene delivery vector. Human Gene Therapy. 2014;**25**(1):3-11

[67] McGrory WJ, Bautista DS, Graham FL. A simple technique for the rescue of early region I mutations into infectious human adenovirus type 5. Virology. 1988;**163**(2):614-617

[68] Yang Y, Nunes FA, Berencsi K, Furth EE, Gonczol E, Wilson JM. Cellular immunity to viral antigens limits E1-deleted adenoviruses for gene therapy. Proceedings of the National Academy of Sciences of the United States of America. 1994;**91**(10):4407-4411

[69] Wang Q, Finer MH. Second-generation adenovirus vectors. Nature Medicine. 1996;**2**(6):714-716

[70] Atchison RW, Casto BC, Hammon WM. Adenovirus-Associated Defective Virus Particles. Science. 1965;**149**(3685):754-756

[71] Flotte T, Carter B, Conrad C, Guggino W, Reynolds T, Rosenstein B, et al. A phase I study of an adeno-associated virus-CFTR gene vector in adult CF patients with mild lung disease. Human Gene Therapy. 1996;**7**(9):1145-1159

[72] Ylä-Herttuala S. Endgame: Glybera Finally Recommended for Approval as the First Gene Therapy Drug in the European Union. Molecular Therapy. 2012;**20**(10):1831-1832

[73] Wang D, Tai PWL, Gao G. Adeno-associated virus vector as a platform for gene therapy delivery. Nature Reviews Drug Discovery. 2019;**18**(5):358-378

[74] McCarty DM, Self-complementary AAV. Vectors. Advances and Applications. Molecular Therapy. 2008;**16**(10):1648-1656

[75] Wu Z, Asokan A, Samulski RJ. Adeno-associated Virus Serotypes: Vector Toolkit for Human Gene Therapy. Molecular Therapy. 2006;**14**(3):316-327

[76] Chen YH, Chang M, Davidson BL. Molecular signatures of disease brain endothelia provide new sites for CNS-directed enzyme therapy. Nature Medicine. 2009;**15**(10):1215-1218

[77] Bish LT, Morine K, Sleeper MM, Sanmiguel J, Wu D, Gao G, et al. Adeno-associated virus (AAV) serotype 9 provides global cardiac gene transfer superior to AAV1, AAV6, AAV7, and AAV8 in the mouse and rat. Human Gene Therapy. 2008;**19**(12):1359-1368

[78] Zincarelli C, Soltys S, Rengo G, Rabinowitz JE. Analysis of AAV serotypes 1-9 mediated gene expression and tropism in mice after systemic injection. Molecular Therapy. 2008;**16**(6):1073-1080

[79] Gabisonia K, Prosdocimo G, Aquaro GD, Carlucci L, Zentilin L, Secco I, et al. MicroRNA therapy stimulates uncontrolled cardiac repair after myocardial infarction in pigs. Nature. 2019;**569**(7756):418-422

[80] Gao G, Bish LT, Sleeper MM, Mu X, Sun L, Lou Y, et al. Transendocardial delivery of AAV6 results in highly efficient and global cardiac gene transfer in rhesus macaques. Human Gene Therapy. 2011;**22**(8):979-984

[81] Piacentino V, Milano CA, Bolanos M, Schroder J, Messina E, Cockrell AS, et al. X-linked inhibitor of apoptosis protein-mediated attenuation of apoptosis, using a novel cardiac-enhanced adeno-associated viral vector. Human gene therapy. 2012;**23**(6):635-646

[82] Mingozzi F, High KA. Immune responses to AAV vectors: Overcoming barriers to successful gene therapy. Blood. 2013;**122**(1):23-36

[83] Bertin B, Veron P, Leborgne C, Deschamps JY, Moullec S, Fromes Y, et al. Capsid-specific removal of circulating antibodies to adeno-associated virus vectors. Scientific Reports. 2020;**10**(1):864

[84] Leborgne C, Barbon E, Alexander JM, Hanby H, Delignat S, Cohen DM, et al. IgG-cleaving endopeptidase enables in vivo gene therapy in the presence of anti-AAV neutralizing antibodies. Nature Medicine. 2020;**26**(7):1096-1101

[85] Maheshri N, Koerber JT, Kaspar BK, Schaffer DV. Directed evolution of adeno-associated virus yields enhanced gene delivery vectors. Nature Biotechnology. 2006;**24**(2):198-204

[86] Bartel M, Schaffer D, Büning H. Enhancing the Clinical Potential of AAV Vectors by Capsid Engineering to Evade Pre-Existing Immunity. Frontiers in Microbiology. 2011;**2**:204

[87] Grimm D, Lee JS, Wang L, Desai T, Akache B, Storm TA, et al. In Vitro and In Vivo Gene Therapy Vector Evolution via Multispecies Interbreeding and Retargeting of Adeno-Associated Viruses. Journal of Virology. 2008;**82**(12):5887-5911

[88] Biswas M, Marsic D, Li N, Zou C, Gonzalez-Aseguinolaza G, Zolotukhin I, et al. Engineering and In Vitro Selection of a Novel AAV3B Variant with High Hepatocyte Tropism and Reduced Seroreactivity. Molecular Therapy - Methods & Clinical Development. 2020;**19**:347-361

[89] Naldini L, Blomer U, Gallay P, Ory D, Mulligan R, Gage FH, et al. In vivo gene delivery and stable transduction of

nondividing cells by a lentiviral vector. Science. 1996;**272**(5259):263-267

[90] Kieserman JM, Myers VD, Dubey P, Cheung JY, Feldman AM. Current Landscape of Heart Failure Gene Therapy. Journal of the American Heart Association. 2019;**8**(10):e012239

[91] Yu X, Zhan X, D'Costa J, Tanavde VM, Ye Z, Peng T, et al. Lentiviral vectors with two independent internal promoters transfer high-level expression of multiple transgenes to human hematopoietic stem-progenitor cells. Molecular Therapy. 2003;7(6):827-838

[92] Tian J, Andreadis ST. Independent and high-level dual-gene expression in adult stem-progenitor cells from a single lentiviral vector. Gene Therapy. 2009;**16**(7):874-884

[93] Di Pasquale E, Latronico MVG, Jotti GS, Condorelli G. Lentiviral vectors and cardiovascular diseases: a genetic tool for manipulating cardiomyocyte differentiation and function. Gene Therapy. 2012;**19**(6):642-648

[94] Papayannakos C, Daniel R. Understanding lentiviral vector chromatin targeting: working to reduce insertional mutagenic potential for gene therapy. Gene Therapy. 2013;**20**(6):581-588

[95] Kaiser RA, Mao SA, Glorioso J, Amiot B, Nicolas CT, Allen KL, et al. Lentiviral Vector-mediated Gene Therapy of Hepatocytes Ex Vivo for Autologous Transplantation in Swine. Journal of Visualized Experiments. 2018;**141**:58399

[96] Kohn DB, Booth C, Shaw KL, Xu-Bayford J, Garabedian E, Trevisan V, et al. Autologous Ex Vivo Lentiviral Gene Therapy for Adenosine Deaminase Deficiency. The New England Journal of Medicine. 2021;**384**(21):2002-2013

[97] Ramamoorth M, Narvekar A. Non viral vectors in gene therapy- an overview. Journal of Clinical and Diagnostic Research. 2015;**9**(1):GE01-GGE6

[98] Kawabata K, Takakura Y, Hashida M. The fate of plasmid DNA after intravenous injection in mice: involvement of scavenger receptors in its hepatic uptake. Pharmaceutical Research. 1995;**12**(6):825-830

[99] Zangi L, Hajjar RJ. Synthetic MicroRNAs Stimulate Cardiac Repair. Circulation Research. 2017;**120**(8):1222-1223

[100] Zhang Q, Li Y, Shi Y, Zhang Y. HVJ envelope vector, a versatile delivery system: Its development, application, and perspectives. Biochemical and Biophysical Research Communications. 2008;**373**(3):345-349

[101] Yonemitsu Y, Kaneda Y. Hemagglutinating virus of Japan liposome-mediated gene delivery to vascular cells. Methods Mol Med. 1999;**30**:295-306. DOI: 10.1385/1-59259-247-3:295. PM ID: 21341034

[102] Kaneda Y, Nakajima T, Nishikawa T, Yamamoto S, Ikegami H, Suzuki N, et al. Hemagglutinating Virus of Japan (HVJ) Envelope Vector as a Versatile Gene Delivery System. Molecular Therapy. 2002;**6**(2):219-226

[103] Guzman RJ, Lemarchand P, Crystal RG, Epstein SE, Finkel T. Efficient gene transfer into myocardium by direct injection of adenovirus vectors. Circulation Research. 1993;**73**(6):1202-1207

[104] Fortuin FD, Vale P, Losordo DW, Symes J, DeLaria GA, Tyner JJ, et al.

One-year follow-up of direct myocardial gene transfer of vascular endothelial growth factor-2 using naked plasmid deoxyribonucleic acid by way of thoracotomy in no-option patients**Drs. Isner and Schatz are stockholders of Vascular Genetics, Inc., the sponsor of this trial. The American Journal of Cardiology. 2003;**92**(4):436-439

[105] Grossman PM, Han Z, Palasis M, Barry JJ, Lederman RJ. Incomplete retention after direct myocardial injection. Catheterization and Cardiovascular Interventions. 2002;**55**(3):392-397

[106] Shirley JL, De Jong YP, Terhorst C, Herzog RW. Immune Responses to Viral Gene Therapy Vectors. Molecular Therapy. 2020;**28**(3):709-722

[107] Pellegrini C. Influence of temperature on adenovirus-mediated gene transfer. European Journal of Cardio-Thoracic Surgery. 1998;**13**(5):599-603

[108] Van Raemdonck D, Rega F, Rex S, Neyrinck A. Machine perfusion of thoracic organs. Journal of Thoracic Disease. 2018;**10**(Suppl 8):S910-SS23

[109] Ragalie WS, Ardehali A. Current status of normothermic ex-vivo perfusion of cardiac allografts. Current Opinion in Organ Transplantation. 2020;**25**(3):237-240

[110] Kypson AP, Peppel K, Akhter SA, Lilly RE, Glower DD, Lefkowitz RJ, et al. Ex vivo adenovirus-mediated gene transfer to the adult rat heart. The Journal of Thoracic and Cardiovascular Surgery. 1998;**115**(3):623-630